Deep Brain Stimulation for Neurological Disorders

Deep Brain Stimulation for Neurological Disorders

Editor: Roy McClen

AMERICAN
MEDICAL PUBLISHERS
www.americanmedicalpublishers.com

Cataloging-in-Publication Data

Deep brain stimulation for neurological disorders / edited by Roy McClen.
    p. cm.
Includes bibliographical references and index.
ISBN 978-1-63927-651-6
1. Brain stimulation. 2. Neural stimulation. 3. Nervous system--Diseases.
4. Nervous system--Diseases--Treatment. 5. Neurology. I. McClen, Roy.
RC350.B72 D44 2023
616.8--dc23

American Medical Publishers,
41 Flatbush Avenue,
1st Floor, New York,
NY 11217, USA

ISBN 978-1-63927-651-6 (Hardback)

Contents

Preface

The world is advancing at a fast pace like never before. Therefore, the need is to keep up with the latest developments. This book was an idea that came to fruition when the specialists in the area realized the need to coordinate together and document essential themes in the subject. That's when I was requested to be the editor. Editing this book has been an honour as it brings together diverse authors researching on different streams of the field. The book collates essential materials contributed by veterans in the area which can be utilized by students and researchers alike.

The brain is an important organ that controls all the functions in the human body. It regulates everything, including emotions, hunger, thoughts, breathing, motor skills, memory, body temperature, and more. Therefore, even a minor injury, disease or infection in the brain can have a serious impact on a person's life. Neurological disorders are those conditions, which interfere with the normal functioning of the brain and hence the body. They can be caused by a variety of factors, including biochemical, structural and electrical abnormalities in the spinal cord, brain and other nerves. A surgical procedure named deep brain stimulation (DBS) is used for treating various neurological symptoms like slowed movement, tremor, stiffness, walking problems and rigidity. It can also be utilized for treating focal epilepsy, dystonia and tremors. It involves the implantation of electrodes inside the brain. The electrical impulses produced by these electrodes are used for the regulation of abnormal impulses in the diseased brain. This book aims to understand the clinical perspectives of neurological disorders. It is appropriate for students seeking detailed information in this area as well as for experts. Different approaches, evaluations, and advanced studies on deep brain stimulation have been included in this book.

Each chapter is a sole-standing publication that reflects each author's interpretation. Thus, the book displays a multi-facetted picture of our current understanding of application, resources and aspects of the field. I would like to thank the contributors of this book and my family for their endless support.

Editor

Machine Learning's Application in Deep Brain Stimulation for Parkinson's Disease

Jeremy Watts [1], Anahita Khojandi [1], Oleg Shylo [1] and Ritesh A. Ramdhani [2],*

[1] Department of Industrial and Systems Engineering, University of Tennessee, Knoxville, TN 37996, USA; gkm819@vols.utk.edu (J.W.); khojandi@utk.edu (A.K.); oshylo@utk.edu (O.S.)

[2] Department of Neurology, Donald and Barbara Zucker School of Medicine at Hofstra/Northwell, Hempstead, NY 11549, USA

* Correspondence: rramdhani@northwell.edu

Abstract: Deep brain stimulation (DBS) is a surgical treatment for advanced Parkinson's disease (PD) that has undergone technological evolution that parallels an expansion in clinical phenotyping, neurophysiology, and neuroimaging of the disease state. Machine learning (ML) has been successfully used in a wide range of healthcare problems, including DBS. As computational power increases and more data become available, the application of ML in DBS is expected to grow. We review the literature of ML in DBS and discuss future opportunities for such applications. Specifically, we perform a comprehensive review of the literature from PubMed, the Institute for Scientific Information's Web of Science, Cochrane Database of Systematic Reviews, and Institute of Electrical and Electronics Engineers' (IEEE) Xplore Digital Library for ML applications in DBS. These studies are broadly placed in the following categories: (1) DBS candidate selection; (2) programming optimization; (3) surgical targeting; and (4) insights into DBS mechanisms. For each category, we provide and contextualize the current body of research and discuss potential future directions for the application of ML in DBS.

Keywords: machine learning; deep brain stimulation; Parkinson's disease

1. Introduction

Deep brain stimulation (DBS) has evolved into an effective therapeutic agent for Parkinson's disease (PD) patients suffering from medication refractory tremor, motor fluctuations, and/or troublesome dyskinesia. The stimulation is delivered through electrodes that are stereotactically implanted into either the subthalamic nucleus (STN) or the globus pallidus internus (GPi). Targeting is achieved with intraoperative image guidance (magnetic resonance imaging (MRI) or computed tomography (CT)) [1–3]. Neurophysiological mapping via microelectrode recording (MER) is often utilized to improve targeting precision. DBS therapy is engineered by customizing the size, shape, and intensity of the stimulation field with newer electrodes (tripartite-segmented electrodes from Abbott®, Medical Infinity™, Austin TX, USA, and Boston Scientific®, Vercise™, Marlborough, MA, USA), producing larger therapeutic windows and increasing the combinations of programming options [4,5].

Currently, high frequency continuous stimulation drives therapeutic benefit and requires time-consuming programming sessions, often relying on a trained clinician culling from experience and established programming approaches [6,7] to achieve the best clinical outcomes. However, stimulation-related side effects and suboptimal clinical responses can be limiting factors. Adaptive DBS (aDBS), which is a closed loop stimulation system [8] that uses a physiological biomarker of the parkinsonian state to automatically adjust the stimulation level and location, can provide an alternative to traditional DBS. This offers the possibility of more efficiently treating patients while reducing the challenges inherent in the current programming approaches. Furthermore, the recent advances in DBS technology, including improvements in spatial control from segmented electrodes and image guided programming, along with brain sensing (a likely precursor for closed loop DBS) can benefit from the application of data driven modeling to enhance clinical decision making and outcome prediction. In this review, we examine the applications of machine learning approaches for DBS in PD.

Machine learning (ML) is a subfield of artificial intelligence (AI) that identifies patterns within data sets. The application of ML in healthcare is becoming more widespread to augment the work of clinicians [9]. For instance, ML models have been created to identify anatomical structures through medical imaging [10], and to optimize pervasive sensing in healthcare informatics [11]. In the context of PD, much work has been done to successfully use ML/AI. This includes detecting PD symptoms for diagnosis purposes (e.g., [12]), predicting disease progression and patient response to medication using motor symptoms (e.g., [13]), optimizing clinical assessments through leveraging wearable sensors (e.g., [14]), and providing medication regimen planning (e.g., [15]).

Traditionally, computer algorithms execute explicit, specifically written code to interpret data and make decisions. ML is a computer analysis subfield that distinguishes itself from traditional methods by seeking to "learn" the relationships that underscore data without exact instructions [16,17]. Simply put, ML is an automated method that uncovers patterns in the data and utilizes those patterns to make predictions and/or facilitate decisions. ML has a wide domain of uses but excels in tasks that have large and complex data sets [16]. Generally, ML algorithms are categorized into two subtypes, namely, supervised and unsupervised learning.

In supervised learning, the algorithm's general goal is to learn a mapping of inputs to outputs. To accomplish this task, the algorithm is provided a training set of input–output pairs. These inputs are generally multi-dimensional vectors representing features of the data. The response variable, also known as a dependent variable, is the output of interest that is associated with these features. As the true values of the response variable, namely the ground truth, have already been identified by a human, supervised learning algorithms frequently are attempting to approximate human performance [18]. The response variable may be discrete (often called a label) or continuous, resulting in a classification or a regression task, respectively [17]. The performance of a supervised learning algorithm is objectively evaluated on a testing set, a subset of the data that is never examined by the algorithm when training. This allows for quantifying the generalizability of the learned model to unseen data. Dependent on the type of task (classification vs. regression), the model performance is described by diagnostical statistic measurements, such as accuracy, F1 score, or the area under the receiver operating characteristic (AUC) for classification, or metrics such as mean squared error or mean absolute error for regression. The descriptions of these metrics are provided in Appendix A. Examples of supervised learning algorithms include random forests (RF) [19], neural networks (NN) [20], support vector machines (SVM) [21], naïve Bayes (NB) [22], and k-nearest neighbor (KNN) [23].

In unsupervised learning, the algorithm's general goal is to find trends in data given only inputs. Unsupervised learning tends to be a more difficult process, as there are no known ground truths to predict. Examples of unsupervised learning algorithms include clustering [24], density estimation [25], and some neural networks [20]. Each technique requires different methods to determine the model's performance. For instance, in clustering, data is separated into distinct groups that ideally share characteristics. A clustering algorithm's performance may then be analyzed by how close its group members are to one another (intra-cluster distance) or how close the members are to another cluster (inter-cluster distance). While benchmarking unsupervised learning algorithms can be challenging, unsupervised learning allows for the analysis of data sets that are completely incompatible with supervised learning algorithms. Unsupervised learning is well suited for situations where ground truths cannot be identified or in which human experts cannot determine trends. Under these situations, unsupervised learning can propose trends in the data that can lead to meaningful insights when interpreted by experts.

The efficacy of DBS in the treatment of PD is well established [26–29]. Many of the potential benefits of ML in strategic PD treatment planning have been considered [12–14]; however, these reviews do not generally explore the role of ML in DBS. Specific surgical or treatment topics relating to ML in DBS have been explored [30–33]. However, they do not explore all facets of ML in DBS, and frequently only provide brief considerations of its application. As such, identification of the best performing models, as well as gaps in the existing body of literature, could help guide future exploration in using the powerful tool of ML. Here, we review the applications of ML approaches for DBS in PD. We compartmentalize these approaches into four groups: (1) DBS candidate selection; (2) programming approaches; (3) surgical targeting; and (4) insights into DBS mechanisms.

2. Materials and Methods

We performed a comprehensive search for studies that applied ML techniques in conjunction with DBS treatment of PD. This search encompassed all relevant journal, review, and conference publications cataloged on four common computerized database search engines: (1) PubMed, (2) the Institute for Scientific Information's Web of Science, (3) the Cochrane Database of Systematic Reviews, and (4) IEEE's Xplore Digital Library. We utilized the computerized databases' keyword search functions using a combination of three key phrases: (1) "Parkinson's Disease," (2) "Deep Brain Stimulation," and (3) "Machine Learning." We limited our results to publications that were published between January 2010 and August 2020. We further limited our results to English language manuscripts. This initial search identified 76 potential publications. These were evaluated with the predetermined exclusion criteria: (1) PD was not the primary application focus (seven papers were excluded), and (2) papers that contained only published abstracts (one paper was excluded). This process returned 68 publications that were included in this review. The number of publications per year and the number of papers per database are provided in Figures A1 and A2, respectively, in Appendix B.

3. DBS Candidate Selection

A key challenge for clinicians is to properly identify DBS candidates who will receive measurable clinical benefits with minimal surgical and stimulation related risk. A large-scale ML assisted analysis was performed to identify patients who may experience complications from DBS surgery. Specifically, Farrokhi et al. [34] examined a retrospective cohort of 501 DBS patients and determined presurgical features that indicated a greater chance of DBS complications. Logistic regression was applied to evaluate risk factors. The model was able to correctly identify subjects that would have any complications (AUC 0.86) and complications within 12 months (AUC 0.91) following DBS surgery. They found that age body mass index, procedure side, gender, and diagnosis of PD were all prominent features.

The screening of potential DBS patients can be limited through visits conducted virtually. There is a growing body of research that utilizes video recordings and ML to determine symptom scores for use in telemedicine. Das et al. [35] compared DBS patients on and off stimulation and classified severe versus mild symptoms using full-body capture video. This analysis was performed for six DBS subjects and classified through SVM. Yohanandan and colleagues [36] used wearable sensors with RF models and predicted tremor severity following the Bain–Findley tremor rating scale (BTRS) with 81% accuracy for use in telemedicine. These studies not only demonstrate the feasibility of using ML in remote monitoring platforms, but also provide early insights into developing a way to classify symptom severity or patients' phenotypes virtually.

3.1. Predictive Motor Biomarkers

Several studies have deciphered motor classifiers by comparing certain motor response differences between healthy and Parkinson's subjects [37–40]. Kuhner et al. [37,38] used RF algorithms to stratify 14 PD patients with (DBS-ON) or without (DBS-OFF) stimulation from 26 healthy subjects using a variety of motor control tasks. They found a 94.6% accuracy in distinguishing DBS-OFF patients from healthy subjects when using a standing up test. Another study [38] performed 3D motion capture and gait analysis on 26 PD patients (seven with STN-DBS) and 25 healthy subjects. They identified classifiers (a combination of low-order time derivatives) that performed best at distinguishing DBS-OFF patients from healthy subjects. Such classifying features could then be applied to a large-scale study of gait analysis. Similarly, Huo et al. [39] developed a unique multi-sensor motor response test and utilized KNN to classify 33 subjects as either having PD or being healthy with a 96.6% accuracy.

3.2. Non-Motor Considerations in Candidate Selection

Non-motor symptoms (NMS) of PD include neurobehavioral dysfunction, dysautonomia, and sleep dysfunction. NMS treatment response has varied with DBS [41–43], with several of these symptoms (i.e., sleep, pain, impulse control disorders, anxiety, and nonmotor fluctuations) showing some degree of improvement. However, with the limited number of studies investigating NMS changes with DBS, the mechanisms underlying the responses are postulated to be related to direct stimulation effects on the anatomic substrate (i.e., STN), postoperative dopaminergic medication reductions, or indirect relation to motoric benefit. Since NMS impacts the quality of life in PD patients, factoring it into the surgical decision-making process is an important clinical consideration.

Koch et al. [44] studied 40 DBS patients' preoperative electroencephalograms (EEGs) to identify those who would have postoperative cognitive deterioration using an RF algorithm. The data set was balanced in cognitive performance outcomes. The best performing model used both EEG and clinical features and achieved an accuracy of 91%. Chen et al. [45] examined the sleep cycle characteristics of 12 DBS patients. These patients were classified by SVM and decision trees based on local field potential (LFP) signals from the implanted target (STN). They found that alpha, beta, and gamma brain waves were the important predictors in sleep monitoring. Paliwal et al. [46] explored the effect that DBS had on impulsivity in decision making. In this study, 38 PD patients played a virtual slot machine before and after beginning DBS treatment. They applied a hierarchical Gaussian filter model that determined gambling behaviors. They found that DBS patients had increased volatility in relationship to impulsivity. Further, Chrabaszcz et al. [47] examined the LFP signals of 11 patients with STN-DBS while they read three-phoneme words. They were able to identify tongue or lip articulation, specific to DBS patients, that showed that DBS affected some patients' speech patterns.

4. Programming Optimization

Once potential DBS patients have been identified, the optimization of stimulation oftentimes requires frequent and time-consuming programming sessions conducted over 3–6 months from implantation. The programming strategies, coupled with simultaneous medication adjustments, rely a great deal on clinical trial and error. The efficient optimization of strategic DBS treatment planning using ML has been investigated. For example, Khojandi et al. [48] performed a retrospective analysis on 20 STN-DBS patients' Unified Parkinson's Disease Rating Scale (UPDRS) III scores. UPDRS [49] is a standard, subjective clinical measurement of PD symptom severity. Khojandi et al. developed an RF algorithm based on preoperative patient and disease characteristics to distinguish patients' optimized stimulation frequency (high and 60 Hz) with 95% accuracy. Such a model could enable more efficient optimization of DBS parameters. Additionally, Shamir et al. [50] predicted the expected stimulation and medication dosage based on three ML methods, specifically SVM, NB, and RF, for ten patients using 89 post-DBS surgical visits. These visits were used to create a clinical decision support system. This system enabled the correct prediction of motor improvement scores one year after surgery at 86% accuracy. The best performing model that classified individual symptoms varied. For example, SVM predicted tremor and speech outcomes with up to 100% and 93% accuracy, respectively, whereas RF outperformed SVM in terms of axial akinetic symptom prediction, with 86% accuracy.

Khodakarami et al. [51] examined the role of wearable sensors, specifically the personal kinetigraph, in an on/off stimulation classification problem. Their linear regression models determined classification with an AUC of 0.92. Baumgarten et al. [52] examined ten patients with GPi implanted DBS for pyramidal tract side effects (PTSE). An NN classified PTSE in patients whose parameters had been designed to trigger PTSE by clinicians. Each PTSE event was identified by professionals. A positive predictive value (PPV) of over 0.8 was achieved in this study.

Due to the clinical significance of the UPDRS, several publications explored the prediction of the UPDRS score as a response variable. Przybyszewski et al. [53,54] used data mining and decision tree approaches to predict UPDRS III scores based on reflexive saccades with 76% accuracy for 41 PD patients (18 with STN-DBS), and consequently using UPRDRS predictions, they estimated the disease progression in a cohort of PD-DBS patients. Candamil et al. [55] successfully categorized four subjects' UPDRS scores through linear machine learning based on a copy/draw test that could be applied to calibrate stimulation parameters. A study [56] that applied KNN on seven DBS subjects was able to predict UPDRS symptom severity with over 90% accuracy using wearable sensors on the most affected arm. The authors determined the potential benefit for home-based objective sensor measurements for improving DBS parameter optimization.

Adaptive DBS

Adaptive DBS (aDBS) refers to automated stimulation based on the real-time feedback of electrophysiology or wearable sensor signals [8,57]. Validated input signals, including basal ganglia local field potentials and especially beta band activity [8,58–60], are deemed to be associated with rigidity and bradykinesia (further review of electrophysiology-based aDBS is provided in [61]). Alternative input signals rely on wearable sensors [55,56,62–64] that can measure tremor, bradykinesia, dyskinesia, and gait [62]. The fidelity of tremor detection in calibrating a closed loop adaptive system has been demonstrated in several studies [65,66]. The use of ML in tremor classification for DBS patients was also explored and deemed as a useful tool for adaptive, patient-specific optimization [49,62,63,67–71]. Khobragade et al. [62] examined the surface electromyography of two patients (one PD-DBS) over two sessions and analyzed the signals using an NN. They achieved over 80% accuracy when detecting tremor using an NN trained on the same session. However, there was a nearly 50% decrease in performance for repeat patient measurement taken a week apart, which indicated the high variability of tremor symptoms and the benefits from aDBS, which is capable of real-time performance. To that point, LeMoyne et al. [67] surveyed the use of the BioStamp nPoint, a data acquisition device for tremor detection, specifically with the use of an NN, to identify stimulation parameters based on tremor response for future use in aDBS. Camara et al. [63] examined four STN DBS patients and classified tremor based on LFP signals. The authors suggested that a simple threshold would be insufficient to classify tremors. Therefore, they instead used ε-recurrence networks to classify tremors, and consequently applied an SVM to adaptively start or stop stimulation. This process averaged over 90% accuracy at stopping stimulation and over 78% accuracy at starting the stimulation. Shah et al. [49] used a logistic regression algorithm to classify tremor and non-tremor periods in seven DBS subjects using wearable sensor (accelerometer) data. The data set was labeled based on the frequency and duration of accelerometer events. The model achieved an AUC of 0.78 ± 0.11 for the identification of tremor periods. Additionally, Yao et al. [68,69] showcased the benefits of Kalman filtering when applied to tremor classification using multiple ML methods (SVM, RF, KNN, etc.), with as high as 11% classification improvement.

Additionally, ML has been applied to freezing of gait (FoG) [64], boundary decisions [72,73], and PD stages [74] for use in aDBS. However, the clinical feasibility of detecting these non-tremor motor symptoms have yet to be clinically validated in such a system.

Classifying human behavior from brain signals has also been explored in developing closed loop aDBS [75–78]. The real-time classification of human behaviors would allow for adaptively optimizing stimulation parameters per task. Golshan et al. [50] used variants of SVM classifiers to predict a variety of human behaviors, including speech, mouth movements, arm movements, finger movements, and a button press, with 70% accuracy, and demonstrated the effects of medication on STN-LFP [77]. Mamun et al. [79] decoded movement behaviors from LFPs of the STN and GPi from 12 PD and dystonia subjects with DBS by conducting a finger-clicking task with an accuracy of 99.8%. Furthermore, Niketeghad et al. [80] used SVM from 14 patients' LFPs to recognize speech, motor, and random type tasks with 73.2% accuracy. Additionally, several other studies examined the classification of behavioral actions using hidden Markov models (HMMs) in combination with the ML techniques [81–83]. For example, Jiang et al [83] created an HMM in combination with ML for the classification of motor, language, and motor/language combination tasks. They examined the LFP signals of nine DBS patients using their HMM model, and achieved over 80% accuracy at distinguishing between a combination of any two tasks.

5. Surgical Targeting

The surgical implantation of DBS electrodes necessitates accurate real-time identification of a specific brain region. Image guidance with direct magnetic resonance imaging (MRI) based targeting or co-registration of computed tomography (CT) with a 3-Tesla MRI are currently used to localize anatomic targets (i.e, STN and GPi) [28,84,85]. The selection of targets and surgical approaches varies among DBS centers, with microelectrode recording (MER) and intraoperative stimulation effects used to refine electrode placement [86]. ML techniques have been proposed to utilize microelectrode recordings to aid in subthalamic nucleus classification and thereby facilitate electrode placement. Cardona et al. [87,88] performed a retrospective analysis of MER region localization of 10 patients. They compared traditional ML classifiers (NB, SVM, KNN, etc.) with a multi-output Gaussian approach. The relative performance of the classifiers varied by task, but each achieved an accuracy of over 70%. The classification of other specific brain regions through MER signals has also been explored. For example, Khosravi et al. [89–91] analyzed the MERs of electrode trajectories with ML techniques over several studies. They retrospectively analyzed 100 DBS subjects' physicians determinations of optimal implantation trajectory's MERs with a deep NN and obtained an accuracy of 92% in localizing specific brain regions. Additionally, they utilized unsupervised machine learning techniques on 50 subjects' MERs and determined the dorsal border of the STN region with 80% accuracy. Finally, a fast Fourier transform was applied to the MERs of 20 DBS surgeries, and a logistic regression algorithm and SVM were applied to localize STN depth. This achieved an accuracy of 85% in detecting the borders of STN. High accuracy region SVM classification models were used by Guillén et al. [92,93] with a 99.5% accuracy at stratifying MERs between the STN, thalamus nucleus, and the substantia nigra. Similarly, Lu et al. [94] applied SVM to 16 subjects' MERs guided by 3-Tesla MRIs. This model achieved an AUC of 0.87. It is important to consider that MER measurements can be confounded based on the patient's state of sedation: minimal (awake), light, or deep (general anesthesia).

Alternative approaches, such as the utilization of traditional MRIs [50] and state-of-the-art 7-Tesla MRIs [95,96] or magnetoencephalography (MEG) [97] in conjunction with ML techniques, have been rarely explored. Ozturk et al. [98] examined ten patients' LFP signals and determined STN localization by an online linear discriminant classifier. Similarly, Darbin et al. [99] used LFP signals in a Tree Bagger algorithm to identify regions in non-human primates. Stuart et al. [100] examined 16 subjects' EEGs with multiple stimulation regions specifically: GPI, VIM, or STN. The fast Fourier transform was used to extract features. They compared the performance of several ML classifiers in determining the stimulation region. A decision tree based gradient booster paired with principal component analysis (PCA) performed the best at region identification (F1 0.62, precision 0.68).

ML has also been used in conjunction with HMMs to model surgical planning. For example, Valsky et al. [101] developed a real-time ML classification of the subthalamic border for accurate detection of the STN in DBS surgery. They examined 58 STN trajectories using an SVM and achieved an accuracy of 97.6%. They used the SVM results to inform an HMM for real-time identification, and this model was tested on an additional 73 trajectories, achieving an accuracy of 94%. Valsky et al. then continued this work in [102] for the identification of the striatopallidal border site to the GPi. They applied a similar SVM/HMM algorithm to 116 trajectories over three patient types: awake PD patients, lightly anesthetized genetic, and non-genetic dystonia subjects. Their algorithm had similar performance to clinical experts at GPi border identification across all patient types considered.

6. Insights into DBS Mechanisms

A small body of work exists that aims to better understand the underlying biological and chemical signals that impact DBS performance. Trevathan and colleagues [103] used NN and Volterra kernels to characterize stimulation-evoked neurochemical releases. They compared their proposed frameworks of stimulation-evoked dopamine releases in several animal models. This allowed for a neurochemical signaling comparison of healthy and diseased brains, which theoretically could be used to develop strategies for controlling DBS systems. In another study, Khawaldeh et al. [104] examined the off medication LFPs of 18 STN-DBS patients. They used NB classifiers for movement predictions and determined the band frequency of oscillatory synchronization associated with motor impairment in PD.

Finally, ML techniques have been utilized in the design of DBS systems. Jovanov et al. [105] developed a unique aDBS system hardware platform that allowed for the real-time optimization of DBS treatments by utilizing a genetic algorithm to identify patterns in treatment planning. Other studies that concentrate on hardware limitations include: Zhu et al. [106], which focused on performance, memory, and hardware requirements for seizure detection tasks in PD using EEG/ECoG (electrocorticography) as inputs to a custom decision tree algorithm; and De La Pava et al. [107], which applied hierarchical KNN to reduce the computational load of tissue-activated visualization in DBS modeling.

7. Discussion

The application of ML in DBS treatment for PD is a rapidly growing, interdisciplinary field that has unprecedented potential to transform all aspects of DBS. If considered and executed appropriately, ML will prove a tremendously beneficial tool for clinicians. This review examined the role of ML in DBS in the broadest terms, performing an exhaustive review and considering nearly a decade of publications. We found compelling applications for ML in (1) DBS candidate selection; (2) programming optimization; (3) surgical targeting; and (4) insights into DBS mechanisms. Even within a specific category, there was large heterogeneity among the studies regarding feature type, ML models, and practicality of implementation. Broadly speaking, the clinical features utilized in ML studies benefited from objectiveness. As such, ML research favors LFP, wearable sensors, MERs, and similar unbiased measurements.

The identification of PD patients whose motor control symptoms would be more effectively managed under DBS than medication-based therapies is a clear target for ML. Predicting which patients may have adverse effects from DBS therapies is crucial to ensuring optimal patient outcomes. Non-motor symptoms present further complexity to the PD phenotype, which has implications on disease progression, response to therapy (medication and stimulation), and surgical risk. Recent publications have offered methods to predict neurobehavioral changes preoperatively, hence possibly influencing the DBS decision-making process. Measuring motor and non-motor symptomatology through objective means will permit the expansion and robustness of these ML-based decision models. Additionally, patient phenotyping through unsupervised methods may reveal trends in patient data that have not been incorporated into current predictions. The automatic classification of potential DBS patients could efficiently determine an optimized treatment plan, thus dramatically improving patients' quality of life.

Adaptive DBS has a significant scope of clinical impact on a patient's quality of life. The use of LFPs and/or wearable sensors serve as robust measurement instruments for the classification of specific behavioral tasks, severity, and/or tremor. However, a large portion of these studies utilized assessments obtained in a clinical setting. Further work is needed to identify motor control symptoms in real-world environments. Tremor detection using wearable sensors appears to be one of the nearest methods to application in the clinical field. Additionally, the development of HMMs that accurately describe a DBS would have a great impact on strategic treatment planning. To that end, dynamic treatment planning would require a further assessment as to the practicality of adaptively tuning DBS parameters.

Surgical targeting utilizing ML to interpret intraoperative signals can be used to enhance the targeting of anatomic substrates, providing immediate clinical relevance as a support tool to assist in surgical planning. However, while many of the studies reviewed and utilized MER signals in classifying or delineating surgical targets to enhance optimal electrode placement, it is important to note that few studies have robustly examined clinically relevant outcomes related to these approaches. Image-based training of surrounding anatomy in ML modeling to enhance surgical target localization is expanding and showing greater precision and adaptability than current direct (image guided) or indirect (Talaraich coordinates) methods [108,109].

Although ML's application in DBS is relatively early in its development, the preliminary evidence is remarkably promising. Its ability to determine underlying patterns within patient data offers the potential to enhance candidate selection, facilitate surgical targeting, and more efficiently optimize programming approaches to yield rapid and robust clinical outcomes. In general, ML models that have interpretable data structures (explainable AI) should be favored in future studies. This allows experts to translate ML decision-making criteria, and could potentially provide insights into the fundamental nature of DBS. Additional insights may be found in the growing body of literature that proposes using PD-related genetic mutations and genetic profiles to identify DBS therapy effectiveness [110,111]. Furthermore, ML methods generally benefit from large data sets. The majority of studies considered in this review are limited by their small number of patients. Before any of the presented methods can be applied in a clinical setting, large-scale, randomized, multi-center studies are necessary to ensure an expansive data set while minimizing differences in target selection and surgical planning.

Author Contributions: J.W. drafted the paper and completed a review of the literature, A.K., O.S., and R.A.R. conceptualized the manuscript and outlined its content. J.W., A.K., and R.A.R. extensively reviewed and edited the manuscript to shape its final form. All authors have read and agreed to the published version of the manuscript.

Appendix A

Several statistical metrics are frequently calculated to measure model performance in classification tasks. These include:

- Precision: the measurement of positive and negative results that are truly positive
- Recall: the proportion of positives that are correctly identified
- Accuracy: the measurement of correct predictions out of all predictions
- PPV: the proportion of positive predictions that are true positives
- F1 Score: the harmonic average of precision and recall
- AUC under the receiver operating characteristic: the aggregate comparison of the true positive rate and the false positive rate at different classification thresholds, providing an overall performance metric

Similarly, several statistical metrics are frequently used to measure model performance in regressions tasks. These include:

- MSE: the average squared difference between the predicted and actual values
- MAE: the average of absolute errors between the predicted and actual values
- MAPE: the average percentage error between the predicted and actual values

Appendix B

After exclusion criteria were applied, we reviewed 68 publications from four databases. The number of publications that explore machine learning's role in deep brain stimulation as a treatment of Parkinson's disease is rapidly expanding. Figure A1 shows the number of publications within our review, segmented by publication year.

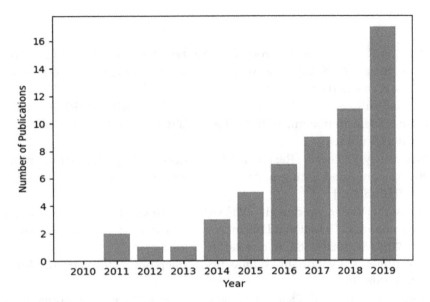

Figure A1. The number of publications examined within the review, segmented by the original publication date up to the last full year. There were 12 publications reviewed between January 2020 and August 2020.

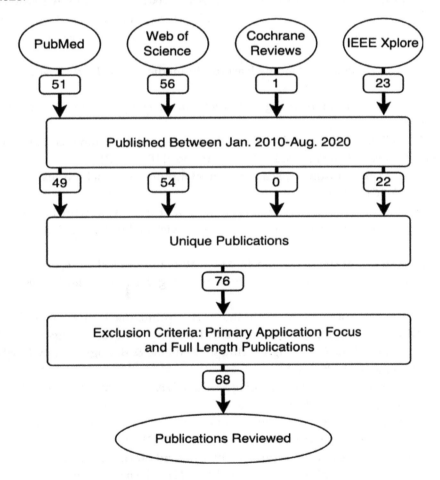

Figure A2. The description of the database keyword search results per database. Each number located within a square indicates the number of returned publications. The exclusion criteria are described in Section 2.

References

1. Machado, A.; Rezai, A.R.; Kopell, B.H.; Gross, R.E.; Sharan, A.D.; Benabid, A.L. Deep brain stimulation for Parkinson's disease: Surgical technique and perioperative management. *Mov. Disord. Off. J. Mov. Disord. Soc.* **2006**, *21*, S247–S258. [CrossRef] [PubMed]
2. Patel, N.; Plaha, P.; O'sullivan, K.; McCarter, R.; Heywood, P.; Gill, S. MRI directed bilateral stimulation of the subthalamic nucleus in patients with Parkinson's disease. *J. Neurol. Neurosurg. Psychiatry* **2003**, *74*, 1631–1637. [CrossRef] [PubMed]
3. Burchiel, K.J.; McCartney, S.; Lee, A.; Raslan, A.M. Accuracy of deep brain stimulation electrode placement using intraoperative computed tomography without microelectrode recording. *J. Neurosurg.* **2013**, *119*, 301–306. [CrossRef] [PubMed]
4. Dembek, T.A.; Reker, P.; Visser-Vandewalle, V.; Wirths, J.; Treuer, H.; Klehr, M.; Roediger, J.; Dafsari, H.S.; Barbe, M.T.; Timmermann, L. Directional DBS increases side-effect thresholds—A prospective, double-blind trial. *Mov. Disord.* **2017**, *32*, 1380–1388. [CrossRef] [PubMed]
5. Steigerwald, F.; Matthies, C.; Volkmann, J. Directional deep brain stimulation. *Neurotherapeutics* **2019**, *16*, 100–104. [CrossRef] [PubMed]
6. Volkmann, J.; Herzog, J.; Kopper, F.; Deuschl, G. Introduction to the programming of deep brain stimulators. *Mov. Disord. Off. J. Mov. Disord. Soc.* **2002**, *17*, S181–S187. [CrossRef] [PubMed]
7. Moro, E.; Esselink, R.; Xie, J.; Hommel, M.; Benabid, A.; Pollak, P. The impact on Parkinson's disease of electrical parameter settings in STN stimulation. *Neurology* **2002**, *59*, 706–713. [CrossRef]
8. Little, S.; Pogosyan, A.; Neal, S.; Zavala, B.; Zrinzo, L.; Hariz, M.; Foltynie, T.; Limousin, P.; Ashkan, K.; FitzGerald, J. Adaptive deep brain stimulation in advanced Parkinson disease. *Ann. Neurol.* **2013**, *74*, 449–457. [CrossRef]
9. Rajkomar, A.; Dean, J.; Kohane, I. Machine learning in medicine. *N. Engl. J. Med.* **2019**, *380*, 1347–1358. [CrossRef]
10. Shen, D.; Wu, G.; Suk, H.-I. Deep learning in medical image analysis. *Annu. Rev. Biomed. Eng.* **2017**, *19*, 221–248. [CrossRef]
11. Ravì, D.; Wong, C.; Deligianni, F.; Berthelot, M.; Andreu-Perez, J.; Lo, B.; Yang, G.-Z. Deep learning for health informatics. *IEEE J. Biomed. Health* **2016**, *21*, 4–21. [CrossRef] [PubMed]
12. Ahlrichs, C.; Lawo, M. Parkinson's disease motor symptoms in machine learning: A review. *arXiv* **2013**, arXiv:1312.3825. [CrossRef]
13. Belić, M.; Bobić, V.; Badža, M.; Šolaja, N.; Đurić-Jovičić, M.; Kostić, V.S. Artificial intelligence for assisting diagnostics and assessment of Parkinson's disease—A review. *Clin. Neurol. Neurosurg.* **2019**, *184*, 105442. [CrossRef]
14. Ramdhani, R.A.; Khojandi, A.; Shylo, O.; Kopell, B.H. Optimizing clinical assessments in Parkinson's disease through the use of wearable sensors and data driven modeling. *Front. Comput. Neurosci.* **2018**, *12*. [CrossRef] [PubMed]
15. Watts, J.; Khojandi, A.; Vasudevan, R.; Ramdhani, R. Optimizing Individualized Treatment Planning for Parkinson's Disease Using Deep Reinforcement Learning. In Proceedings of the 2020 42nd Annual International Conference of the IEEE Engineering in Medicine & Biology Society (EMBC), Montreal, QC, Canada, 20–24 July 2020; pp. 5406–5409.
16. Shalev-Shwartz, S.; Ben-David, S. *Understanding Machine Learning: From Theory to Algorithms*; Cambridge University Press: Cambridge, UK, 2014.
17. Murphy, K.P. *Machine Learning: A Probabilistic Perspective*; MIT Press: Cambridge, MA, USA, 2012.
18. Deo, R.C. Machine learning in medicine. *Circulation* **2015**, *132*, 1920–1930. [CrossRef]
19. Liaw, A.; Wiener, M. Classification and regression by randomForest. *R News* **2002**, *2*, 18–22.
20. Hansen, L.K.; Salamon, P. Neural network ensembles. *IEEE Trans. Pattern Anal. Mach. Intell.* **1990**, *12*, 993–1001. [CrossRef]
21. Suykens, J.A.; Vandewalle, J. Least squares support vector machine classifiers. *Neural Process. Lett.* **1999**, *9*, 293–300. [CrossRef]
22. Rish, I. An empirical study of the naive Bayes classifier. In Proceedings of the IJCAI 2001 Workshop on Empirical Methods in Artificial Intelligence, Seattle, DC, USA, 4–6 August 2001; pp. 41–46.

Machine Learning's Application in Deep Brain Stimulation for Parkinson's Disease										11

23.	Dudani, S.A. The distance-weighted k-nearest-neighbor rule. *IEEE Trans. Syst. ManCybern.* **1976**, 325–327. [CrossRef]
24.	Grira, N.; Crucianu, M.; Boujemaa, N. Unsupervised and semi-supervised clustering: A brief survey. *A Rev. Mach. Learn. Tech. Process. Multimed. Content* **2004**, *1*, 9–16.
25.	Biba, M.; Esposito, F.; Ferilli, S.; Di Mauro, N.; Basile, T.M.A. Unsupervised Discretization Using Kernel Density Estimation. In Proceedings of the IJCAI, Hyderabad, India, 6–12 January 2007; pp. 696–701.
26.	Deuschl, G.; Schade-Brittinger, C.; Krack, P.; Volkmann, J.; Schäfer, H.; Bötzel, K.; Daniels, C.; Deutschländer, A.; Dillmann, U.; Eisner, W. A randomized trial of deep-brain stimulation for Parkinson's disease. *N. Engl. J. Med.* **2006**, *355*, 896–908. [CrossRef]
27.	Volkmann, J. Deep brain stimulation for the treatment of Parkinson's disease. *J. Clin. Neurophysiol.* **2004**, *21*, 6–17. [CrossRef] [PubMed]
28.	Benabid, A.L. Deep brain stimulation for Parkinson's disease. *Curr. Opin. Neurobiol.* **2003**, *13*, 696–706. [CrossRef] [PubMed]
29.	Kumar, R.; Lozano, A.; Kim, Y.; Hutchison, W.; Sime, E.; Halket, E.; Lang, A. Double-blind evaluation of subthalamic nucleus deep brain stimulation in advanced Parkinson's disease. *Neurology* **1998**, *51*, 850–855. [CrossRef] [PubMed]
30.	Cerasa, A.; Novellino, F.; Quattrone, A. Connectivity changes in Parkinson's disease. *Curr. Neurol. Neurosci. Rep.* **2016**, *16*, 91. [CrossRef]
31.	Hebb, A.O.; Zhang, J.J.; Mahoor, M.H.; Tsiokos, C.; Matlack, C.; Chizeck, H.J.; Pouratian, N. Creating the feedback loop: Closed-loop neurostimulation. *Neurosurg. Clin.* **2014**, *25*, 187–204. [CrossRef]
32.	Wan, K.R.; Maszczyk, T.; See, A.A.Q.; Dauwels, J.; King, N.K.K. A review on microelectrode recording selection of features for machine learning in deep brain stimulation surgery for Parkinson's disease. *Clin. Neurophysiol.* **2019**, *130*, 145–154. [CrossRef]
33.	Prange, S.; Metereau, E.; Thobois, S. Structural imaging in Parkinson's disease: New developments. *Curr. Neurol. Neurosci. Rep.* **2019**, *19*, 50. [CrossRef]
34.	Farrokhi, F.; Buchlak, Q.D.; Sikora, M.; Esmaili, N.; Marsans, M.; McLeod, P.; Mark, J.; Cox, E.; Bennett, C.; Carlson, J. Investigating risk factors and predicting complications in deep brain stimulation surgery with machine learning algorithms. *World Neurosurg.* **2020**, *134*, e325–e338. [CrossRef]
35.	Das, S.; Trutoiu, L.; Murai, A.; Alcindor, D.; Oh, M.; De la Torre, F.; Hodgins, J. Quantitative measurement of motor symptoms in Parkinson's disease: A study with full-body motion capture data. In Proceedings of the 2011 Annual International Conference of the IEEE Engineering in Medicine and Biology Society, Boston, MA, USA, 30 August–3 September 2011; pp. 6789–6792.
36.	Yohanandan, S.A.; Jones, M.; Peppard, R.; Tan, J.L.; McDermott, H.J.; Perera, T. Evaluating machine learning algorithms estimating tremor severity ratings on the Bain–Findley scale. *Meas. Sci. Technol.* **2016**, *27*, 125702. [CrossRef]
37.	Kuhner, A.; Schubert, T.; Cenciarini, M.; Wiesmeier, I.K.; Coenen, V.A.; Burgard, W.; Weiller, C.; Maurer, C. Correlations between motor symptoms across different motor tasks, quantified via random forest feature classification in Parkinson's disease. *Front. Neurol.* **2017**, *8*, 607. [CrossRef] [PubMed]
38.	Kuhner, A.; Wiesmeier, I.K.; Cenciarini, M.; Maier, T.L.; Kammermeier, S.; Coenen, V.A.; Burgard, W.; Maurer, C. Motion Biomarkers Showing Maximum Contrast Between Healthy Subjects and Parkinson's Disease Patients Treated With Deep Brain Stimulation of the Subthalamic Nucleus. A Pilot Study. *Front. Neurosci.* **2019**, *13*, 1450. [CrossRef] [PubMed]
39.	Huo, W.; Angeles, P.; Tai, Y.F.; Pavese, N.; Wilson, S.; Hu, M.T.; Vaidyanathan, R. A Heterogeneous Sensing Suite for Multisymptom Quantification of Parkinson's Disease. *IEEE Trans. Neural Syst. Rehabil. Eng.* **2020**, *28*, 1397–1406. [CrossRef] [PubMed]
40.	Oliveira, F.H.M.; Machado, A.R.; Andrade, A.O. On the Use of *t*-Distributed Stochastic Neighbor Embedding for Data Visualization and Classification of Individuals with Parkinson's Disease. *Comput. Math. Methods Med.* **2018**, *2018*, 8019232. [CrossRef]
41.	Seppi, K.; Weintraub, D.; Coelho, M.; Perez-Lloret, S.; Fox, S.H.; Katzenschlager, R.; Hametner, E.M.; Poewe, W.; Rascol, O.; Goetz, C.G. The Movement Disorder Society evidence-based medicine review update: Treatments for the non-motor symptoms of Parkinson's disease. *Mov. Disord.* **2011**, *26*, S42–S80. [CrossRef] [PubMed]

42. Chaudhuri, K.R.; Schapira, A.H. Non-motor symptoms of Parkinson's disease: Dopaminergic pathophysiology and treatment. *Lancet Neurol.* **2009**, *8*, 464–474. [CrossRef]

43. Fasano, A.; Daniele, A.; Albanese, A. Treatment of motor and non-motor features of Parkinson's disease with deep brain stimulation. *Lancet Neurol.* **2012**, *11*, 429–442. [CrossRef]

44. Koch, M.; Geraedts, V.; Wang, H.; Tannemaat, M.; Bäck, T. Automated Machine Learning for EEG-Based Classification of Parkinson's Disease Patients. In Proceedings of the 2019 IEEE International Conference on Big Data (Big Data), Los Angeles, CA, USA, 9–12 December 2019; pp. 4845–4852.

45. Chen, Y.; Gong, C.; Hao, H.W.; Guo, Y.; Xu, S.J.; Zhang, Y.H.; Yin, G.P.; Cao, X.; Yang, A.C.; Meng, F.G.; et al. Automatic Sleep Stage Classification Based on Subthalamic Local Field Potentials. *IEEE Trans. Neural Syst. Rehabil. Eng.* **2019**, *27*, 118–128. [CrossRef]

46. Paliwal, S.; Mosley, P.E.; Breakspear, M.; Coyne, T.; Silburn, P.; Aponte, E.; Mathys, C.; Stephan, K.E. Subjective estimates of uncertainty during gambling and impulsivity after subthalamic deep brain stimulation for Parkinson's disease. *Sci. Rep.* **2019**, *9*, 1–16. [CrossRef]

47. Chrabaszcz, A.; Neumann, W.-J.; Stretcu, O.; Lipski, W.J.; Bush, A.; Dastolfo-Hromack, C.A.; Wang, D.; Crammond, D.J.; Shaiman, S.; Dickey, M.W. Subthalamic nucleus and sensorimotor cortex activity during speech production. *J. Neurosci.* **2019**, *39*, 2698–2708. [CrossRef]

48. Khojandi, A.; Shylo, O.; Mannini, L.; Kopell, B.H.; Ramdhani, R.A. Stratifying Parkinson's Patients With STN-DBS Into High-Frequency or 60 Hz-Frequency Modulation Using a Computational Model. *Neuromodulation* **2017**, *20*, 450–455. [CrossRef] [PubMed]

49. Shah, S.A.; Tinkhauser, G.; Chen, C.C.; Little, S.; Brown, P. Parkinsonian tremor detection from subthalamic nucleus local field potentials for closed-loop deep brain stimulation. In Proceedings of the 2018 40th Annual International Conference of the IEEE Engineering in Medicine and Biology Society (EMBC), Honolulu, HI, USA, 17–21 July 2018; pp. 2320–2324.

50. Shamir, R.R.; Dolber, T.; Noecker, A.M.; Walter, B.L.; McIntyre, C.C. Machine learning approach to optimizing combined stimulation and medication therapies for Parkinson's disease. *Brain Stimul.* **2015**, *8*, 1025–1032. [CrossRef] [PubMed]

51. Khodakarami, H.; Ricciardi, L.; Contarino, M.F.; Pahwa, R.; Lyons, K.E.; Geraedts, V.J.; Morgante, F.; Leake, A.; Paviour, D.; De Angelis, A. Prediction of the Levodopa Challenge Test in Parkinson's Disease Using Data from a Wrist-Worn Sensor. *Sensors -Basel* **2019**, *19*, 5153. [CrossRef]

52. Baumgarten, C.; Zhao, Y.; Sauleau, P.; Malrain, C.; Jannin, P.; Haegelen, C. Image-guided preoperative prediction of pyramidal tract side effect in deep brain stimulation: Proof of concept and application to the pyramidal tract side effect induced by pallidal stimulation. *J. Med. Imaging* **2016**, *3*, 025001. [CrossRef] [PubMed]

53. Przybyszewski, A.W.; Szlufik, S.; Habela, P.; Koziorowski, D.M. Rough Set Rules Determine Disease Progressions in Different Groups of Parkinson's Patients. In Proceedings of the International Conference on Pattern Recognition and Machine Intelligence, Kolkata, India, 5–8 December 2017; pp. 270–275.

54. Przybyszewski, A.W.; Szlufik, S.; Habela, P.; Koziorowski, D.M. Rules Found by Multimodal Learning in One Group of Patients Help to Determine Optimal Treatment to Other Group of Parkinson's Patients. In Proceedings of the Asian Conference on Intelligent Information and Database Systems, Kanazawa, Japan, 3–5 April 2017; pp. 359–367.

55. Castaño-Candamil, S.; Piroth, T.; Reinacher, P.; Sajonz, B.; Coenen, V.A.; Tangermann, M. An Easy-to-Use and Fast Assessment of Patient-Specific DBS-Induced Changes in Hand Motor Control in Parkinson's Disease. *IEEE Trans. Neural Syst. Rehabil. Eng.* **2019**, *27*, 2155–2163. [CrossRef]

56. Angeles, P.; Tai, Y.; Pavese, N.; Wilson, S.; Vaidyanathan, R. Automated assessment of symptom severity changes during deep brain stimulation (DBS) therapy for Parkinson's disease. In Proceedings of the 2017 International Conference on Rehabilitation Robotics (ICORR), London, UK, 17–20 July 2017; pp. 1512–1517.

57. Habets, J.G.; Heijmans, M.; Kuijf, M.L.; Janssen, M.L.; Temel, Y.; Kubben, P.L. An update on adaptive deep brain stimulation in Parkinson's disease. *Mov. Disord.* **2018**, *33*, 1834–1843. [CrossRef]

58. Maurer, A.; Hanrahan, S.; Nedrud, J.; Hebb, A.O.; Papandreou-Suppappola, A. Suppression of neurostimulation artifacts and adaptive clustering of Parkinson's patients behavioral tasks using EEG. In Proceedings of the 2016 50th Asilomar Conference on Signals, Systems and Computers, Pacific Grove, CA, USA, 6–9 November 2016; pp. 851–855.

59. Little, S.; Pogosyan, A.; Kuhn, A.; Brown, P. Beta band stability over time correlates with Parkinsonian rigidity and bradykinesia. *Exp. Neurol.* **2012**, *236*, 383–388. [CrossRef]

60. Amoozegar, S.; Pooyan, M.; Roughani, M. Toward a closed-loop deep brain stimulation in Parkinson's disease using local field potential in parkinsonian rat model. *Med. Hypotheses* **2019**, *132*, 109360. [CrossRef]

61. Neumann, W.-J.; Turner, R.S.; Blankertz, B.; Mitchell, T.; Kühn, A.A.; Richardson, R.M. Toward electrophysiology-based intelligent adaptive deep brain stimulation for movement disorders. *Neurotherapeutics* **2019**, *16*, 105–118. [CrossRef]

62. Khobragade, N.; Tuninetti, D.; Graupe, D. On the need for adaptive learning in on-demand Deep Brain Stimulation for Movement Disorders. In Proceedings of the 2018 40th Annual International Conference of the IEEE Engineering in Medicine and Biology Society (EMBC), Honolulu, HI, USA, 17–21 July 2018; pp. 2190–2193.

63. Camara, C.; Subramaniyam, N.P.; Warwick, K.; Parkkonen, L.; Aziz, T.; Pereda, E. Non-Linear Dynamical Analysis of Resting Tremor for Demand-Driven Deep Brain Stimulation. *Sensors (Basel)* **2019**, *19*, 2507. [CrossRef]

64. Tahafchi, P.; Molina, R.; Roper, J.A.; Sowalsky, K.; Hass, C.J.; Gunduz, A.; Okun, M.S.; Judy, J.W. Freezing-of-Gait detection using temporal, spatial, and physiological features with a support-vector-machine classifier. In Proceedings of the 2017 39th Annual International Conference of the IEEE Engineering in Medicine and Biology Society (EMBC), Jeju Island, Korea, 11–15 July 2017; pp. 2867–2870.

65. Herron, J.A.; Thompson, M.C.; Brown, T.; Chizeck, H.J.; Ojemann, J.G.; Ko, A.L. Chronic electrocorticography for sensing movement intention and closed-loop deep brain stimulation with wearable sensors in an essential tremor patient. *J. Neurosurg.* **2016**, *127*, 580–587. [CrossRef] [PubMed]

66. Graupe, D.; Khobragade, N.; Tuninetti, D.; Basu, I.; Slavin, K.V.; Verhagen Metman, L. Who may benefit from on-demand control of deep brain stimulation? Noninvasive evaluation of Parkinson patients. *Neuromodul. Technol. Neural Interface* **2018**, *21*, 611–616. [CrossRef] [PubMed]

67. LeMoyne, R.; Mastroianni, T.; Whiting, D.; Tomycz, N. Parametric evaluation of deep brain stimulation parameter configurations for Parkinson's disease using a conformal wearable and wireless inertial sensor system and machine learning. In Proceedings of the 2020 42nd Annual International Conference of the IEEE Engineering in Medicine & Biology Society (EMBC), Montreal, QC, Canada, 20–24 July 2020; pp. 3606–3611.

68. Yao, L.; Brown, P.; Shoaran, M. Resting Tremor Detection in Parkinson's Disease with Machine Learning and Kalman Filtering. In Proceedings of the 2018 IEEE Biomedical Circuits and Systems Conference (BioCAS), Cleveland, OH, USA, 17–19 October 2018; pp. 1–4.

69. Yao, L.; Brown, P.; Shoaran, M. Improved detection of parkinsonian resting tremor with feature engineering and kalman filtering. *Clin. Neurophysiol.* **2020**, *131*, 274–284. [CrossRef]

70. Livi, L.; Sadeghian, A.; Sadeghian, H. Discrimination and characterization of Parkinsonian rest tremors by analyzing long-term correlations and multifractal signatures. *IEEE Trans. Biomed. Eng.* **2016**, *63*, 2243–2249. [CrossRef] [PubMed]

71. Mohammed, A.; Bayford, R.; Demosthenous, A. A framework for adapting deep brain stimulation using Parkinsonian state estimates. *Front. Neurosci.* **2020**, *14*, 499. [CrossRef]

72. Mohammed, A.; Zamani, M.; Bayford, R.; Demosthenous, A. Patient specific Parkinson's disease detection for adaptive deep brain stimulation. In Proceedings of the 2015 37th Annual International Conference of the IEEE Engineering in Medicine and Biology Society (EMBC), Milano, Italy, 25–29 August 2015; pp. 1528–1531.

73. Mohammed, A.; Zamani, M.; Bayford, R.; Demosthenous, A. Toward on-demand deep brain stimulation using online Parkinson's disease prediction driven by dynamic detection. *IEEE Trans. Neural Syst. Rehabil. Eng.* **2017**, *25*, 2441–2452. [CrossRef]

74. Connolly, A.T.; Jensen, A.L.; Baker, K.B.; Vitek, J.L.; Johnson, M.D. Classification of pallidal oscillations with increasing parkinsonian severity. *J. Neurophysiol.* **2015**, *114*, 209–218. [CrossRef]

75. Golshan, H.M.; Hebb, A.O.; Hanrahan, S.J.; Nedrud, J.; Mahoor, M.H. A multiple kernel learning approach for human behavioral task classification using STN-LFP signal. In Proceedings of the 2016 38th Annual International Conference of the IEEE Engineering in Medicine and Biology Society (EMBC), Orlando, FL, USA, 16–20 August 2016; pp. 1030–1033.

76. Golshan, H.M.; Hebb, A.O.; Hanrahan, S.J.; Nedrud, J.; Mahoor, M.H. A hierarchical structure for human behavior classification using STN local field potentials. *J. Neurosci. Methods* **2018**, *293*, 254–263. [CrossRef]

77. Golshan, H.M.; Hebb, A.O.; Nedrud, J.; Mahoor, M.H. Studying the Effects of Deep Brain Stimulation and Medication on the Dynamics of STN-LFP Signals for Human Behavior Analysis. In Proceedings of the 2018 40th Annual International Conference of the IEEE Engineering in Medicine and Biology Society (EMBC), Honolulu, HI, USA, 18–21 July 2018; pp. 4720–4723.

78. Golshan, H.M.; Hebb, A.O.; Mahoor, M.H. LFP-Net: A deep learning framework to recognize human behavioral activities using brain STN-LFP signals. *J. Neurosci. Methods* **2020**, *335*, 108621. [CrossRef]

79. Mamun, K.; Mace, M.; Lutman, M.; Stein, J.; Liu, X.; Aziz, T.; Vaidyanathan, R.; Wang, S. Movement decoding using neural synchronization and inter-hemispheric connectivity from deep brain local field potentials. *J. Neural Eng.* **2015**, *12*, 056011. [CrossRef]

80. Niketeghad, S.; Hebb, A.O.; Nedrud, J.; Hanrahan, S.J.; Mahoor, M.H. Single trial behavioral task classification using subthalamic nucleus local field potential signals. In Proceedings of the 2014 36th Annual International Conference of the IEEE Engineering in Medicine and Biology Society, Chicago, IL, USA, 26–30 August 2014; pp. 3793–3796.

81. Zaker, N.; Dutta, A.; Maurer, A.; Zhang, J.J.; Hanrahan, S.; Hebb, A.O.; Kovvali, N.; Papandreou-Suppappola, A. Adaptive learning of behavioral tasks for patients with Parkinson's disease using signals from deep brain stimulation. In Proceedings of the 2014 48th Asilomar Conference on Signals, Systems and Computers, Pacific Grove, CA, USA, 2–5 November 2014; pp. 208–212.

82. Zaker, N.; Zhang, J.; Hanrahan, S.; Nedrud, J.; Hebb, A.O. A new approach for automated detection of behavioral task onset for patients with Parkinson's disease using subthalamic nucleus local field potentials. In Proceedings of the 2015 49th Asilomar Conference on Signals, Systems and Computers, Pacific Grove, CA, USA, 8–11 November 2015; pp. 780–784.

83. Jiang, H.G.; Zhang, J.J.; Hebb, A.; Mahoor, M.H. Time-frequency Analysis of Brain Electrical Signals for behvior Recognition in Patients with Parkinson's Disease. *Conf Rec Asilomar C* **2013**, 1843–1847.

84. Foltynie, T.; Zrinzo, L.; Martinez-Torres, I.; Tripoliti, E.; Petersen, E.; Holl, E.; Aviles-Olmos, I.; Jahanshahi, M.; Hariz, M.; Limousin, P. MRI-guided STN DBS in Parkinson's disease without microelectrode recording: Efficacy and safety. *J. Neurol. Neurosurg. Psychiatry* **2011**, *82*, 358–363. [CrossRef] [PubMed]

85. Neumann, J.-O.; Giese, H.; Biller, A.; Nagel, A.M.; Kiening, K. Spatial distortion in MRI-guided stereotactic procedures: Evaluation in 1.5-, 3-and 7-Tesla MRI Scanners. *Stereotact. Funct. Neurosurg.* **2015**, *93*, 380–386. [CrossRef]

86. Hariz, M.I. Safety and risk of microelectrode recording in surgery for movement disorders. *Stereotact. Funct. Neurosurg.* **2002**, *78*, 146–157. [CrossRef]

87. Cardona, H.D.V.; Orozco, A.A.; Alvarez, M.A. Multi-patient learning increases accuracy for Subthalamic nucleus identification in deep brain stimulation. In Proceedings of the 2012 Annual International Conference of the IEEE Engineering in Medicine and Biology Society, San Diego, CA, USA, 28 August –1 September 2012; pp. 4341–4344.

88. Cardona, H.D.V.; Álvarez, M.A.; Orozco, Á.A. Multi-task learning for subthalamic nucleus identification in deep brain stimulation. *Int. J. Mach. Learn. Cybern.* **2018**, *9*, 1181–1192. [CrossRef]

89. Khosravi, M.; Atashzar, S.F.; Gilmore, G.; Jog, M.S.; Patel, R.V. Electrophysiological signal processing for intraoperative localization of subthalamic nucleus during deep brain stimulation surgery. In Proceedings of the 2018 IEEE Global Conference on Signal and Information Processing (GlobalSIP), Anaheim, CA, USA, 26–28 November 2018; pp. 424–428.

90. Khosravi, M.; Atashzar, S.F.; Gilmore, G.; Jog, M.S.; Patel, R.V. Unsupervised Clustering of Micro-Electrophysiological Signals for localization of Subthalamic Nucleus during DBS Surgery. In Proceedings of the 2019 9th International IEEE/EMBS Conference on Neural Engineering (NER), San Francisco, CA, USA, 20–23 March 2019; pp. 17–20.

91. Khosravi, M.; Atashzar, S.F.; Gilmore, G.; Jog, M.S.; Patel, R.V. Intraoperative Localization of STN During DBS Surgery Using a Data-Driven Model. *IEEE J. Transl. Eng. Health Med.* **2020**, *8*, 1–9. [CrossRef]

92. Guillén-Rondon, P.; Robinson, M.D. Deep brain stimulation signal classification using deep belief networks. In Proceedings of the 2016 International Conference on Computational Science and Computational Intelligence (CSCI), Las Vegas, NV, USA, 15–17 December 2016; pp. 155–158.

93. Guillén, P.; Martinez-de-Pison, F.; Sanchez, R.; Argáez, M.; Velázquez, L. Characterization of subcortical structures during deep brain stimulation utilizing support vector machines. In Proceedings of the 2011 Annual International Conference of the IEEE Engineering in Medicine and Biology Society, Boston, MA, USA, 30 August–3 September 2011; pp. 7949–7952.

94. Lu, C.W.; Malaga, K.A.; Chou, K.L.; Chestek, C.A.; Patil, P.G. High density microelectrode recording predicts span of therapeutic tissue activation volumes in subthalamic deep brain stimulation for Parkinson disease. *Brain Stimul.* **2020**, *13*, 412–419. [CrossRef]

95. Shamir, R.R.; Duchin, Y.; Kim, J.; Patriat, R.; Marmor, O.; Bergman, H.; Vitek, J.L.; Sapiro, G.; Bick, A.; Eliahou, R.; et al. Microelectrode Recordings Validate the Clinical Visualization of Subthalamic-Nucleus Based on 7T Magnetic Resonance Imaging and Machine Learning for Deep Brain Stimulation Surgery. *Neurosurgery* **2019**, *84*, 749–756. [CrossRef]

96. Kim, J.; Duchin, Y.; Shamir, R.R.; Patriat, R.; Vitek, J.; Harel, N.; Sapiro, G. Automatic localization of the subthalamic nucleus on patient-specific clinical MRI by incorporating 7 T MRI and machine learning: Application in deep brain stimulation. *Hum. Brain Mapp.* **2019**, *40*, 679–698. [CrossRef]

97. Boring, M.J.; Jessen, Z.F.; Wozny, T.A.; Ward, M.J.; Whiteman, A.C.; Richardson, R.M.; Ghuman, A.S. Quantitatively validating the efficacy of artifact suppression techniques to study the cortical consequences of deep brain stimulation with magnetoencephalography. *Neuroimage* **2019**, *199*, 366–374. [CrossRef]

98. Ozturk, M.; Telkes, I.; Jimenez-Shahed, J.; Viswanathan, A.; Tarakad, A.; Kumar, S.; Sheth, S.A.; Ince, N.F. Randomized, Double-Blind Assessment of LFP Versus SUA Guidance in STN-DBS Lead Implantation: A Pilot Study. *Front. Neurosci.* **2020**, *14*, 611. [CrossRef] [PubMed]

99. Darbin, O.; Hatanaka, N.; Takara, S.; Kaneko, M.; Chiken, S.; Naritoku, D.; Martino, A.; Nambu, A. Local field potential dynamics in the primate cortex in relation to parkinsonism reveled by machine learning: A comparison between the primary motor cortex and the supplementary area. *Neurosci. Res.* **2020**, *156*, 66–79. [CrossRef] [PubMed]

100. Stuart, M.; Wickramasinghe, C.S.; Marino, D.L.; Kumbhare, D.; Holloway, K.; Manic, M. Machine Learning for Deep Brain Stimulation Efficacy using Dense Array EEG. In Proceedings of the 2019 12th International Conference on Human System Interaction (HSI), Richmond, VA, USA, 25–27 June 2019; pp. 143–150.

101. Valsky, D.; Marmor-Levin, O.; Deffains, M.; Eitan, R.; Blackwell, K.T.; Bergman, H.; Israel, Z. Stop! Border Ahead: Automatic Detection of Subthalamic Exit During Deep Brain Stimulation Surgery. *Mov. Disord.* **2017**, *32*, 70–79. [CrossRef]

102. Valsky, D.; Blackwell, K.T.; Tamir, I.; Eitan, R.; Bergman, H.; Israel, Z. Real-time machine learning classification of pallidal borders during deep brain stimulation surgery. *J. Neural Eng.* **2020**, *17*, 016021. [CrossRef]

103. Trevathan, J.K.; Yousefi, A.; Park, H.O.; Bartoletta, J.J.; Ludwig, K.A.; Lee, K.H.; Lujan, J.L. Computational modeling of neurotransmitter release evoked by electrical stimulation: Nonlinear approaches to predicting stimulation-evoked dopamine release. *ACS Chem. Neurosci.* **2017**, *8*, 394–410. [CrossRef] [PubMed]

104. Khawaldeh, S.; Tinkhauser, G.; Shah, S.A.; Peterman, K.; Debove, I.; Nguyen, T.K.; Nowacki, A.; Lachenmayer, M.L.; Schuepbach, M.; Pollo, C. Subthalamic nucleus activity dynamics and limb movement prediction in Parkinson's disease. *Brain* **2020**, *143*, 582–596. [CrossRef]

105. Jovanov, I.; Nauman, M.; Kumaravelu, K.; Lesi, V.; Zutshi, A.; Grill, W.M.; Pajic, M. Learning-based control design for deep brain stimulation. In Proceedings of the 2018 ACM/IEEE 9th International Conference on Cyber-Physical Systems (ICCPS), Porto, Portugal, 11–13 April 2018; pp. 349–350.

106. Zhu, B.; Farivar, M.; Shoaran, M. ResOT: Resource-Efficient Oblique Trees for Neural Signal Classification. *IEEE Trans. Biomed. Circuits Syst.* **2020**, *14*, 692–704. [CrossRef]

107. De La Pava, I.; Mejía, J.; Álvarez-Meza, A.; Álvarez, M.; Orozco, A.; Henao, O. A hierarchical K-nearest neighbor approach for volume of tissue activated estimation. In Proceedings of the Iberoamerican Congress on Pattern Recognition, Lima, Peru, 8–11 November 2016; pp. 125–133.

108. Bermudez, C.; Rodriguez, W.; Huo, Y.; Hainline, A.E.; Li, R.; Shults, R.; D'Haese, P.D.; Konrad, P.E.; Dawant, B.M.; Landman, B.A. Towards machine learning prediction of deep brain stimulation (DBS) intra-operative efficacy maps. In Proceedings of the Medical Imaging 2019: Image Processing, San Diego, CA, USA, 16–21 February 2019; p. 1094922.

109. Park, S.-C.; Cha, J.H.; Lee, S.; Jang, W.; Lee, C.S.; Lee, J.K. Deep learning-based deep brain stimulation targeting and clinical applications. *Front. Neurosci.* **2019**, *13*, 1128. [CrossRef]

110. Ligaard, J.; Sannæs, J.; Pihlstrøm, L. Deep brain stimulation and genetic variability in Parkinson's disease: A review of the literature. *npj Parkinson's Dis.* **2019**, *5*, 1–10. [CrossRef]

111. de Oliveira, L.M.; Barbosa, E.R.; Aquino, C.C.; Munhoz, R.P.; Fasano, A.; Cury, R.G. Deep Brain Stimulation in Patients With Mutations in Parkinson's Disease–Related Genes: A Systematic Review. *Mov. Disord. Clin. Pract.* **2019**, *6*, 359–368. [CrossRef]

## 2

Thalamic Deep Brain Stimulation in Essential Tremor Plus is as Effective as in Essential Tremor

Julia K. Steffen [1,*], Hannah Jergas [1], Jan N. Petry-Schmelzer [1], Till A. Dembek [1](iD),
Tabea Thies [1](iD), Stefanie T. Jost [1], Haidar S. Dafsari [1], Josef Kessler [1], Jochen Wirths [2],
Gereon R. Fink [1,3], Veerle Visser-Vandewalle [2] and Michael T. Barbe [1]

[1] Department of Neurology, Faculty of Medicine and University Hospital Cologne, University of Cologne,
    50937 Cologne, Germany; Hannah.jergas@ul-koeln.de (H.J.); jan.petry-schmelzer@uk-koeln.de (J.N.P.-S.);
    till.dembek@uk-koeln.de (T.A.D.); tabea.thies@uk-koeln.de (T.T.); stefanie.jost@uk-koeln.de (S.T.J.);
    haidar.dafsari@uk-koeln.de (H.S.D.); josef.kessler@uk-koeln.de (J.K.); gereon.fink@uk-koeln.de (G.R.F.);
    michael.barbe@uk-koeln.de (M.T.B.)
[2] Department of Stereotactic and Functional Neurosurgery, Faculty of Medicine and University Hospital
    Cologne, University of Cologne, 50937 Cologne, Germany; jochen.wirths@uk-koeln.de (J.W.);
    veerle.visser-vandewalle@uk-koeln.de (V.V.-V.)
[3] Cognitive Neuroscience, Research Center Jülich, Institute of Neuroscience and Medicine (INM-3),
    52428 Jülich, Germany
*   Correspondence: Julia.steffen@uk-koeln.de

Abstract: The new essential tremor (ET) classification defined ET-plus (ET-p) as an ET subgroup with additional neurological signs besides action tremor. While deep brain stimulation (DBS) is effective in ET, there are no studies specifically addressing DBS effects in ET-p. 44 patients with medication-refractory ET and thalamic/subthalamic DBS implanted at our center were postoperatively classified into ET and ET-p according to preoperative documentation. Tremor suppression with DBS (stimulation ON vs. preoperative baseline and vs. stimulation OFF), measured via the Fahn–Tolosa–Marin tremor rating scale (TRS), stimulation parameters, and the location of active contacts were compared between patients classified as ET and ET-p. TRS scores at baseline were higher in ET-p. ET-p patients showed comparable tremor reduction as patients with ET, albeit higher stimulation parameters were needed in ET-p. Active electrode contacts were located more dorsally in ET-p of uncertain reason. Our data show that DBS is similarly effective in ET-p compared to ET. TRS scores were higher in ET-p preoperatively, and higher stimulation parameters were needed for tremor reduction compared to ET. The latter may be related to a more dorsal location of active electrode contacts in the ET-p group of this cohort. Prospective studies are warranted to investigate DBS in ET-p further.

Keywords: essential tremor; deep brain stimulation; ET plus; tremor classification; thalamic DBS

1. Introduction

Essential tremor (ET) is characterized by bilateral upper limb action tremor but may include other neurological symptoms. In 2017, the Movement Disorder Society (MDS) published a tremor classification with new diagnostic criteria [1]. In this classification, ET with additional neurological signs, such as ataxia, rest tremor, or cognitive impairment, was defined as ET plus (ET-p). Retrospective studies suggest that ET-p is more common than ET [2,3]. However, there is an ongoing debate on the validity of the new classification [4].

Deep brain stimulation (DBS) of the thalamic ventral intermediate nucleus (VIM) and the posterior subthalamic area (PSA) is an effective treatment for medication-refractory ET. It reduces tremors up to 90% [5]. Previous studies on DBS in ET did not differentiate between ET and ET-p. Since in those studies, where patients were not systematically grouped in ET with and without plus signs, DBS response varies [6,7], this study aimed to investigate the effect of DBS in the ET-p group.

2. Materials and Methods

2.1. Patients

Patients with ET according to the previous MDS tremor classification [8], who had received VIM/PSA DBS between February 2009 and May 2019 at our center were retrospectively reclassified as either ET or ET-p. Indication for DBS and DBS implantation had been determined beforehand and independently of this study according to established criteria (medication refractory ET without contraindications for surgery, e.g., relevant cerebral atrophy, relevant cognitive impairment, ...). Surgery was performed with microelectrode recordings. The final target of the DBS lead was determined after intraoperative clinical testing of effects and side effects. Retrospective classification in ET and ET-p was based on preoperative documentation (medical reports, neuropsychological testing) and, if available, on preoperative videos. Following the new MDS criteria [1], patients with plus signs were classified as ET-p. Cognitive impairment was defined as a deterioration of ≥ 1.5 standard-deviations in the memory domain of a neuropsychological testing battery compared to a standardized control group [9]. Inclusion criteria were DBS for at least three months before enrollment and sufficient preoperative documentation for valid classification in either ET or ET-p. In case of insufficient documentation, patients were excluded from the analysis.

2.2. Protocol Approval, Registration, and Consent

This investigator-initiated study was approved by the local Ethics Committee of the University of Cologne (study-no: 19-258) and conducted under the Declaration of Helsinki. Patients gave written informed consent for postoperative videos taken explicitly for this study. The study was registered at the German Clinical Trials Register (Registration -No: DRKS00021068).

2.3. Data Acquisition and Tremor Analysis

Age and disease duration at the time of DBS implantation were determined. Postural, kinetic, and rest tremor of upper and lower limbs, as well as head-tremor, were evaluated using the Fahn–Tolosa–Marin Tremor rating scale part A and B [10], reported as a sum score of part A and B. TRS-evaluation was based on video documentation, if available, before DBS surgery (baseline) and at follow-up in the ON-stimulation (ON, chronic stimulation with best clinical parameters) and the OFF-stimulation (OFF, stimulation in both hemispheres switched off) state. There was no defined time range between DBS implantation and follow-up videos, nor was there a standardized time from switching off stimulation and video taking in the OFF state. Most of the videos had been recorded independently of the study, implemented in our clinical routine. Additionally, patients were invited for follow-up postoperative video documentation as part of this study. TRS scores were assessed by an experienced, unblinded rater (JKS).

2.4. Active Contact Location and Stimulation Parameters

Locations of active contacts were determined with the LEAD DBS toolbox 2.3.2 (Berlin, Germany) [11] as described previously [12] and are reported in relation to the midcommissural point (MCP) in standardized MNI space. All contacts were mirrored to the right hemisphere. To compare stimulation settings, we calculated the total electric energy delivered per second (TEED) [13].

2.5. Statistical Analysis

TRS scores at baseline and follow-up (ON and OFF) were in a non-parametric distribution and were therefore compared via the Wilcoxon signed-rank test with a significance threshold of $p < 0.05$. Other pre-

and postoperative scores and data on age and disease duration at the time of DBS implantation in patients with ET-p compared to ET were analyzed using the Mann–Whitney U test. The significance level of $p < 0.05$ were Bonferroni-corrected for multiple comparisons. Variance analysis was conducted using Levene's test with a significance threshold of $p < 0.05$. Active contact location and TEED were compared via unpaired t-test or Mann–Whitney U test. Results are shown as means ± standard deviation. Statistical analyses were conducted using IBM SPSS Statistics 26 (Armonk, NY, USA) and MATLAB 2018b (Natick, MA, USA).

3. Results

3.1. Patient Characteristics

Forty-four patients (15 female) were included, of whom 31 patients (70%) were reclassified as ET-p, 13 as ET. For 17 patients (6 ET, 11 ET-p), reclassification was not only based on written documentation but also on visual evaluation of preoperative videos. The most frequent plus-sign was rest tremor ($n = 14$), followed by mild cognitive impairment (MCI, $n = 13$), dystonic posturing ($n = 9$), and gait ataxia ($n = 5$). Twelve patients showed more than one plus-sign. Patient characteristics are provided in Table 1.

3.2. DBS Effect and Tremor-Scores

3.2.1. TRS in Stimulation-OFF and -ON

For 40 patients (28 ET-p) postoperative TRS-videos existed and TRS scores in OFF and ON were assessed from video documentation. Mean time between DBS implantation and follow-up was comparable for both groups (ET: 28.25 ± 26.20 months, ET-p: 23.68 ± 25.74 months, $p = 0.850$). TRS-OFF scores (ET: 25.83 ± 17.16, ET-p: 41.89 ± 15.56, $p = 0.007$) as well as TRS-ON scores (ET: 7.42 ± 5.20, ET-p: 15.68 ± 11.24, $p = 0.019$) were higher in ET-p than in ET, and ON scores additionally showed higher variance in ET-p (Levene test ON: F = 7.721, $p = 0.008$, OFF: F = 0.233, $p = 0.632$). Both groups showed significant (ET: $p = 0.002$; ET-p: 0.000) and comparable tremor reduction due to DBS, of 68.9% in ET (± 14.62%) and 62.0% in ET-p (± 19.60%; $p = 0.224$, Levene test: F = 1.629, $p = 0.210$, Figure 1a).

3.2.2. TRS at Baseline and Follow-Up

For 17 patients (6 ET, 11 ET-p) pre- and postoperative TRS scores could be assessed. Follow-up periods were comparable (ET: 20.83 ± 17.71 months; ET-p: 13.27 ± 12.40 months; $p = 0.256$). Groups further showed comparable TRS scores at baseline (ET: 20.33 ± 5.47, ET-p: 29.27 ± 12.63, $p = 0.180$), albeit variance was again higher in ET-p (Levene test: F = 6.557, $p = 0.022$). Comparing baseline to ON DBS, significant tremor reduction was observed in both groups (ET: $p = 0.028$; ET-p: $p = 0.006$) with a comparable reduction of 75.03% (± 17.43%) in ET and 56.27% (± 22.84%) in ET-p ($p = 0.122$, Levene test: F = 0.581, $p = 0.458$). Groups showed comparable TRS scores in ON (ET: 5.00 ± 3.35, ET-p: 13.22 ± 10.22, $p = 0.027$, Levene test: F = 2.809, $p = 0.114$, Figure 1b).

3.2.3. Active Contact Location

Mean coordinates of active contacts in ET were x = 11.81 ± 2.26 mm, y = −4.77 ± 1.97 mm, and z = −2.16 mm ± 1.55. In ET-p mean coordinates were x = 12.18 ± 2.51 mm, y = −4.8 ± 2.05 mm, and z = −0.63 ± 2 mm. Mean x- and y-coordinates did not differ between groups (x: $p = 0.11$, y: $p = 0.9$, Figure 1), while active contacts were located more dorsally in ET-p ($p < 0.01$, Figure 2).

3.2.4. Stimulation Parameters

Stimulation parameters were available for all, but one ET-p-patient. Stimulation amplitude (ET: 1.7 ± 0.5 mA, ET-p: 2.9 ± 1.13 mA, $p < 0.001$) and TEED (ET: 30.4 ± 20.8 µJ, ET-p: 120 ± 133.2 µJ, $p = 0.0001$) were significantly higher in ET-p.

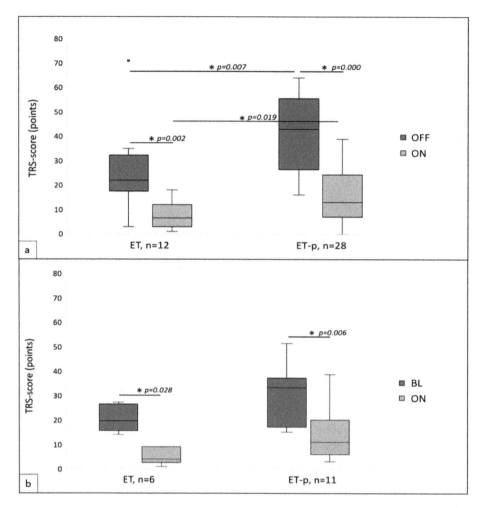

Figure 1. (a) Postoperative Fahn–Tolosa–Marin tremor rating scale (TRS) scores in essential tremor (ET) and ET-plus (ET-p) in stimulation switched OFF (OFF) and in stimulation switched ON (ON). (b) TRS scores in ET and ET-p at preoperative baseline (BL) and postoperative in ON. * indicates statistical significance, $p < 0.05$.

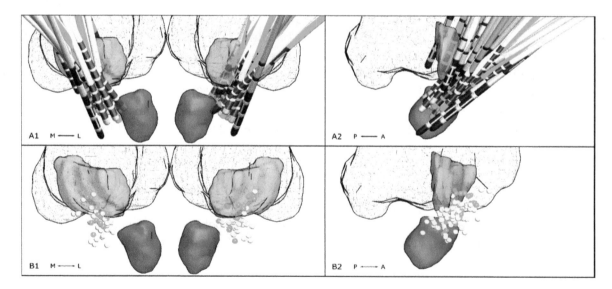

Figure 2. Lead locations in relation to the VIM (turquoise), the red nucleus (red) and thalamus (fishnet structure) taken from the DISTAL atlas implemented in LEAD DBS. In the top row, electrode locations of patients with ET (green) and ET-p (yellow) are shown bilaterally (**A1**) and mirrored to the right hemisphere (**A2**). Electrode contacts are marked in gray. In the bottom row, locations of active electrode contacts are shown bilaterally (**B1**) and mirrored on the right hemisphere (**B2**).

Table 1. Patient characteristics and individual TRS scores. Abbreviations: f = female; m = male; age = age at DBS implantation; DD = disease duration at DBS implantation; y = years; FU = follow-up (time between DBS implantation and TRS-scoring in months, m); RT = rest tremor; MCI = mild cognitive impairment; BL = baseline; OFF = stimulation OFF; ON = stimulation ON; % (BL) = tremor reduction in percent in ON compared to baseline; % (OFF) = tremor reduction in percent in ON compared to OFF.

Pat-ID	Sex	Age (y)	DD (y); FU (m)	Syndrome	Plus-Sign	BL-TRS	OFF-TRS	ON-TRS	% (BL)	% (OFF)	Clinical Stimulation Settings Left Hemisphere	Clinical Stimulation Settings Right Hemisphere
1	f	78	9;11	ET	-	27	-	9	66.67	-	C+, 0-100%, 60 µs, 130 Hz, 2.5 mA	C+, 8-100%, 60 µs, 130 Hz, 1 mA
2	m	67	37;54	ET	-	16	20	5	68.75	75	C+, 2-50%, 4-50%, 60 µs, 223 Hz, 2.5 mA	C+, 10-50%, 12-50%, 60 µs, 223 Hz, 2.2 mA
3	m	71	39;10	ET	-	22	21	3	86.36	85.71	C+, 5-34%, 6-33%, 7-33%; 60 µs; 174 Hz; 2 mA	C+, 10-24%, 11-23%, 12-23%, 13-10%, 14-10%, 15-10%; 60 µs; 130 Hz; 1.3 mA
4	m	26	9;18	ET	-	14	3	1	92.86	66.67	C+, 3-100%, 60 µs, 174 Hz, 1.3 mA	C+, 11-100%, 60 µs, 174 Hz, 0.7 mA
5	m	56	46;26	ET	-	17	71	9	47.06	87.32	C+, 3-100%, 60 µs, 130 Hz, 3 mA	C+, 11-100%, 60 µs, 174 Hz, 2 mA
6	m	72	11;6	ET	-	26	19	3	88.46	84.21	C+, 1-100%, 60µs, 130 Hz, 1.1 mA	C+, 9-100%, 60µs, 130 Hz, 1 mA
7	m	64	32;6	ET	-	-	23	7	-	69.57	C+, 0-100%, 60 µs, 130 Hz, 2.0 V	C+, 8-100%, 60 µs, 130 Hz, 1.8 V
8	m	68	30;61	ET	-	-	33	14	-	57.58	C+, 0-50%, 1-50%, 90µs, 150 Hz, 2 V	C+, 10-100%, 90µs, 150 Hz, 2.2 V
9	m	60	44;3	ET	-	-	30	18	-	40.0	C+, 1-100%, 60 µs, 130 Hz, 1.6 mA	C+, 9-100%, 60 µs, 130 Hz, 1.7 mA
10	m	53	44;3	ET	-	-	17	7	-	58.82	C+, 2-34%, 3-33%, 4-33%, 60 µs, 130 Hz, 1.4 mA	C+, 10-34%,11-33%, 12-33%; 60 µs, 130 Hz, 0.7 mA
11	m	48	34;67	ET	-	-	8	3	-	62.5	VIM 1: C+, 1-0.3 V, 60µs, 120 Hz VIM 2:2-1.1 V, 60µs, 120 Hz	C+, 9-50%, 10-50%, 60µs, 120 Hz, 1.3 V
12	m	62	29;67	ET	-	-	35	6	-	82.86	VIM 1: C+, 0-3.1 V, 60µs, 120 Hz VIM 2: C+, 1-1.3 V, 60 µs, 120 Hz	VIM 1: C+, 9-2.1 V, 60 µs, 120 Hz VIM 2:10-2.8 V, 60 µs, 120 Hz
13	m	54	45;18	ET	-	-	30	13	-	56.67	C+, 2-34%, 3-33%, 4-33%, 204 Hz, 50 µs, 1.3 mA	C+, 10-34%, 11-33%, 12-33%, 204 Hz, 50 µs, 1.7 mA
14	f	72	61;12	ET-p	RT	34	-	3	91.18	-	C+, 0-100%, 60 µs, 130 Hz, 2.2 V	C+, 8-100%, 60 µs, 130 Hz, 2.4 V
15	m	22	13;11	ET-p	Dystonia, MCI	51	-	21	58.82	-	C+, 3-30% 4-60% 5-10%, 60 µs 174 Hz, 5.7 mA	C+, 11-25% 12-75% 60 µs 174 Hz, 4 mA
16	f	61	15;11	ET-p	RT, MCI	37	-	20	45.95	-	C+, 2-100% 60 µs, 130 Hz, 3.9 mA	C+, 10-100%, 60 µs, 130 Hz, 3.9 mA
17	m	60	29;10	ET-p	Dystonia	21	32	10	52.38	68.75	C+, 1-30%, 2-35%, 3-35%, 60 µs, 130 Hz, 1.9 mA	C+, 13-33%, 14-33%, 15-34%, 60 µs, 130 Hz, 1.6 mA
18	m	66	16;9	ET-p	RT	33	58	28	15.15	51.72	C+, 1-100%, 60 µs, 208 Hz, 4.2 mA	C+, 11-100%, 60 µs, 208 Hz, 2.5 mA
19	m	66	49;43	ET-p	Dystonia	46	48	14	69.57	70.83	C+, 3-100% 60 µs, 130 Hz, 3.8 mA	C+, 11-, 100% 60 µs, 130 Hz, 2.9 mA
20	f	61	60;4	ET-p	MCI	17	26	11	35.29	57.69	C+, 2-100%, 60 µs, 130 Hz, 6.5 mA	C+, 10-100%, 60 µs, 130 Hz, 4 mA
21	m	70	29;5	ET-p	RT, MCI	16	21	11	31.25	47.62	C+;1-100% 60 µs, 130 Hz, 1 mA	C+, 9-100%, 60 µs, 130 Hz, 1 mA
22	f	63	21;3	ET-p	MCI	15	20	4	73.33	80.0	C+, 1-100%, 60 µs, 130 Hz, 1.4 mA	C+, 9-100%, 60 µs, 130 Hz, 1.2 mA
23	f	77	27;8	ET-p	RT, MCI	34	42	7	79.41	83.33	C+, 1-62% 2-14%, 3-12% 4-12%, 50 µs, 174 Hz, 1.8 mA	C+, 9-75%, 10-9%, 11-8%, 12-8%, 50 µs, 174 Hz, 1.7 mA

Table 1. *Cont.*

Pat-ID	Sex	Age (y)	DD (y); FU (m)	Syndrome	Plus-Sign	BL-TRS	OFF-TRS	ON-TRS	% (BL)	% (OFF)	Clinical Stimulation Settings Left Hemisphere	Clinical Stimulation Settings Right Hemisphere
24	f	68	31;31	ET-p	RT, Ataxia	18	25	6	66.67	76.0	2-70%, 3-30%, 5 + 100%, 60 µs, 174 Hz, 2.0 mA	10-70%, 11-30%, 13 + 100%, 60 Hz, 174 Hz, 2.0 mA
25	f	70	56;38	ET-p	RT	-	64	39	-	39.06	C+, 1-100%, 60 us, 185 Hz, 2.8 mA	C+, 9-100%, 60 us, 185 Hz, 2.8 mA
26	m	52	41;98	ET-p	MCI	-	51	13	-	74.51	C+, 1-100%, 60 µs, 200 Hz, 2.0 V	C+, 9-100%m, 60 µs, 200 Hz, 3.3 V
27	m	77	16;13	ET-p	RT	-	41	18	-	56.1	C+, 1-100%, 60 µs, 200 Hz, 2.0 V	C+, 9-100%m, 60 µs, 200 Hz, 3.3 V
28	f	75	10;28	ET-p	RT	-	41	2	-	95.12	C+, 2-100%, 60 µs, 125 Hz, 3.2 mA	VIM 1: C+, 8-50% 9-50%, 60 µs, 125 Hz, 3.6 mA Vim 2: C+, 9-100%, 60 µs, 125 Hz, 3.2 mA
29	m	64	5;15	ET-p	Ataxia	-	53	36	-	32.08	5 + 34%, 6 + 33%, 7 + 33%, 1-90%, 2-5%, 4-5% 40 µs, 204 Hz, 5 mA	13 + 34%, 14 + 33%, 15 + 33%, 9-80%, 11-10%, 40 µs, 204 Hz, 4.7 mA
30	f	65	24;12	ET-p	Ataxia	-	33	5	-	84.85	C+, 2-21% 3-5% 4-29%, 5-17%,6-5%,7-23%, 60 µs, 149 Hz, 2.3 mA	C+, 10-17%, 11-26% 12-27%, 13-10%, 14-10%, 15-10%, 60 µs, 149 Hz, 2.3 mA
31	m	58	11;12	ET-p	MCI	-	47	22	-	53.19	C+, 0-100%, 60 µs, 130 Hz, 3.3 V	C+, 8-100%, 60 µs, 130 Hz, 3.3 V
32	m	69	6;111	ET-p	RT	-	64	36	-	43.75	C+, 0-100%, 60 µs, 180 Hz, 3.5 V	C+, 8-100%, 60 µs, 180 Hz, 3.1 V
33	f	57	43;32	ET-p	Dystonia	-	58	0	-	100.0	VIM 1:C+; 2-100%, 2.4 V 90µs, 120 Hz VIM 2:3-100% 90µs, 120 Hz, 1.8 V	C+, 10-100%, 60µs, 120 Hz, 2.8 V
34	m	79	3;37	ET-p	MCI	-	58	13	-	48.0	C+, 1-100%, 80 µs, 149 Hz, 2.7 mA	C+, 9-100%, 60 µs, 149 Hz, 2.1 mA
35	m	63	13;17	ET-p	Dystonia, ataxia	-	54	7	-	87.04	C+ 10%, 1-100%, 2 + 30%, 3 + 30%, 4 + 30%, 50 µs, 179 Hz, 2.8 mA	C+ 20%, 12-60%, 15-40%, 10 + 19%, 11 + 19%, 13 + 21%, 14 + 21% G + 20%, 50 µs, 179 Hz, 3.5 mA
36	m	63	44;9	ET-p	RT, dystonia	-	52	28	-	46.15	1-100%, 2 + 34%, 3 + 33%, 4 + 33%, 60 µs, 179 Hz, 3.1 mA	9-100%, 10 + 34%, 11 + 33%, 12 + 33%, 70 µs, 179 Hz, 3.4 mA
37	m	75	66;7	ET-p	RT, MCI	-	28	8	-	71.43	C+, 2-34%, 3-33%, 4-33%, 60 µs, 130 Hz, 2.1 mA	C+, 2-34%, 3-33%, 4-33%, 60 µs, 130 Hz, 2.1 mA
38	m	67	18;8	ET-p	Ataxia	-	22	18	-	18.18	-	-
39	f	66	9;14	ET-p	Dystonia, MCI	-	16	4	-	75.0	VIM 1: C+, 8-100%, 90 µs, 125 Hz, 1.3 V VIM 2: C+, 9-100%, 90 µs, 125 Hz, 2.1 V	VIM 1: C+, 1-100%, 90 µs, 125 Hz, 2.1 V; VIM 2: C+, 0-100%, 90 µs, 125 Hz, 1.3 V
40	f	77	47;11	ET-p	Dystonia	-	16	7	-	56.25	C+, 2-100%, 60 µs, 130 Hz, 3.6 mA	C+, 10-29%, 11-43% 12-28%, 60 µs, 130 Hz, 1.9 mA
41	f	80	20;34	ET-p	Dystonia, ataxia	-	56	33	-	41.07	C+, 5-32%, 6-29%, 7-29% 8-10% 40 µs 170 Hz 3.3 mA	C+, 13-45%, 14-40%, 15-15% 40 µs 170 Hz 4.1 mA
42	f	70	7;4	ET-p	RT	-	44	15	-	65.91	C+, 1-100%, 60 µs, 130 Hz, 1.2 mA	C+, 9-100%, 60 µs, 130 Hz, 1.2 mA
43	m	72	14;25	ET-p	RT	-	64	25	-	60.94	VIM1: C+, 2-100%, 60 µs, 125 Hz, 2.9 VVIM 2: C+, 1-100%, 60 µs, 125 Hz, 1.8 V	C+, 8, 100%, 60 us, 125 Hz 3.0
44	m	55	10;26	ET-p	MCI	-	39	0	-	51.28	VIM 1: C+, 1-100%, 125 µs, 60 Hz, 0.5 V; VIM 2: C+, 2-100%, 125 µs, 60 Hz, 3.5 V	VIM1: C+, 9-100%, 125 µs, 60 Hz, 0.5 V VIM 2: C+, 10-100%, 125 µs, 60 Hz, 3.8 V

4. Discussion

Our data suggest that VIM/PSA DBS is effective in ET-p, with effects comparable to those observed in ET. ET-p (70.45%) was more common in our cohort, with rest tremor being the most common plus-sign. This is in line with a previous retrospective analysis reclassifying ET-patients to ET-p in 83% of cases [3]. Another study reclassified 54% of ET patients as ET-p [2]. When comparing studies on ET-p, one must consider that due to a lack of strictly defined research criteria of ET-p, inconsistencies in classification may occur, especially when comparing analyses from different study groups [4]. There is also an ongoing debate about the new tremor classification and its validity, not only because there is room for interpretation regarding certain plus signs but also because of a strong heterogeneity of ET-p-patients and a lack of consideration of the underlying etiology [4]. Further, as previous studies found ET-p-patients being older than ET-patients, the possibility remains that ET-p may represent an advanced state of ET [14]. In our cohort, VIM/PSA DBS was effective in ET-p with a mean TRS-reduction of 62.0%, comparable to the one in ET in our cohort (68.9%) and in previous ET-studies [6,15]. However, a higher TEED was applied in ET-p-patients, suggesting that a higher current was needed to achieve comparable DBS effects. This effect may be due to higher preoperative TRS scores in ET-p but could further be influenced by the location of the active electrode contacts. Several studies found that stimulation of the more ventral subthalamic area may be more efficient [16–19] so that, regarding our data, higher stimulation parameters in ET-p may partly be due to a more dorsal stimulation. The reason for the more dorsal stimulation in the ET-p subgroup is unknown and could not be investigated in this cohort in detail due to the retrospective nature of the study and the lack of electronic documentation of side effects during each clinical testing. One may speculate that more side effects (such as gait ataxia or dysarthria) occurred during ventral stimulation in the ET-p-group, potentially due to worsening of preexisting cerebellar signs. Comparing TRS scores in ET and ET-p, one must consider further that rest tremor, as a plus-sign only represented in ET-p, automatically augments TRS scores in ET-p with rest tremor and thereby in the overall ET-p subgroup. Due to the retrospective character of this study and a missing standardized time range between switching off stimulation and TRS-rating, we cannot report on a potential tremor rebound effect as it is described in previous studies [20,21]. This study further does not provide any standardized evaluation of long-term effects of DBS or tremor habituation in ET-p as only one follow-up period per patient after DBS implantation was analyzed.

5. Conclusions

This study shows that VIM/PSA DBS is effective in ET-p with a similar tremor suppression as observed in ET. The higher TEED needed in ET-p patients may be related to the different locations of active contacts in this cohort. For valid long-term outcomes, prospective, multicenter registries on ET-p-patients as well as defined research criteria for ET-p are needed. Future trials on DBS in tremor should include the new classification criteria for ET and ET-p.

Author Contributions: J.K.S.—conceptualization and study design, methodology, data acquisition, analysis, drafting of the manuscript; H.J.—data acquisition, data analysis, critical revision of the manuscript, visualization; J.N.P.-S.—critical revision of the manuscript; T.A.D.—critical revision of the manuscript; T.T.—data analysis, critical revision of the manuscript; S.T.J.—data analysis, critical revision of the manuscript; H.S.D.—critical revision of the manuscript; J.K.—data acquisition, critical revision of the manuscript; J.W.—critical revision of the manuscript; G.R.F.—critical revision of the manuscript; V.V.-V.—critical revision of the manuscript; M.T.B.—supervision, conceptualization and study design, critical revision of the manuscript. All authors have read and agreed to the published version of the manuscript.

References

1. Bhatia, K.P.; Bain, P.; Bajaj, N.; Elble, R.J.; Hallett, M.; Louis, E.D.; Raethjen, J.; Stamelou, M.; Testa, C.M.; Deuschl, G.; et al. Consensus Statement on the classification of tremors. from the task force on tremor of the International Parkinson and Movement Disorder Society. *Mov. Disord.* **2017**, *33*, 75–87. [CrossRef] [PubMed]

2. Prasad, S.; Pal, P.K. Reclassifying essential tremor: Implications for the future of past research. *Mov. Disord.* **2019**, *34*, 437. [CrossRef] [PubMed]

3. Rajalingam, R.; Breen, D.P.; Lang, A.E.; Fasano, A. Essential tremor plus is more common than essential tremor: Insights from the reclassification of a cohort of patients with lower limb tremor. *Parkinsonism Relat. Disord.* **2018**, *56*, 109–110. [CrossRef] [PubMed]

4. Louis, E.D. 'Essential Tremor Plus': A Problematic Concept: Implications for Clinical and Epidemiological Studies of Essential Tremor. *Neuroepidemiology* **2020**, 1–5. [CrossRef] [PubMed]

5. Deuschl, G.; Raethjen, J.; Hellriegel, H.; Elble, R. Treatment of patients with essential tremor. *Lancet Neurol.* **2011**, *10*, 148–161. [CrossRef]

6. Zhang, K.; Bhatia, S.; Oh, M.Y.; Cohen, D.; Angle, C.; Whiting, D. Long-term results of thalamic deep brain stimulation for essential tremor. *J. Neurosurg.* **2009**, *112*, 1271–1276. [CrossRef] [PubMed]

7. Koller, W.C.; Lyons, K.E.; Wilkinson, S.B.; Troster, A.I.; Pahwa, R. Long-term safety and efficacy of unilateral deep brain stimulation of the thalamus in essential tremor. *Mov. Disord.* **2001**, *16*, 464–468. [CrossRef] [PubMed]

8. Deuschl, G.; Bain, P.; Brin, M. Consensus statement of the Movement Disorder Society on Tremor. Ad Hoc Scientific Committee. *Mov. Disord.* **1998**, *13* (Suppl. 3), 2–23. [CrossRef] [PubMed]

9. Petersen, R.C.; Smith, E.G.; Waring, S.C.; Ivnik, R.J.; Tangalos, E.G.; Kokmen, E. Mild Cognitive Impairment: Clinical Characterization and Outcome. *Arch. Neurol.* **1999**, *56*, 303–308. [CrossRef] [PubMed]

10. Fahn, S.; Tolosa, E.; Concepcion, M. Clinical Rating Scale for Tremor. In *Parkinson's Disease and Movement Disorders*; Jankovic, J., Tolosa, E., Eds.; Williams & Wilkins: Philadelphia, PA, USA, 1993.

11. Horn, A.; Li, N.; Dembek, T.A.; Kappel, A.; Boulay, C.; Ewert, S.; Tietze, A.; Husch, A.; Perera, T.; Neumann, W.J.; et al. Lead-DBS v2: Towards a comprehensive pipeline for deep brain stimulation imaging. *Neuroimage* **2019**, *184*, 293–316. [CrossRef] [PubMed]

12. Dembek, T.A.; Roediger, J.; Horn, A.; Reker, P.; Oehrn, C.; Dafsari, H.S.; Li, N.; Kühn, A.A.; Fink, G.R.; Visser-Vandewalle, V.; et al. Probabilistic sweet spots predict motor outcome for deep brain stimulation in Parkinson disease. *Ann. Neurol.* **2019**, *86*, 527–538. [CrossRef] [PubMed]

13. Koss, A.M.; Alterman, R.L.; Tagliati, M.; Shils, J.L. Calculating total electrical energy delivered by deep brain stimulation systems. *Ann. Neurol.* **2005**, *58*, 168. [CrossRef]

14. Huang, H.; Yang, X.; Zhao, Q.; Ning, P.; Shen, Q.; Wang, H.; Xie, D.; Lu, H.; Xu, Y. Clinical characteristics of patients with essential tremor or essential tremor plus. *Acta Neurol. Scand.* **2020**, *141*, 335–341. [CrossRef]

15. Paschen, S.; Forstenpointner, J.; Becktepe, J.; Heinzel, S.; Hellriegel, H.; Witt, K.; Helmers, A.-K.; Deuschl, G. Long-term efficacy of deep brain stimulation for essential tremor: An observer-blinded study. *Neurology* **2019**, *92*, e1378–e1386. [CrossRef] [PubMed]

16. Herzog, J.; Hamel, W.; Wenzelburger, R.; Pötter, M.; Pinsker, M.O.; Bartussek, J.; Morsnowski, A.; Steigerwald, F.; Deuschl, G.; Volkmann, J. Kinematic analysis of thalamic versus subthalamic neurostimulation in postural and intention tremor. *Brain* **2007**, *130*, 1608–1625. [CrossRef]

17. Barbe, M.T.; Liebhart, L.; Runge, M.; Deyng, J.; Florin, E.; Wojtecki, L.; Schnitzler, A.; Allert, N.; Sturm, V.; Fink, G.R.; et al. Deep brain stimulation of the ventral intermediate nucleus in patients with essential tremor: Stimulation below intercommissural line is more efficient but equally effective as stimulation above. *Exp. Neurol.* **2011**, *230*, 131–137. [CrossRef] [PubMed]

18. Sandvik, U.; Koskinen, L.-O.; Lundquist, A.; Blomstedt, P. Thalamic and Subthalamic Deep Brain Stimulation for Essential Tremor: Where Is the Optimal Target? *Neurosurgery* **2012**, *70*, 840–846. [PubMed]

19. Barbe, M.T.; Franklin, J.; Kraus, D.; Reker, P.; Dembek, T.A.; Allert, N.; Wirths, J.; Voges, J.; Timmermann, L.; Visser-Vandewalle, V. Deep brain stimulation of the posterior subthalamic area and the thalamus in patients with essential tremor: Study protocol for a randomized controlled pilot trial. *Trials* **2016**, *17*. [CrossRef] [PubMed]

20. Hariz, M.I.; Shamsgovara, P.; Johansson, F.; Hariz, G.-M.; Fodstad, H. Tolerance and Tremor Rebound following Long-Term Chronic Thalamic Stimulation for Parkinsonian and Essential Tremor. *Stereotact. Funct. Neurosurg.* **2000**, *72*, 208–218. [CrossRef] [PubMed]

21. Patel, N.; Ondo, W.; Jimenez-Shahed, J. Habituation and rebound to thalamic deep brain stimulation in long-term management of tremor associated with demyelinating neuropathy. *Int. J. Neurosci.* **2014**, *124*, 919–925. [CrossRef] [PubMed]

## 3

Applying a Sensing-Enabled System for Ensuring Safe Anterior Cingulate Deep Brain Stimulation for Pain

Yongzhi Huang [1] [ORCID], Binith Cheeran [1], Alexander L. Green [1], Timothy J. Denison [2],*
and Tipu Z. Aziz [1],*

[1]   Oxford Functional Neurosurgery Group, Nuffield Departments of Surgical Sciences, University of Oxford, Oxford OX3 9DU, UK
[2]   Institute of Biomedical Engineering, University of Oxford, Oxford OX3 7DQ, UK
*   Correspondence: timothy.denison@eng.ox.ac.uk (T.J.D.); tipu.aziz@nds.ox.ac.uk (T.Z.A.)

Abstract: Deep brain stimulation (DBS) of the anterior cingulate cortex (ACC) was offered to chronic pain patients who had exhausted medical and surgical options. However, several patients developed recurrent seizures. This work was conducted to assess the effect of ACC stimulation on the brain activity and to guide safe DBS programming. A sensing-enabled neurostimulator (Activa PC + S) allowing wireless recording through the stimulating electrodes was chronically implanted in three patients. Stimulation patterns with different amplitude levels and variable ramping rates were tested to investigate whether these patterns could provide pain relief without triggering after-discharges (ADs) within local field potentials (LFPs) recorded in the ACC. In the absence of ramping, AD activity was detected following stimulation at amplitude levels below those used in chronic therapy. Adjustment of stimulus cycling patterns, by slowly ramping on/off (8-s ramp duration), was able to prevent ADs at higher amplitude levels while maintaining effective pain relief. The absence of AD activity confirmed from the implant was correlated with the absence of clinical seizures. We propose that AD activity in the ACC could be a biomarker for the likelihood of seizures in these patients, and the application of sensing-enabled techniques has the potential to advance safer brain stimulation therapies, especially in novel targets.

Keywords: deep brain stimulation; anterior cingulate cortex; seizures; after-discharge; local field potential; chronic pain

1. Introduction

Deep brain stimulation (DBS) is an established therapy for movement disorders. It has several advantages over lesioning techniques. For example, therapy-induced side effects are considered to be reversible, and DBS can be 'dosed' as symptoms evolve [1]. Interestingly, the first DBS surgeries were performed for chronic post-stroke pain [2]. Cingulotomy has historically been used to target the affective component of pain, for example intractable pain associated with terminal cancer [3–5]. However, side effects are common, such as impairments of attention and cognition [6,7]. As an alternative to destructive lesioning, anterior cingulate cortex (ACC) DBS implants were offered to patients with severe, medically-refractory pain, where established targets, such as sensory thalamus and periventricular/periaqueductal grey, had failed or where pain was too poorly localized to consider these targets [8,9].

The success of ACC stimulation in patients deemed refractory to other medical and surgical interventions was tempered by the onset of recurrent stereotyped neurological events after 12–60 months of active stimulation in approximately 18% of the patients [10]. Some patients experienced recurrent seizures, and stimulation had to be markedly reduced or switched off completely as a conservative solution to ameliorate side effects; at these settings, effective pain relief was lost [10]. However, how ACC stimulation affects brain function and induces seizures remains unclear.

Studies have suggested several neurophysiological biomarkers potentially associated with seizures, e.g., stimulation-elicited after-discharges (ADs) [11,12]. Cortical stimulation can induce ADs, sometimes followed by clinical seizures, whether or not those regions are known to cause spontaneous seizures [11,13,14]. Stimulation parameters for inducing ADs have shown considerable within- and between-subject variability, but in general ADs can be elicited with sufficient stimulus intensity and duration [15–17].

With the advent of recent implant technologies, the effects of DBS on brain neural activities can be chronically investigated by measurements of local field potentials (LFPs) in the brain. Prior animal studies have demonstrated the ability to detect AD activity in LFPs using implanted DBS leads in various brain regions [18,19]. Here, we applied this technology to investigate the effect of ACC stimulation on brain activity in patients with chronic pain and aimed to elucidate safe stimulation parameters that maintained adequate pain relief without inducing seizures.

2. Materials and Methods

2.1. Subjects

Three patients with chronic pain who experienced recurrent seizures during the course of DBS therapy were investigated. All patients initially underwent bilateral implantation of DBS electrodes (Model 3387, Medtronic®, Minneapolis, MN, USA) into the ACC at The John Radcliffe Hospital, Oxford, UK. The surgical procedure has been previously described [8]. Details of the patients are reported in Table 1. None of the patients had suffered seizures prior to their initial surgery. Pre-operative MRI and post-operative CT scans did not reveal any relevant structural abnormalities or complications, such as hemorrhage or ischemia.

However, stereotyped neurological events, clinically diagnosed as seizures, were reported in these patients after some period of effective therapy. Medical management with multiple anti-epileptics was only transiently effective (weeks to months) before seizures recurred. Patient 2 did not take anti-epileptic drugs as he preferred altering the stimulation settings rather than medication. Video-electroencephalograph telemetry (vEEG) was used to investigate and detect seizures, initially in the first case (Figure 1). Reducing stimulation amplitude to levels below the threshold for seizure induction, based on multiple vEEG tests and clinical review, eliminated both the clinical seizures and the benefit of pain relief. Despite the risk of seizure induction, the patients requested reinstatement of stimulation to re-capture pain relief.

Table 1. Demographics, etiologies, stimulation parameters, and clinical events of patients.

Patient	Age at Surgery/Sex	Etiology	Onset of Seizure after Surgery	Seizure Symptoms	DBS Settings at Onset of Seizures	Anti-Epileptic Drugs	DBS Settings with Seizure Free	Follow-Up
1	46/F	Whole spine pain secondary to multiple spinal interventions	20 months	1) Focal non-motor onset with impaired awareness 2) Nocturnal generalized tonic-clonic seizures (maximum frequency reported: 1 event per month, lasting up to 45 min)	5 V 130 Hz 450 μs	Levetiracetam Clobazam Sodium valproate	6 V 130 Hz 450 μs 8-s ramp 3 min ON/ 11 min OFF	Seizure free for 17 months
2	51/M	Whole body pain secondary to excision of ependymoma of cervical spinal cord	60 months	Focal non-motor onset with impaired awareness (maximum frequency reported: 1 event per h)	8.5 V 130 Hz 450 μs	no	6 V 130 Hz 450 μs 8-s ramp1 min ON/ 1 min OFF	Seizure free for 6 months
3	49/M	Right hemi body pain secondary to posterior fossa decompression for Arnold–Chiari malformation	12 months	Focal non-motor onset with impaired awareness (maximum frequency reported: 50 events per day)	8.5 V 130 Hz 450 μs	Levetiracetam Oxcarbazepine	6 V 130 Hz 450 μs 8-s ramp1 min ON/ 1 min OFF	Seizure free for 1 month (then system removed due to infection)

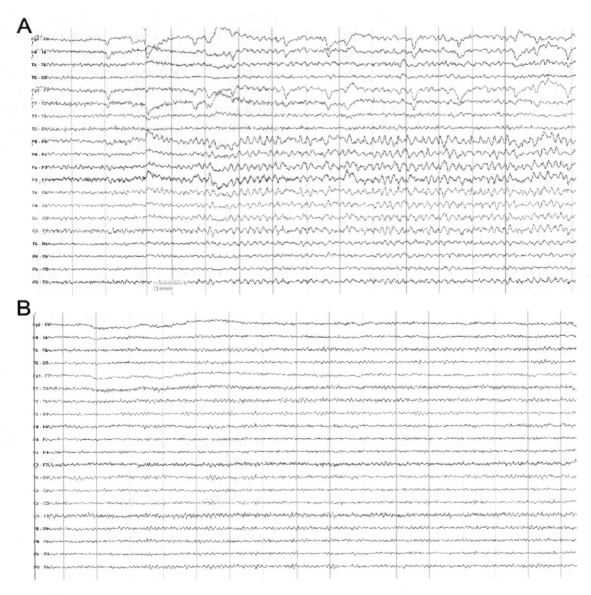

Figure 1. Example EEG recordings from patient 1. (**A**) Ictal EEG showing rhythmical, symmetrical 6 Hz theta slow wave activity across the frontocentral regions. (**B**) EEG showing normal background activity.

2.2. Stimulation and Local Field Potential Recordings

To further investigate the relationship between the stimulation and clinical events, a sensing-enabled neurostimulation system (Activa PC + S, Medtronic®) was implanted chronically, under the Medicines and Healthcare Products Regulatory Agency (MHRA) humanitarian exemption approval. This system allows for concurrent stimulation and recording from implanted DBS leads, and was used in a prior study to measure AD activity in an animal model, exploring network behavior in epilepsy [19].

Stimulation titration tests were systematically performed in patient 1 to investigate the effect of stimulation intensity on ACC neural activity. In particular, we explored whether ADs could be induced by ACC stimulation. Unilateral stimulation was increased from 0 V to target voltage (from 1 V to 6 V, 1 V steps) and then immediately switched off, with a stimulation-off interval of several seconds between steps. Ipsilateral and contralateral LFPs were recorded simultaneously during the same period. In addition, bilateral stimulation was also tested. The implantable pulse generator (IPG) was replaced with a second Activa PC + S system 13 months after the first implant of the Activa PC + S system due to depleted battery. Thereafter, bilateral stimulation at therapeutic amplitudes, using cycled stimulation with ramping, was explored to re-capture pain relief whilst minimizing seizures. Cycled stimulation on/off durations were selected based on results from the stimulation testing trials indicating that pain relief could be achieved with 3 min of stimulation, using therapeutic amplitudes, but could be lost 11 min later in this patient (Table 1). LFPs in the ACC were measured to investigate whether these stimulation patterns would induce ADs. Additional LFP recordings were collected during periods of chronic stimulation at home using the embedded loop recorder in the device [20,21].

The know-how learned in patient 1 was applied to patients 2 and 3. As unilateral ACC stimulation was found to be ineffective, bilateral stimulation without ramp, and with slowly ramped on/off, was tested, and LFPs were measured simultaneously. Subsequently, the stimulation pattern using cycling with ramp, shown through LFP measurements to avoid ADs, was applied for chronic treatment. Unfortunately, a month after IPG implant surgery, the sensing-enabled stimulation system had to be removed because of an infection in patient 3. During this period, the stimulation was clinically effective for pain relief without inducing seizures.

In all tests, electrical stimulation was delivered using a bipolar configuration between electrode contacts 0 (the deepest contact) and 3. Stimulation frequency and pulse width (typical therapy parameters 130 Hz, 450 µs) were fixed. All LFPs were recorded in a bipolar mode using the middle two contacts (1–2) of the electrodes (0.5 Hz pre-amplifier high-pass filtering, 100 Hz pre-amplifier low-pass filtering, 422 Hz sampling rate).

2.3. Data Analysis

LFP data were analyzed using custom scripts written in MATLAB (Version 9.1, MathWorks, Natick, MA, USA). To characterize the dynamic changes of neural activity, time-frequency representations of LFPs were performed using the short-time Fourier transform with a Hanning time window of 0.5 s and overlap of 0.45 s. These parameters provided a time resolution of 0.5 s and a frequency resolution of 2 Hz. Stimulation onset was identified as a period where observable high amplitude artifacts in the raw LFPs were accompanied by obvious 130 Hz stimulation frequency in the spectrograms. An AD episode was defined as the state with a sustained high amplitude, seizure-like activities in the raw LFPs and confirmed through elevated power across multiple frequency bands in the spectrograms.

Sensing channel saturation with large stimulation was a concern. To ensure a robust LFP measurement, a continuous monitoring approach was used to determine the reliability of the received signals [22]. Briefly, a continuous test tone at a discrete frequency (105 Hz) outside of the physiological band of interest was injected into the signal chain during recording through a parallel channel. If this tone's amplitude was compromised due to amplifier saturation, alternative signal chain parameters would be chosen, such as reducing the amplifier gain. For example, in our study, if the test tone shows amplifier saturation then the signal artifact following stimulation can look like a seizure activity (Figure 2A). In such cases, the amplifiers' gain was reduced to ensure the recording of reliable LFPs (Figure 2B).

Figure 2. The use of a test tone to monitor the integrity of the bioelectric amplifier in measuring local field potentials (LFPs). (**A**) LFP measurement using an amplifier with a gain of 2000. The line box illustrates an example of distortion of signals induced by the amplifier recovering. (**B**) LFP measurement using an amplifier with a gain of 250.

3. Results

3.1. AD Activity in ACC LFPs Is Induced Following Stimulation

Stimulation titration tests revealed that the characteristics of LFP changes in the ACC were dependent upon the stimulation amplitudes. Figure 3 provides an illustration of the effects of unilateral stimulation amplitudes on ACC LFPs from patient 1. The ADs were induced following a stimulation at a threshold of 5 V on the left lead and 4 V on the right lead, respectively (Figure 3). Bilateral stimulation with 6 V amplitude on both leads also induced significant ADs in right ACC and slight ADs in left ACC (Figure 4A). The ADs in the ACC could also be observed when we repeated the titration tests after 1 month of bilateral therapeutic stimulation at 3.5 V (not shown). The AD threshold to stimulation was determined based on these tests. During the periods of measuring these LFPs, no clinical seizures were reported. Based on these LFP measurements, bilateral stimulation therapy with amplitudes below the AD threshold level was applied to attempt to prevent seizures and obtain pain relief. However, pain relief was inadequate, although no seizures were reported for approximately 12 months.

Figure 3. Effects of different unilateral stimulation amplitudes on the LFP recordings in the anterior cingulate cortex (ACC) from patient 1. (**A**) Bipolar LFP recordings and corresponding spectrograms from the left ACC during unilateral stimulation with increasing amplitudes. (**B**) Bipolar LFP recordings and corresponding spectrograms from the right ACC during unilateral stimulation with increasing amplitudes. Bottom panels show greater details illustrating several examples of after-discharges that occurred following cessation of stimulation.

Figure 4. Effects of bilateral stimulation with/without a stimulus ramp on the LFP recordings in the bilateral ACC from patient 1. (**A**) Raw LFP recordings and corresponding spectrograms in the left (top panels) and right ACC (bottom panels) during stimulation without a stimulus ramp. (**B**) Raw LFP recordings and corresponding spectrograms in the left (top panels) and right ACC (bottom panels) during stimulation with a 4 s stimulus ramp. (**C**) Raw LFP recordings and corresponding spectrograms in the left (top panels) and right ACC (bottom panels) during stimulation with an 8 s stimulus ramp.

3.2. Stimulation with Slowly Ramped on/off during Cycling Successfully Eliminates ADs

Subsequently, based on the rationale detailed in the discussion, we tested a programming feature that allowed stimulation to be slowly ramped on/off during the cycling, rather than stimulation being started or stopped abruptly. When stimulation was delivered, using a pattern consisting of cycled stimulation, stimulation ramped down from the maximum amplitude to 0 V in 8 s and a high amplitude (6 V) that previously resulted in ADs, we did not observe the typical AD activities following the stimulation in patient 1 (Figure 4C). With these stimulation patterns for therapy, good pain relief was again reported, and the patient was discharged with the device programmed to collect additional LFP recordings over time.

LFPs recordings from patient 2 also showed that ADs were observed in the right ACC when using cycled stimulation patterns without a stimulus ramp and with a 4 s ramp; however, the AD activity disappeared when using stimulation with an 8 s ramp (Figure 5). The patient gained pain relief and no seizures during the test, using the cycled stimulation pattern at 6 V amplitude with an 8 s ramp. Therefore, we applied this stimulation pattern for chronic therapy in the patient.

Figure 5. Effects of bilateral stimulation with/without a stimulus ramp on the LFP recordings in the bilateral ACC from patient 2. (**A**) Raw LFP recordings and corresponding spectrograms in the left (top panels) and right ACC (bottom panels) during stimulation without a stimulus ramp. (**B**) Raw LFP recordings and corresponding spectrograms in the left (top panels) and right ACC (bottom panels) during stimulation with a 4 s stimulus ramp. (**C**) Raw LFP recordings and corresponding spectrograms in the left (top panels) and right ACC (bottom panels) during stimulation with an 8 s stimulus ramp.

Although the system in patient 3 was removed due to infection at one month, the limited LFP recordings also revealed that there were no ADs using cycled stimulation with a ramp. Interestingly, in this case, we also did not observe the ADs when using stimulation without a ramp (Figure 6). Before system removal, the patient achieved pain relief and was seizure free.

Figure 6. Effects of bilateral stimulation with/without a stimulus ramp on the LFP recordings in the bilateral ACC from patient 3. (**A**) Raw LFP recordings and corresponding spectrograms in the left (top panels) and right ACC (bottom panels) during stimulation without a stimulus ramp. (**B**) Raw LFP recordings and corresponding spectrograms in the left (top panels) and right ACC (bottom panels) during stimulation with a 4 s stimulus ramp. (**C**) Raw LFP recordings and corresponding spectrograms in the left (top panels) and right ACC (bottom panels) during stimulation with an 8 s stimulus ramp. Note that the after-effects observed during 3–6 s were confirmed to be due to sensing channel recovery using the test-tone method.

3.3. The Use of Cycled Stimulation with Slow Ramps Provides Sustained Pain Relief without Seizures

At the follow up, the parameter settings of stimulation that provided pain relief without ADs resulted in sustained therapeutic benefit without side-effects. The long-term LFP recordings, obtained during periods of chronic stimulation at home in patient 1, also showed no indication of ADs being triggered by chronic-cycled stimulation with a ramp (Figure 7). At the last follow-up, patient 1 had been seizure free (self-reported) for 17 months and patient 2 had been seizure free (self-reported) for 6 months.

Figure 7. Long-term effects of bilateral therapeutic stimulation with an 8 s ramp on the LFP recordings in the bilateral ACC from patient 1. (**A**) Raw LFP recordings and corresponding spectrograms in the left (top panels) and right ACC (bottom panels) during stimulation for 5 months. (**B**) Raw LFP recordings and corresponding spectrograms in the left (top panels) and right ACC (bottom panels) during stimulation for 9 months.

4. Discussion

Neuromodulation can be an effective approach to pain management in patients that have exhausted medical therapies. However, the risk of adverse events with cortical stimulation, as reported here, needs to be addressed. For example, epidural motor cortex stimulation and repetitive transcranial magnetic stimulation have been explored for a variety of pain syndromes with variable success, but the induction of seizures has been reported as one of the more serious adverse events [23–25]. Stimulation induced ADs are common during cortical mapping for epilepsy surgery, yet, despite decades of clinical observation, the cellular and network mechanisms underlying their generation remain areas of active investigation [26]. However, it is generally agreed that a disruption in excitatory-inhibitory balance results in the hyperexcitable state associated with these phenomena. During stimulation, the inhibitory drive on the post-synaptic neurons is increased, resulting in hyperpolarization. However, upon termination of the stimulus train, a phenomenon known as "post-inhibitory rebound excitation" can occur [27]. This rebound depolarization leads to a strong excitatory discharge in the primary neurons and may be one of the cellular mechanisms responsible for the generation of ADs. Using the same implantable device described here, this pattern of inhibition during stimulation, followed by strong excitatory bursts upon stimulus termination, has been observed in LFPs, chronically recorded from the sheep hippocampus [19].

This study indicates that AD activity in the ACC could be a biomarker for the likelihood of seizures. The relationship between the generation of ADs and the initial appearance of clinical seizures in these patients is unclear. Their recurrent seizures developed during a period where DBS was delivered in a continuous (not cycled) manner and could more likely be related to a kindling-like phenomenon. In animal models, classical kindling typically involves the application of periodic subthreshold stimuli to evoke network synchronization, which gradually induces long-lasting neuronal changes that eventually lead to spontaneous seizures. However, other kindling models employ higher level, more continuous stimulation, above the AD threshold, and result in a more rapid induction of epileptogenesis [28].

Stimulation with the cycle mode, rather than the prolonged continuous stimulation, has been proposed to reduce the risk of seizures [29]. Moreover, in an attempt to minimize the likelihood of ADs, a stimulation cycle that was slowly ramped off, rather than stopped abruptly, was evaluated in these patients. When stimulation was delivered using this pattern, the typical post-stimulation burst of spiking activity was not observed, even at intensity levels above those that earlier produced ADs, using the sensing capability of the implanted brain-machine-interface. Due to the large stimulus artifact, it was not possible to conclusively determine whether any spiking/ictal activity was present during stimulation. However, the stimulation pattern with a ramp appeared to avoid the generation of ADs following stimulation, possibly due to a reduction in the post-inhibitory rebound. Importantly, it has allowed for two patients to achieve long-term seizure freedom and pain relief.

Future systems would benefit from continuous monitoring of neural activity. Our data suggests that the likelihood of AD occurrence can fluctuate depending on the functional state of the stimulated network at that time [16]. This may explain why the LFPs recorded from patient 3 did not show ADs when using a stimulus without a ramp, which also suggests the importance of long-term monitoring and adaptive algorithms. Implanted sensing-enabled interfaces have the capability to chronically monitor for AD/ictal types of activity, based on spectral characteristics, and options to reduce or turn off stimulation, if detected [21,30]. Moreover, the sensing-enabled interfaces could be easily automated and run in the background and allow for more automated processing in the future. This type of closed-loop approach may potentially minimize or prevent stimulation-induced adverse events, such as those observed in this study.

New applications of DBS of new targets for therapy delivery continue to be explored; however, in most cases, the default stimulation parameters selected are based upon those that have been effective in the currently approved movement disorder therapies [31]. When exploring new therapies, a commonly accepted concept in neuromodulation is that side-effects and adverse events can be eliminated by simply turning off the device. However, the patients then fail to obtain symptomatic relief, and, as illustrated in this case series, there is a potential for sustained adverse events, even in the absence of stimulation. This caveat is important, as several recent large trials of DBS for new indications have not yielded positive outcomes [32–34] and a post-hoc review questioned whether stimulation parameters were adequately dosed. The unique opportunity to directly observe stimulation effects on the implanted structure [35,36] or neural network [37–39] targeted for therapy provided by sensing-enabled systems may usher in a new era, where DBS programming is informed by objective electrophysiological measures in conjunction with clinical observations, hopefully leading to safer and more effective therapies.

5. Conclusions

The events of unforeseen consequences following ACC DBS serve as a clarion call to those working in the field of neuromodulation. This report revealed that use of sensing-enabled systems could help to understand relationship between ACC stimulation and side-effects (seizures in these series), suggesting sensing-enabled techniques have the potential to advance safer brain stimulation therapies, especially in novel targets.

Author Contributions: Conceptualization, T.J.D. and T.Z.A.; methodology, Y.H., B.C., T.J.D., and T.Z.A.; formal analysis, Y.H.; investigation, Y.H., B.C., T.J.D., and T.Z.A.; data curation, Y.H.; writing—original draft preparation, Y.H., B.C., A.L.G., T.J.D., and T.Z.A.; writing—review and editing, Y.H., B.C., A.L.G., T.J.D., and T.Z.A.; visualization, Y.H.; supervision, T.J.D. and T.Z.A.; project administration, T.J.D. and T.Z.A.

Acknowledgments: The authors thank Gaetano Leogrande, Paul Stypulkowski, and Scott Stanslaski for their help in data collection and manuscript review for technical accuracy. A.L.G. is supported by the National Institute for Health Research (NIHR) Oxford Biomedical Research Centre, based at Oxford University Hospitals NHS Trust and the University of Oxford.

References

1.   Lozano, A.M.; Lipsman, N.; Bergman, H.; Brown, P.; Chabardes, S.; Chang, J.W.; Matthews, K.; McIntyre, C.C.; Schlaepfer, T.E.; Schulder, M.; et al. Deep brain stimulation: Current challenges and future directions. *Nat. Rev. Neurol.* **2019**, *15*, 148–160. [CrossRef] [PubMed]

2.   Hariz, M.I.; Blomstedt, P.; Zrinzo, L. Deep brain stimulation between 1947 and 1987: The untold story. *Neurosurg. Focus* **2010**, *29*, E1. [CrossRef] [PubMed]

3.   Foltz, E.L.; White, L.E., Jr. Pain "relief" by frontal cingulumotomy. *J. Neurosurg.* **1962**, *19*, 89–100. [CrossRef] [PubMed]

4.   Hassenbusch, S.J.; Pillay, P.K.; Barnett, G.H. Radiofrequency cingulotomy for intractable cancer pain using stereotaxis guided by magnetic resonance imaging. *Neurosurgery* **1990**, *27*, 220. [CrossRef] [PubMed]

5.   Viswanathan, A.; Harsh, V.; Pereira, E.A.C.; Aziz, T.Z. Cingulotomy for medically refractory cancer pain. *Neurosurg. Focus* **2013**, *35*, E1. [CrossRef]

6.   Cohen, R.A.; Kaplan, R.F.; Moser, D.J.; Jenkins, M.A.; Wilkinson, H. Impairments of attention after cingulotomy. *Neurology* **1999**, *53*, 819. [CrossRef] [PubMed]

7.   Ochsner, K.N.; Kosslyn, S.M.; Cosgrove, G.; Cassem, E.H.; Price, B.H.; Nierenberg, A.A.; Rauch, S.L. Deficits in visual cognition and attention following bilateral anterior cingulotomy. *Neuropsychoogy* **2001**, *39*, 219–230. [CrossRef]

8.   Boccard, S.G.; Fitzgerald, J.J.; Pereira, E.A.; Moir, L.; Van Hartevelt, T.J.; Kringelbach, M.L.; Green, A.L.; Aziz, T.Z. Targeting the affective component of chronic pain: A case series of deep brain stimulation of the anterior cingulate cortex. *Neurosurgery* **2014**, *74*, 628–635. [CrossRef]

9. Pereira, E.A.; Green, A.L.; Aziz, T.Z. Deep brain stimulation for pain. *Handbook Clin. Neurol.* **2013**, *116*, 277–294.

10. Maslen, H.; Cheeran, B.; Pugh, J.; Pycroft, L.; Boccard, S.; Prangnell, S.; Green, A.L.; FitzGerald, J.; Savulescu, J.; Aziz, T. Unexpected Complications of Novel Deep Brain Stimulation Treatments: Ethical Issues and Clinical Recommendations. *Neuromodulation* **2018**, *21*, 135–143. [CrossRef]

11. Blume, W.T.; Jones, D.C.; Pathak, P. Properties of after-discharges from cortical electrical stimulation in focal epilepsies. *Clin. Neurophysiol.* **2004**, *115*, 982–989. [CrossRef] [PubMed]

12. Gollwitzer, S.; Hopfengärtner, R.; Rössler, K.; Müller, T.; Olmes, D.G.; Lang, J.; Köhn, J.; Onugoren, M.D.; Heyne, J.; Schwab, S.; et al. Afterdischarges elicited by cortical electric stimulation in humans: When do they occur and what do they mean? *Epilepsy Behav.* **2018**, *87*, 173–179. [CrossRef] [PubMed]

13. Wieser, H.G.; Bancaud, J.; Talairach, J.; Bonis, A.; Szikla, G. Comparative Value of Spontaneous and Chemically and Electrically Induced Seizures in Establishing the Lateralization of Temporal Lobe Seizures. *Epilepsia* **1979**, *20*, 47–59. [CrossRef] [PubMed]

14. Lesser, R.P.; Kim, S.H.; Beyderman, L.; Miglioretti, D.L.; Webber, W.R.S.; Bare, M.; Cysyk, B.; Krauss, G.; Gordon, B. Brief bursts of pulse stimulation terminate afterdischarges caused by cortical stimulation. *Neurology* **1999**, *53*, 2073. [CrossRef]

15. Lesser, R.P.; Lüders, H.; Klem, G.; Dinner, D.S.; Morris, H.H.; Hahn, J. Cortical Afterdischarge and Functional Response Thresholds: Results of Extraoperative Testing. *Epilepsia* **1984**, *25*, 615–621. [CrossRef] [PubMed]

16. Lesser, R.P.; Lee, H.W.; Webber, W.R.S.; Prince, B.; Crone, N.E.; Miglioretti, D.L. Short-term variations in response distribution to cortical stimulation. *Brain* **2008**, *131*, 1528–1539. [CrossRef] [PubMed]

17. Lee, H.W.; Webber, W.; Crone, N.; Miglioretti, D.L.; Lesser, R.P. When is electrical cortical stimulation more likely to produce afterdischarges? *Clin. Neurophysiol.* **2010**, *121*, 14–20. [CrossRef]

18. Stypulkowski, P.; Stanslaski, S.; Denison, T.; Giftakis, J. Chronic Evaluation of a Clinical System for Deep Brain Stimulation and Recording of Neural Network Activity. *Ster. Funct. Neurosurg.* **2013**, *91*, 220–232. [CrossRef]

19. Stypulkowski, P.H.; Stanslaski, S.R.; Jensen, R.M.; Denison, T.J.; Giftakis, J.E. Brain Stimulation for Epilepsy—Local and Remote Modulation of Network Excitability. *Brain Stimul.* **2014**, *7*, 350–358. [CrossRef]

20. Rouse, A.G.; Stanslaski, S.R.; Cong, P.; Jensen, R.M.; Afshar, P.; Ullestad, D.; Gupta, R.; Molnar, G.F.; Moran, D.W.; Denison, T.J.; et al. A Chronic Generalized Bi-directional Brain-Machine Interface. *J. Neural Eng.* **2011**, *8*, 036018. [CrossRef]

21. Stanslaski, S.; Afshar, P.; Cong, P.; Giftakis, J.; Stypulkowski, P.; Carlson, D.; Linde, D.; Ullestad, D.; Avestruz, A.-T.; Denison, T. Design and Validation of a Fully Implantable, Chronic, Closed-Loop Neuromodulation Device With Concurrent Sensing and Stimulation. *IEEE Trans. Neural Syst. Rehabil. Eng.* **2012**, *20*, 410–421. [CrossRef] [PubMed]

22. Denison, T.J.; Afshar, P.; Stanslaski, S.R. Simultaneous Physiological Sensing and Stimulation with Saturation Detection. Google Patents 2016. Available online: https://patents.patsnap.com/v/US10080898-simultaneous-physiological-sensing-and-stimulation-with-saturation-detection.html (accessed on 25 September 2018).

23. Fontaine, D.; Hamani, C.; Lozano, A. Efficacy and safety of motor cortex stimulation for chronic neuropathic pain: Critical review of the literature. *J. Neurosurg.* **2009**, *110*, 251–256. [CrossRef] [PubMed]

24. Klein, M.M.; Treister, R.; Raij, T.; Pascual-Leone, A.; Park, L.; Nurmikko, T.; Lenz, F.; Lefaucheur, J.-P.; Lang, M.; Hallett, M.; et al. Transcranial magnetic stimulation of the brain: Guidelines for pain treatment research. *Pain* **2015**, *156*, 1601–1614. [CrossRef] [PubMed]

25. Cruccu, G.; Aziz, T.Z.; Garcia-Larrea, L.; Hansson, P.; Jensen, T.S.; Lefaucheur, J.-P.; Simpson, B.A.; Taylor, R.S. EFNS guidelines on neurostimulation therapy for neuropathic pain. *Eur. J. Neurol.* **2007**, *14*, 952–970. [CrossRef] [PubMed]

26. Kalamangalam, G.P.; Tandon, N.; Slater, J.D. Dynamic mechanisms underlying afterdischarge: A human subdural recording study. *Clin. Neurophysiol.* **2014**, *125*, 1324–1338. [CrossRef] [PubMed]

27. Llinás, R. The intrinsic electrophysiological properties of mammalian neurons: Insights into central nervous system function. *Science* **1988**, *242*, 1654–1664. [CrossRef]

28. Morales, J.C.; Roncagliolo, M.; Fuenzalida, M.; Wellmann, M.; Nualart, F.J.; Bonansco, C.; Álvarez-Ferradas, C. A new rapid kindling variant for induction of cortical epileptogenesis in freely moving rats. *Front. Cell. Neurosci.* **2014**, *8*, 200. [CrossRef]

29. De Ridder, D.; De Mulder, G.; Verstraeten, E.; Van Der Kelen, K.; Sunaert, S.; Smits, M.; Kovacs, S.; Verlooy, J.; Van De Heyning, P.; Moller, A.R. Primary and Secondary Auditory Cortex Stimulation for Intractable Tinnitus. *ORL* **2006**, *68*, 48–55. [CrossRef] [PubMed]

30. Afshar, P.; Khambhati, A.; Stanslaski, S.; Carlson, D.; Jensen, R.; Linde, D.; Dani, S.; Lazarewicz, M.; Cong, P.; Giftakis, J.; et al. A translational platform for prototyping closed-loop neuromodulation systems. *Front. Neural. Circuits* **2012**, *6*, 117. [CrossRef] [PubMed]

31. Miocinovic, S.; Somayajula, S.; Chitnis, S.; Vitek, J.L. History, Applications, and Mechanisms of Deep Brain Stimulation. *JAMA Neurol.* **2013**, *70*, 163. [CrossRef]

32. Dougherty, D.D.; Rezai, A.R.; Carpenter, L.L.; Howland, R.H.; Bhati, M.T.; O'Reardon, J.P.; Eskandar, E.N.; Baltuch, G.H.; Machado, A.D.; Kondziolka, D.; et al. A Randomized Sham-Controlled Trial of Deep Brain Stimulation of the Ventral Capsule/Ventral Striatum for Chronic Treatment-Resistant Depression. *Boil. Psychiatry* **2015**, *78*, 240–248. [CrossRef] [PubMed]

33. Lozano, A.M.; Fosdick, L.; Chakravarty, M.M.; Leoutsakos, J.-M.; Munro, C.; Oh, E.; Drake, K.E.; Lyman, C.H.; Rosenberg, P.B.; Anderson, W.S.; et al. A Phase II Study of Fornix Deep Brain Stimulation in Mild Alzheimer's Disease. *J. Alzheimer's Dis.* **2016**, *54*, 777–787. [CrossRef] [PubMed]

34. Holtzheimer, P.E.; Husain, M.M.; Lisanby, S.H.; Taylor, S.F.; A Whitworth, L.; McClintock, S.; Slavin, K.V.; Berman, J.; McKhann, G.M.; Patil, P.G.; et al. Subcallosal cingulate deep brain stimulation for treatment-resistant depression: A multisite, randomised, sham-controlled trial. *Lancet Psychiatry* **2017**, *4*, 839–849. [CrossRef]

35. Quinn, E.J.; Blumenfeld, Z.; Velisar, A.; Koop, M.M.; Shreve, L.A.; Trager, M.H.; Hill, B.C.; Kilbane, C.; Henderson, J.M.; Bronte-Stewart, H. Beta oscillations in freely moving Parkinson's subjects are attenuated during deep brain stimulation. *Mov. Disord.* **2015**, *30*, 1750–1758. [CrossRef] [PubMed]

36. Velisar, A.; Syrkin-Nikolau, J.; Blumenfeld, Z.; Trager, M.H.; Afzal, M.F.; Prabhakar, V.; Bronte-Stewart, H. Dual threshold neural closed loop deep brain stimulation in Parkinson disease patients. *Brain Stimul.* **2019**, *12*, 868–876. [CrossRef] [PubMed]

37. Van Gompel, J.J.; Klassen, B.T.; Worrell, G.A.; Lee, K.H.; Shin, C.; Zhao, C.Z.; Brown, D.A.; Goerss, S.J.; Kall, B.A.; Stead, M. Anterior nuclear deep brain stimulation guided by concordant hippocampal recording. *Neurosurg. Focus* **2015**, *38*, E9. [CrossRef] [PubMed]

38. Shute, J.B.; Okun, M.S.; Opri, E.; Molina, R.; Rossi, P.J.; Martinez-Ramirez, D.; Foote, K.D.; Gunduz, A. Thalamocortical network activity enables chronic tic detection in humans with Tourette syndrome. *NeuroImage Clin.* **2016**, *12*, 165–172. [CrossRef]

39. Swann, N.C.; De Hemptinne, C.; Miocinovic, S.; Qasim, S.; Ostrem, J.L.; Galifianakis, N.B.; Luciano, M.S.; Wang, S.S.; Ziman, N.; Taylor, R.; et al. Chronic multisite brain recordings from a totally implantable bidirectional neural interface: Experience in 5 patients with Parkinson's disease. *J. Neurosurg.* **2018**, *128*, 605–616. [CrossRef]

## 4

Illness Representations and Coping Strategies in Patients Treated with Deep Brain Stimulation for Parkinson's Disease

Marc Baertschi [1,2,*], Nicolas Favez [1], João Flores Alves Dos Santos [3], Michalina Radomska [1], François Herrmann [4], Pierre R. Burkhard [5], Alessandra Canuto [6], Kerstin Weber [6] and Paolo Ghisletta [1,7,8]

[1] Faculty of Psychology and Educational Sciences, University of Geneva, Boulevard du Pont-d'Arve 40, 1205 Geneva, Switzerland; nicolas.favez@unige.ch (N.F.); Michalina.Radomska@etu.unige.ch (M.R.); Paolo.Ghisletta@unige.ch (P.G.)

[2] Nant Foundation, Service of General Psychiatry and Psychotherapy, Avenue des Alpes 66, 1820 Montreux, Switzerland

[3] Service of Liaison Psychiatry and Crisis Intervention, Geneva University Hospitals, Rue Gabrielle-Perret-Gentil 4, 1205 Geneva, Switzerland; Joao.FloresAlvesDosSantos@hcuge.ch

[4] Division of Geriatrics, Geneva University Hospitals, Chemin du Pont-Bochet 3, 1226 Thônex, Switzerland; Francois.Herrmann@hcuge.ch

[5] Service of Neurology, Geneva University Hospitals, Rue Gabrielle-Perret-Gentil 4, 1205 Geneva, Switzerland; Pierre.Burkhard@hcuge.ch

[6] Faculty of Medicine, University of Geneva, Rue Michel Servet 1, 1206 Geneva, Switzerland; Alessandra.Canuto@unige.ch (A.C.); kerstin.weber@hcuge.ch (K.W.)

[7] Swiss Distance Learning University, Überlandstrasse 12, 3900 Brig, Switzerland

[8] Swiss National Centre of Competence in Research LIVES—Overcoming Vulnerability: Life Course Perspectives, Universities of Lausanne and of Geneva, CH-1015 Lausanne, Switzerland

* Correspondence: Marc.Baertschi@nant.ch

Abstract: There is a debate on possible alterations of self-identity following deep brain stimulation for neurological disorders including Parkinson's disease. Among the psychological variables likely to undergo changes throughout such a medical procedure, illness representations and coping strategies have not been the target of much research to this day. In order to remedy this, we investigated the dynamics of illness representations and coping strategies in an 18-month longitudinal study involving 45 patients undergoing deep brain stimulation for idiopathic Parkinson's disease. Two research hypotheses were formulated and investigated through repeated measures of ANOVAs and structural equation modelling with full information maximum likelihood and Bayesian estimations. Representations of Parkinson's disease as a cyclical condition and perception of control over the disease diminished after surgery. Use of instrumental coping strategies was not modified after deep brain stimulation. These changes were identified by SEM but not ANOVAs; their magnitude was nevertheless relatively small, implying general stability in representations. These findings suggest that psychological variables do not undergo major changes after deep brain stimulation for Parkinson's disease.

Keywords: deep brain stimulation; Parkinson's disease; illness representations; illness perceptions; coping strategies

1. Introduction

A chronic and degenerative condition without a widely available curative treatment, Parkinson's disease (PD) is characterized by a complex constellation of motor and non-motor symptoms [1,2].

Preferential treatment targets motor symptoms and consists in substitutive dopaminergic therapy. Yet, when disabling symptoms persist despite optimal medical treatment, patients may be proposed to undergo deep brain stimulation (DBS), a stereotactic neurosurgical procedure during which electrodes are implanted into strategic deep nuclei of the brain [3]. DBS results in rapid motor improvement, in some cases immediately observable after the stimulation is switched on [4]. In addition, DBS allows neurologists to drastically decrease patients' dopaminergic medication, leading to a positive impact on drug-induced motor and non-motor symptoms [5,6]. Beneficial effects on motor symptoms and medication decrease for patients treated with DBS over those only treated with medication had large size effects with a Cohen's d approaching 1.35 in both cases [7].

As illustrated by the therapeutic objectives of DBS, there is a medical focus on motor symptoms in PD that underscores the under-appreciation of health professionals and researchers regarding non-motor symptoms [8]. This factual situation is nevertheless paradoxical as, in the long run, patients consider non-motor symptoms as more disabling than motor symptoms [9]. In this regard, it should be mentioned that recent research points out the importance to consider non-motor symptoms along with motor symptoms in the development of future treatments such as closed-loop DBS [10]. Among the numerous non-motor symptoms of PD identified in the literature, some are related to mental health such as depression, apathy, anxiety, or hallucinations [1,8]. Although a leading treatment like DBS provides moderate improvement ($d \approx 0.30$) on variables related to mental health and quality of life [7], it is unsurprising that a range of non-motor symptoms remain in the patients' clinical picture even after a medically successful DBS.

The paradox of patients experiencing a medically successful DBS, objectively assessed in measuring the pre/post-operative difference of motor functioning, but nevertheless, a psychosocially unsuccessful DBS characterized by dissatisfaction regarding the everyday life was pictured as a 'burden of health' by Burkhard et al. [11]. Progressively, the concept of social or psychosocial adjustment has emerged as a pivotal theme in the post-DBS rehabilitation of PD patients [12,13]. More recently, a study has provided empirical data supporting the beneficial effects of designing specific rehabilitation programs based on psychosocial adjustment [14]. In this context, researchers have suggested that the burden of normality, a model of psychosocial adjustment initially developed for epilepsy surgery [15,16], could relevantly describe the ins and outs of psychosocial adjustment difficulties throughout the DBS process provided that characteristics inherent to PD (e.g., symptoms continuing to develop post-surgery) are taken into account [17–19]. Among the various difficulties listed in the burden of normality regarding the post-surgical adjustment process, patients may encounter psychological changes and notably feelings of self-transformation [16]. In PD, patients have indeed reported identity-related complains following DBS surgery, such as feelings of strangeness, loss of body control and dehumanization [12,20–23], which were associated with life adjustment difficulties. As patients undergoing DBS for PD expect improvement of their motor symptoms, unexpected side effects of brain surgery leading to psychological changes would constitute, in addition to adjustment problems, an ethical issue: Indeed, such involuntary changes would possibly induce more harm than benefits and therefore be experienced negatively because they are undesired [24–26]. In a recent literature review, Gilbert et al. [27] have nevertheless pointed out the lack of empirical data supporting changes after DBS in variables that could labelled 'psychological' such as personality, self-identity, agency, authenticity and autonomy. This publication has given rise to a scientific debate that is still ongoing [28,29]. Among similar psychological types of variables, neither illness representations nor coping strategies have been widely studied in the context of DBS, notably for PD.

Both illness representations and coping strategies are psychological constructs pivotal to understand the dynamics that are in play in the patients' subjective perception of their clinical condition. The common sense model [30,31] indeed posits that internal or external stimuli (e.g., appearance of clinical symptoms) generate cognitive and emotional representations of what is associated with a potential danger (e.g., an illness). These representations are addressed with coping strategies, whose efficiency in the symptom/illness management is appraised, leading to possible changes to better adapt the situation. Thus, patients' subjective representations of their illness are closely intertwined with the way they attempt to cope with the stress related to their clinical condition, as both illness representations and coping strategies are likely to be modified depending on the perceived outcome on health [30–32]. From this perspective, one may wonder whether DBS could constitute a life experience disruptive enough to elicit psychological changes in patients; such kinds of changes would besides have a potential impact on psychosocial adjustment as illness representations and coping strategies have been associated to a variety of adaptive and maladaptive outcomes in terms of well-being and social functioning [33].

To our knowledge, no research has been published on the illness representations of patients undergoing DBS for PD. Nevertheless, based on the common sense model, one might expect that DBS would bring in changes in patients' feelings of personal control over their symptoms. Indeed, in advanced PD, patients look to gain a certain degree of control over their symptoms, including motor and non-motor fluctuations, by managing themselves medication intake [12,22,34–37]. Yet, DBS requires active and regular neurologist intervention to adjust stimulation parameters to PD continuous development, which might lead patients to experience feelings of increased dependence on external intervention in their postsurgical disease management. In line with this, one may wonder whether DBS would lead patients to consider PD as more cyclical with regard to the regular search for stimulation adjustment. On the other hand, it is likely that PD would remain identified as such and associated with severe consequences despite the motor improvement brought in by DBS, as the diseased continues to develop and is frequently associated with psychosocial symptoms [20,23,38].

In contrast, a limited number of studies have longitudinally addressed coping strategies before and after surgery, yielding contradictory findings. While some found that patients use more frequently instrumental coping strategies (i.e., task-oriented responses, such as looking for information or for efficient treatment) before than after surgery [14,39,40], others noted that coping strategies were not employed differently over this period [41]. When observed, changes in coping strategies were associated with patients' situation regarding their illness. Those about to undergo surgery or who could possibly be treated by DBS in the future sought out further information on this procedure, hence a more frequent recourse to instrumental strategies. Yet, patients already operated appeared to be concerned by new life issues and, accordingly, adjusted their ways of coping; they nevertheless kept using more instrumental strategies than those not selected for DBS, who employed predominantly emotional coping strategies (e.g., avoidance, emotional preoccupation) [39,40].

In light of the above, the present study aimed to address, at least partially, the current lack of empirical data regarding potential changes in the psychological experience of patients undergoing DBS highlighted by Gilbert et al. [27]. This study focused on two specific aspects, namely illness representations and coping strategies, in patients treated with DBS for idiopathic PD through an 18-month longitudinal investigation. Taking limitations of our methodological design into account, we decided to preferentially test hypotheses underlying potential pre/post-DBS changes. Thus, based on the existing literature, we assumed that patients should consider PD after surgery as more cyclical and less controllable in comparison with the pre-DBS period (Hypothesis 1). Second, as all patients included in the study knew that they were about to undergo surgery, they should have resorted to instrumental strategies more frequently before DBS than after (Hypothesis 2).

2. Materials and Methods

2.1. Procedure

Forty-five patients diagnosed with PD and treated at the Geneva University Hospitals were included between 31 January 2013 and 8 June 2017 in a global study investigating the possible determinants of quality of life after DBS. The study procedure consisted in filling out a series of self-reported questionnaires 2 weeks before DBS surgery (T0), as well as 6 (T1), 12 (T2) and 18 (T3) months after. Inclusion criteria were a DBS medical indication for idiopathic PD collaboratively established by senior neurologist, neurosurgeon, neuropsychologist and consultation-liaison psychiatrist; a sufficient French level to read and understand a series of self-administered questionnaires; and agreement to sign a consent form. Participation was proposed to all patients clinically accepted for DBS, which includes capacity of discernment, and all participants agreed with the study procedure.

The present study received approval from the Canton of Geneva ethics committee under the registration number 14-182.

2.2. Participants

At study inclusion, patients were aged 60.6 ± 8.6 years and most of them (60.0%) were males. The majority (66.7%) had been in a couple relationship for a long time (on average 33.1 ± 13.0 years), and 71.4% had children (1.5 ± 1.2 on average). Patients had a school background of 12.1 ± 5.3 years and had been diagnosed with PD for 9.8 ± 4.0 years. Patients score at the third part of the Movement Disorder Society Unified Parkinson's Disease Rating Scale (MDS-UPDRS), a clinician-administered measurement of motor functioning standard in PD, was 21.105 ± 11.347 at T0, 11.419 ± 7.244 at T2 (corresponding to a 45.9% improvement), and 14.720 ± 6.921 at T3 (corresponding to a 30.3% improvement compared to T0). No measure was available at T1, post-DBS scores correspond to an on-medication and on-stimulation condition.

2.3. Instruments

The revised version of the Illness Perception Questionnaire (IPQ-R) [42] assesses attributes of illness representations based on the common sense model of Leventhal et al. [30,31]. This instrument proposes a self-evaluation of the main attributes defined by the common sense model, that is the identity of the illness (i.e., the observed symptoms, which may form a label—typically, the name of a disease), the possible causes of the illness, the timeline defining an acute, chronic or cyclic perception of the illness course, the consequences of the illness on daily living, the representations of the controllability or curability of the illness, the perception of the illness as a more or less coherent entity, and the emotional impact of illness representations. For the specific need of this study, we focused on two types of illness representations, namely cyclical timeline and curability/controllability.

The IPQ-R proposes scales to measure separately each of these attributes. Timeline is assessed with one scale whereas curability/controllability is evaluated with two scales (i.e., personal control and treatment control). These scales are designed with Likert-type items proposing five response possibilities (score range per item: 1–5). Test-retest reliability for the two illness representations considered in this study (i.e., cyclical timeline, and personal control and treatment control) showed mixed stability at 3 weeks (correlations from 0.46 to 0.72) and 6 months (correlations from 0.35 to 0.57) [42]. A version of the scale in French language is available on its official website (http://www.uib.no/ipq/).

The Brief COPE [43] is a questionnaire assessing 14 coping strategies with two items for each, leading to a total of 28 items. Coping strategies are evaluated using four-point Likert scales. The score range for each coping strategy is 2–8, with high scores indicating frequent use of the strategy in question. In order to investigate the use of instrumental coping strategies before and after DBS (Hypothesis 2), we created a composite variable by adding the scores of three subscales of the Brief COPE, namely active coping (e.g., item 7: "I've been taking action to try to make the situation better"), use of instrumental support (e.g., item 10: "I've been getting help and advice from other people"), and planning (e.g., item 25: "I've been thinking hard about what steps to take"). This composite variable had a score range of 6–24, with higher scores suggesting greater use of instrumental coping strategies. Like the IPQ-R, internal reliability of the Brief COPE scales was mixed with correlations ranging from 0.50 to 0.90 [43].

2.4. Statistical Analyses

After computing descriptive statistics for all variables of interest, we attempted to test our two hypotheses by a series of inferential analyses. As these hypotheses were all based on mean comparisons, we initially conducted repeated measures analyzes of variance (rANOVA). Yet, ANOVA deals with missing data through pairwise or listwise deletion, which increases the likelihood to lose information on participants notably in a longitudinal design. For this reason, we ran additional analyses with structural equation modelling (SEM), a statistical method offering better options with regard to missing data. Three nested models were built for model comparison, namely; a level model assuming no change between before and after DBS (i.e., T0 = T1 = T2 = T3); a step model assuming a change between before and after DBS (i.e., T0 ≠ T1 = T2 = T3), and; a model allowing a free slope estimation so that possible changes within post-DBS measurement times can be taken into consideration. This procedure was repeated to address each research hypothesis.

In the present study, the initial sample size (n = 45) increases to a potential n = 180 because of its longitudinal design comprising four measurement times. Although SEM is generally used with larger sample sizes, it can be applied to smaller samples starting from 30 depending on the model tested [44]. Notably, Bayesian estimation has been found adapted to small samples [45,46]. Thus, we conducted SEM analyses by comparing models estimated; first, with the traditionally used full information maximum likelihood (FIML) and; second, with Bayesian estimation of probability. In order to assess the latter, we examined the following attributes: convergence statistic (acceptable if < 1.002), trace plots stability, convergence in the comparison of first and last third of each parameter's posterior distribution, stability of autocorrelation plots, and comparison of value estimates with those obtained from FIML analyses. In addition, we provided the deviance information criterion (DIC) and the effective number of parameters (enp) in tables.

All statistical analyses were conducted with IBM SPSS Statistics version 25.0 (IBM Corp., Armonk, NY, USA) and IBM SPSS Amos version 25.0 (IBM SPSS, Chicago, IL, USA). A significance threshold of 0.05 was adopted for inferential statistics. All the data were normally distributed.

3. Results

Hypothesis 1. *We tested this hypothesis by using three illness representations variables, that is cyclical timeline, personal control and treatment control.*

First, cyclical timeline representations of PD were stable between pre- and post-DBS assessments as showed by a rANOVA, F (2.025, 32.397) = 0.867, p = 0.431, η^2 = 0.020, ω^2 = 0.000. Because of sphericity violation (Greenhouse-Geisser ε = 0.675), we used Greenhouse-Geisser correction to interpret the analyses.

In contrast with the rANOVA above, SEM analyses showed that patients perceived PD as less cyclical after surgery than before, as demonstrated with significant global mean slope changes in both the step (b = −1.482, SE = 0.536, p = 0.006) and the free (b = −0.556, SE = 0.235, p = 0.018) models. The latter model showed a significant change between T0 and T1 (b = 3.122, SE = 0.523, p < 0.001) with an effect size (d = 0.540) estimated as medium to large according to the criteria of Cohen [47]. In FIML estimation, the free model obtained the best statistical fit to the data as depicted in Table 1; yet using Bayesian estimation the step model was better adjusted. Considering that the magnitude of the T1-T2 change was, although significant, very small (b = 2.804, SE = 0.528, p < 0.001, d = 0.053), our data suggest that the change toward less cyclical representations of PD after DBS does not reinforce but stabilizes in the later post-surgical assessment sessions.

Second, patients did not report change in their representation of personal control over PD between pre- and post-DBS assessments as showed by a rANOVA, F (3, 48) = 0.044, p = 0.987, η^2 = 0.001,

$\omega^2 = 0.000$. Because of sphericity violation (Greenhouse-Geisser $\varepsilon = 0.867$), we used Huynh-Feldt correction to interpret the analyses.

In the SEM analyses, although the three tested models showed good statistical fit (see Table 2), the step model was significantly better than the level, suggesting that representations of personal control over PD decreased after surgery ($b = -1.393$, SE $= 0.627$, $p = 0.026$). The free model specified that this diminution had a small to medium effect size in the DBS pre-post transition ($\beta_{T1} = 1.776$, SE $= 0.687$, $p = 0.010$, $d = 0.267$) and continued after surgery, albeit with a much smaller amplitude, $\beta_{T2} = 2.026$, SE $= 0.774$, $p = 0.009$, $d = 0.039$. Bayesian analyses were adequate for all models, except for the slightly unstable autocorrelation trace plots of the free model.

Third, patients did not report change in their representations of treatment control on PD between pre- and post-DBS assessments as showed by a rANOVA, F $(2.197, 35.146) = 0.1.195$, $p = 0.318$, $\eta^2 = 0.001$, $\omega^2 = 0.000$. Because of sphericity violation (Greenhouse–Geisser $\varepsilon = 0.732$), we used Greenhouse–Geisser correction to interpret the analyses.

In the SEM analyses, the free model best fitted the data, as shown in Table 2, with significant mean slope change ($b = -0.312$, SE $= 0.145$, $p = 0.030$) and interindividual variability ($b = -1.066$, SE $= 0.411$, $p = 0.010$). This suggests that treatment control was perceived as weaker after DBS than before. Yet, slope estimations were not significantly different from 0 at any specific measurement session; in addition, Bayesian analyses showed that the level and step models were better adjusted to the data than the free. Overall, it implies that representations of treatment control did not undergo significant changes over DBS surgery.

Hypothesis 2. *Recourse to instrumental coping was stable over the pre- and post-DBS period, as showed by a rANOVA, F $(23, 51) = 2.774$, $p = 0.051$, $\eta^2 = 0.032$, $\omega^2 = 0.007$. Because of sphericity violation (Greenhouse–Geisser $\varepsilon = 0.851$), we used Huynh–Feldt correction to interpret the analyses.*

In line with this and as summarized in Table 3, the three models designed through SEM did not differ significantly from one another and were very similar in terms of fit indices. However, the Bayesian solution for the free model was not adequate, contrary to these of the level and the step. Detailed analyses of the step model showed that the global mean slope did not change significantly ($b = -0.562$, SE $= 0.501$, $p = 0.262$).

Table 1. Comparisons of latent growth curve models estimating growth trajectory for a cyclical representation of PD over an 18-month follow-up (T0–T3).

#	n	Mean	SD	Skewness	SE Skewness	Excess Kurtosis	SE Kurtosis
T0	39	13.564	3.307	-0.473	0.378	0.357	0.741
T1	30	11.833	3.495	0.144	0.427	-0.693	0.833
T2	20	11.600	3.050	0.065	0.512	-0.616	0.992
T3	23	12.522	3.475	-0.156	0.481	-0.277	0.935

#	Tested models	χ^2	df	p-value	χ^2/df	CFI	TLI	RMSEA (90% CI), pclose	Model comparison	$\Delta \chi^2$	Δ df	p-value	DIC	enp
1	Level	35.053	11	<0.001	3.187	0.281	0.346	0.226 (0.144–0.311), 0.001	1 vs 2	7.385	1	0.007	416.67	2.78
2	Step	27.668	10	0.002	2.767	0.472	0.472	0.203 (0.115–0.295), 0.005	1 vs 3	20.173	5	0.001	411.16	3.78
3	Free	14.880	6	0.021	2.480	0.734	0.557	0.186 (0.067–0.307), 0.036	2 vs 3	12.788	4	0.012	406.08	7.05

Note: SD = standard deviation, SE = standard error, p = probability, $\chi2$ = chi-squared, df = degrees of freedom, CFI = comparative fit index, pclose = probability that the RMSEA value is below .05, TLI = Tucker-Lewis index, RMSEA = root mean square error of approximation, CI = confidence intervals, DIC = deviance information criterion, enp = effective number of parameters

Table 2. (a) Comparisons of latent growth curve models estimating growth trajectory for the representation of a personal control of PD over an 18-month follow-up (T0–T3). **(b)** Comparisons of latent growth curve models estimating growth trajectory for the representation of a control of PD by treatment over an 18-month follow-up (T0–T3).

(a)

#	n	Mean	SD	Skewness	SE Skewness	Excess Kurtosis	SE Kurtosis
T0	39	20.026	4.374	-0.945	0.378	1.274	0.741
T1	30	18.900	4.302	-0.531	0.427	0.745	0.833
T2	20	19.300	4.256	-0.604	0.512	-0.642	0.992
T3	23	17.609	4.356	-0.209	0.481	-0.973	0.935

#	Tested models	χ^2	df	p-value	χ^2/df	CFI	TLI	RMSEA (90% CI), pclose	Model comparison	$\Delta\chi^2$	Δdf	p-value	DIC	emp
1	Level	9.675	11	0.560	0.880	1.000	1.055	0.000 (0.000–0.145), 0.648	1 vs 2	4.799	1	0.028	460.35	2.82
2	Step	4.876	10	0.89	0.488	1.000	1.232	0.000 (0.000–0.072), 0.928	1 vs 3	8.586	5	0.127	457.35	3.76
3	Free	1.089	6	0.982	0.181	1.000	1.371	0.000 (0.000–0.000), 0.986	2 vs 3	3.787	4	0.436	461.72	7.20

(b)

#	N	Mean	SD	Skewness	SE skewness	Excess kurtosis	SE kurtosis
T0	39	16.923	3.800	0.342	0.378	-0.129	0.741
T1	30	15.333	4.063	-0.986	0.427	0.826	0.833
T2	20	16.650	3.588	-0.526	0.512	-0.629	0.992
T3	23	15.739	2.942	-1.139	0.481	2.512	0.935

#	Tested models	χ^2	df	p-value	χ^2/df	CFI	TLI	RMSEA (90% CI), pclose	Model comparison	$\Delta\chi^2$	Δdf	p-value	DIC	emp
1	Level	17.399	11	0.097	1.582	0.649	0.681	0.116 (0.000–0.215), 0.152	1 vs 2	3.094	1	0.079	432.83	2.78
2	Step	14.305	10	0.160	1.431	0.764	0.764	0.100 (0.000–0.207), 0.228	1 vs 3	11.61	5	0.041	431.77	3.79
3	Free	5.789	6	0.447	2.480	0.734	0.557	0.000 (0.000–0.194), 0.516	2 vs 3	8.516	4	0.074	-	-

Table 3. Comparisons of latent growth curve models estimating growth trajectory for a cyclical representation of PD over an 18-month follow-up (T0-T3).

#	n	Mean	SD	Skewness	SE Skewness	Excess Kurtosis	SE Kurtosis
T0	42	14.000	4.283	0.274	0.365	-0.408	0.717
T1	31	13.097	3.581	0.051	0.421	-0.659	0.821
T2	24	14.333	3.795	-0.750	0.472	0.063	0.918
T3	24	13.417	3.944	-0.047	0.472	-0.875	0.918

#	Tested models	χ^2	df	p-value	χ^2/df	CFI	TLI	RMSEA (90% CI), pclose
1	Level	17.093	11	0.105	1.554	0.868	0.955	0.112 (0.000-0.210), 0.164
2	Step	15.848	10	0.104	1.585	0.874	0.874	0.115 (0.000-0.217), 0.160
3	Free	9.767	6	0.135	1.628	0.919	0.551	0.119 (0.000-0.250), 0.185

Model comparison	$\Delta \chi^2$	Δ df	p-value	DIC	emp
1 vs 2	1.245	1	0.265	457.12	2.85
1 vs 3	7.326	5	0.198	457.77	3.80
2 vs 3	6.081	4	0.193	-	-

4. Discussion

In this study, we attempted to provide empirical evidence on the question of whether DBS may induce psychological changes using an empirical, inferential approach with patients diagnosed with idiopathic PD. To this end, we targeted two specific variables, namely illness representations and coping strategies.

Based on the existing literature, we had expectations of various kinds of change that DBS would bring in as formulated in two research hypotheses. Yet, globally, our results did not provide confirmation of these expected changes. The first hypothesis, related to illness representations, was partly invalidated as PD was perceived as less cyclical after surgery than before, although patients had lower representations of personal control on PD post-surgically, this latter finding being expected. Regarding the second hypothesis, we observed that the use of instrumental coping strategies was not modified by DBS, which invalidates our initial assumption.

These results suggest that PD remains globally perceived as the same medical entity after DBS, despite the important reduction of motor symptoms induced by brain surgery. Patients' representations of control on PD decreased after surgery, and this was notably the case for personal control. The notion of control is ethically important as it is associated with autonomy, which, in this context, relates to the patient's right to decide about his/her treatment [26]. In this regard, feelings of self-estrangement reported from testimonies of operated patients were associated with the impression of losing the control over one's emotions and capabilities [48]. More generally, a loss of personal control in illness management was expected as it has been well illustrated by testimonies of operated patients [12,49]. In terms of adjustment, this is problematic as subjective perception of control over a chronic disease was associated with adaptive outcomes [33]. This association was notably established in PD patients not treated with DBS [50]. It was however surprising to observe a diminution in representations of treatment control of PD—although this was weak and suggests that, globally, perceptions of treatment control remain similar before and after surgery. One might have indeed imagined that the necessity to rely on neurologists to adapt stimulation parameters would have led to an impression that health professionals may manage the disease efficiently. Possibly related to this latter issue, patients had a less cyclical representation of PD after DBS than before. This suggests that regular appointments with a neurologist to adapt stimulations parameters are not sufficient to create a cyclical representation of PD; however, stabilization of motor fluctuations induced by DBS surgery [51] may have instilled the feelings of a medical condition having become less cyclical after surgery. Representations of PD as becoming more stable after DBS may be related to better psychological well-being, as it was measured in non-DBS patients diagnosed with PD [52].

Finally, we found that use of instrumental coping strategies to deal with stressful situations was not reduced after DBS. This result, which adds to some previous findings [41] but stands in contradiction to others [14,39,40], suggests that DBS does not deeply modify strategies of stress management, the latter being not exclusively dependent on situational issues (e.g., intensity of motor symptoms before vs. after DBS).

Overall, the findings of this study highlight the stability in illness representations and coping strategies throughout the DBS process and rehabilitation. Although significant changes were found here and there, their magnitude was generally small. The only notable exception was representations of PD as being less cyclical after DBS than before. Yet, even in this specific case, magnitude of change should be interpreted with caution. For instance, the implied mean at T0 retrieved from the free model was 13.515 and that at T1 was 11.779. As representations of cyclical timeline are assessed in the IPQ-R with four items, these means correspond to an item mean score of 3.379 at T0 and 2.945 at T1. In other words, representations of cyclical timeline remain around a mean item score of 3 corresponding to a "neither agree nor disagree" response anchor at each measurement time. Thus, even significant and with a medium to large effect size, changes in representations of cyclical timeline remain globally stable over the DBS process and should not be associated with a major alteration in patients' perception of PD. Interestingly, these small changes were all identified by a critical examination of both FIML and

Bayesian estimations in SEM, a method that does not suppress missing data from analyses; on the contrary, rANOVA analyses did not find any significant difference between measurement sessions. Methodologically, this observation implies that SEM remains discriminant with small-size samples, which is a scenario likely to happen frequently in heavy medical situations such as DBS surgery.

Our results should be considered with caution because of limitations inherent to the study design. First, illness representations and coping strategies are not representative of all psychological aspects of the DBS experience. Besides, we decided to focus our analyses on a limited number of illness representations and coping strategies, based on assumptions from the literature and methodological limitations of our experimental design; it remains nevertheless possible that other kinds of illness representations and coping strategies are significantly altered after DBS. Finally, the findings of the current study stand for patients undergoing DBS for PD; it cannot be ruled out that individuals treated with DBS for other medical conditions would experience different outcomes regarding the variables investigated in this research.

5. Conclusions

In conclusion, our study suggests that DBS does not induce major psychological changes as measured in terms of illness representations and coping strategies. These conclusions are in line with those of Gilbert et al. [27], who pointed out the lack of current empirical data showing significant changes in personality, self-identity, agency, authenticity, autonomy and self after DBS. Yet, we advocate that future studies continue exploring how psychological variables may impact the acceptation process of life with DBS. In this regard, the burden of normality model may be useful to identify and address the non-motor issues occurring after DBS in PD patients [17]. In addition, and as illustrated in a recent qualitative study [53], considering data related to psychological aspects before surgical implantation may be predictive of post-operative outcome. This implies that a complete psychological assessment taking place before surgery would help clinicians identify risks of developing post-surgical psychosocial complications.

Author Contributions: Conceptualization, M.B., N.F. and P.G.; methodology, M.B., N.F., F.H. and P.G.; software, M.B. and P.G.; validation, M.B., N.F. and P.G.; formal analysis, M.B., F.H. and P.G.; investigation, M.B., J.F.A.D.S., M.R., P.R.B., A.C. and K.W. ; resources, M.B., J.F.A.D.S., K.W.; data curation, J.F.A.D.S. and M.R.; writing—Original draft preparation, M.B.; writing—Review and editing, M.B., N.F. and P.G.; visualization, M.B., N.F., K.W. and P.G.; supervision, N.F. and P.G.; project administration, P.R.B., A.C. and K.W.; funding acquisition, P.R.B. and A.C. All authors have read and agreed to the published version of the manuscript.

Acknowledgments: We are thankful to Bernard Baertschi from the Institute for Biomedical Ethics of the University of Geneva for his precious advice during the construction of the manuscript.

References

1.   Chaudhuri, K.R.; Healy, D.G.; Schapira, A.H. Non-motor symptoms of Parkinson's disease: Diagnosis and management. *Lancet Neurol.* **2006**, *5*, 235–245. [CrossRef]

2.   Jankovic, J. Parkinson's disease: Clinical features and diagnosis. *J. Neurol. Neurosurg. Psychiatry* **2008**, *79*, 368–376. [CrossRef] [PubMed]

3.   Pollak, P. Deep brain stimulation for Parkinson's disease—Patient selection. In *Handbook of Clinical Neurology*, 1st ed.; Elsevier: Amsterdam, The Netherlands, 2013; Volume 116. [CrossRef]

4.   Castrioto, A.; Volkmann, J.; Krack, P. Postoperative management of deep brain stimulation in Parkinson's disease. *Handb. Clin. Neurol.* **2013**, *116*, 129–146. [CrossRef] [PubMed]

5.   Lhommée, E.; Klinger, H.; Thobois, S.; Schmitt, E.; Ardouin, C.; Bichon, A.; Krack, P. Subthalamic stimulation in Parkinson's disease: Restoring the balance of motivated behaviours. *Brain J. Neurol.* **2012**, *135*, 1463–1477. [CrossRef]

6.   Thobois, S.; Ardouin, C.; Lhommée, E.; Klinger, H.; Lagrange, C.; Xie, J.; Krack, P. Non-motor dopamine withdrawal syndrome after surgery for Parkinson's disease: Predictors and underlying mesolimbic denervation. *Brain* **2010**, *133*, 1111–1127. [CrossRef]

7.   Perestelo-Pérez, L.; Rivero-Santana, A.; Pérez-Ramos, J.; Serrano-Pérez, P.; Panetta, J.; Hilarion, P. Deep brain stimulation in Parkinson's disease: Meta-analysis of randomized controlled trials. *J. Neurol.* **2014**, *261*, 2051–2060. [CrossRef]

8.   Chaudhuri, K.R.; Odin, P.; Antonini, A.; Martinez-Martin, P. Parkinson's disease: The non-motor issues. *Parkinsonism Relat. Disord.* **2011**, *17*, 717–723. [CrossRef]

9.   Hely, M.A.; Morris, J.G.L.; Reid, W.G.J.; Trafficante, R. Sydney multicenter study of Parkinson's disease: Non-L-dopa-responsive problems dominate at 15 years. *Mov. Disord.* **2005**, *20*, 190–199. [CrossRef]

10. Bouthour, W.; Mégevand, P.; Donoghue, J.; Lüscher, C.; Birbaumer, N.; Krack, P. Biomarkers for closed-loop deep brain stimulation in Parkinson disease and beyond. *Nat. Rev. Neurol.* **2019**, *15*, 343–352. [CrossRef]

11. Burkhard, P.R.; Vingerhoets, F.J.G.G.; Berney, A.; Bogousslavsky, J.; Villemure, J.-G.; Ghika, J. Suicide after successful deep brain stimulation for movement disorders. *Neurology* **2004**, *63*, 2170–2172. [CrossRef]

12. Haahr, A.; Kirkevold, M.; Hall, E.O.C.; Østergaard, K. From miracle to reconciliation: A hermeneutic phenomenological study exploring the experience of living with Parkinson's disease following deep brain stimulation. *Int. J. Nurs. Stud.* **2010**, *47*, 1228–1236. [CrossRef] [PubMed]

13. Meyer, M.; Montel, S.R.; Colnat-Coulbois, S.; Lerond, J.; Potheegadoo, J.; Vidailhet, P.; Schwan, R. Neurosurgery in Parkinson's disease: Social adjustment, quality of life and coping strategies. *Neural Regen. Res.* **2013**, *8*, 2856–2867. [CrossRef]

14. Flores Alves Dos Santos, J.; Tezenas du Montcel, S.; Gargiulo, M.; Behar, C.; Montel, S.; Hergueta, T.; Welter, M.-L. Tackling psychosocial maladjustment in Parkinson's disease patients following subthalamic deep-brain stimulation: A randomised clinical trial. *PLoS ONE* **2017**, *12*, e0174512. [CrossRef] [PubMed]

15. Bladin, P.F. Psychosocial difficulties and outcome after temporal lobectomy. *Epilepsia* **1992**, *33*, 898–907. [CrossRef]

16. Wilson, S.J.; Bladin, P.; Saling, M. The "burden of normality": Concepts of adjustment after surgery for seizures. *J. Neurol. Neurosurg. Psychiatry* **2001**, *70*, 649–656. [CrossRef] [PubMed]

17. Baertschi, M.; Favez, N.; Radomska, M.; Herrmann, F.; Burkhard, P.R.; Weber, K.; Flores Alves Dos Santos, J. An empirical study on the application of the burden of normality to patients undergoing deep brain stimulation for Parkinson's disease. *J. Psychosoc. Rehabil. Ment. Health* **2019**, *6*, 175–186. [CrossRef]

18. Baertschi, M.; Flores Alves Dos Santos, J.; Burkhard, P.; Weber, K.; Canuto, A.; Favez, N. The burden of normality as a model of psychosocial adjustment after deep brain stimulation for Parkinson's disease: A systematic investigation. *Neuropsychology* **2019**, *33*, 178–194. [CrossRef] [PubMed]

19. Gilbert, F. The burden of normality: From "chronically ill" to "symptom free". New ethical challenges for deep brain stimulation postoperative treatment. *J. Med Ethics* **2012**, *38*, 408–412. [CrossRef]

20. Agid, Y.; Schüpbach, M.; Gargiulo, M.; Mallet, L.; Houeto, J.L.; Behar, C.; Welter, M.L. Neurosurgery in Parkinson's disease: The doctor is happy, the patient less so? *J. Neural Transm.* **2006**, (Suppl. 70), 409–414. [CrossRef]

21. Hariz, G.-M.; Hamberg, K. Perceptions of living with a device-based treatment: An account of patients treated with deep brain stimulation for Parkinson's disease. *Neuromodulation J. Int. Neuromodulation Soc.* **2014**, *17*, 272–277, discussion 277–278. [CrossRef]

22. Perozzo, P.; Rizzone, M.; Bergamasco, B.; Castelli, L.; Lanotte, M.; Tavella, A.; Lopiano, L. Deep brain stimulation of subthalamic nucleus: Behavioural modifications and familiar relations. *Neurol. Sci.* **2001**, *22*, 81–82. [CrossRef] [PubMed]

23. Schüpbach, W.M.M.; Gargiulo, M.; Welter, M.L.; Mallet, L.; Béhar, C.; Houeto, J.L.; Agid, Y. Neurosurgery in Parkinson disease: A distressed mind in a repaired body? *Neurology* **2006**, *66*, 1811–1816. [CrossRef] [PubMed]

24. Baertschi, B. Intended changes are not always good, and unintended changes are not always bad—Why? *Am. J. Bioeth.* **2009**, *9*, 39–40. [CrossRef] [PubMed]

25. Baertschi, B.; Hurst, S.A.; Mauron, A. It's not who you are. *AJOB Neurosci.* **2010**, *1*, 18–19. [CrossRef]

26. Müller, S.; Christen, M. Deep brain stimulation in parkinsonian patients—Ethical evaluation of cognitive, affective, and behavioral sequelae. *AJOB Neurosci.* **2011**, *2*, 3–13. [CrossRef]

27. Gilbert, F.; Viaña, J.N.M.; Ineichen, C. Deflating the "DBS causes personality changes" bubble. *Neuroethics* **2018**, 1–17. [CrossRef]

28. Kubu, C.S.; Ford, P.J.; Wilt, J.A.; Merner, A.R.; Montpetite, M.; Zeigler, J.; Racine, E. Pragmatism and the importance of interdisciplinary teams in investigating personality changes following DBS. *Neuroethics* **2019**, 1–10. [CrossRef]

29. Thomson, C.J.; Segrave, R.A.; Carter, A. Changes in personality associated with deep brain stimulation: A qualitative evaluation of clinician perspectives. *Neuroethics* **2019**. [CrossRef]

30. Leventhal, H.; Bodnar-Deren, S.; Breland, J.Y.; Hash-Converse, J.; Phillips, L.A.; Leventhal, E.A.; Cameron, L.D. Modeling health and illness behavior: The approach of the commonsense model. In *Handbook of Health Psychology*, 2nd ed.; Baum, A., Revenson, T.A., Singer, J., Eds.; Taylor Francis Inc.: Philadelphia, PA, USA, 2012; pp. 3–35.

31. Leventhal, H.; Meyer, D.; Nerenz, D. The common sense representation of illness danger. In *Medical Psychology*; Rachman, S., Ed.; Pergamon Press: New York, NY, USA, 1980; Volume 2, pp. 7–30.

32. Leventhal, H.; Benyamini, Y.; Brownlee, S.; Diefenbach, M.; Leventhal, E.A.; Patrick-Miller, L.; Robitaille, C. Illness representations: Theoretical foundations. In *Perceptions of Health and Illness*; Weinman, J., Petrie, K., Eds.; Harwood: London, UK, 1997; pp. 19–45.

33. Hagger, M.S.; Orbell, S. A meta-analytic review of the common-sense model of illness representations. *Psychol. Health* **2003**, *18*, 141–184. [CrossRef]

34. Caap-Ahlgren, M.; Lannerheim, L. Older Swedish women's experiences of living with symptoms related to Parkinson's disease. *J. Adv. Nurs.* **2002**, *39*, 87–95. [CrossRef]

35. Gisquet, E. Cerebral implants and Parkinson's disease: A unique form of biographical disruption? *Soc. Sci. Med.* **2008**, *67*, 1847–1851. [CrossRef]

36. Haahr, A.; Kirkevold, M.; Hall, E.O.C.; Østergaard, K. Living with advanced Parkinson's disease: A constant struggle with unpredictability. *J. Adv. Nurs.* **2011**, *67*, 408–417. [CrossRef]

37. Van der Bruggen, H.; Widdershoven, G. Being a Parkinson's patient: Immobile and unpredictably whimsical. Literature and existential analysis. *Med. Health Care Philos.* **2004**, *7*, 289–301. [CrossRef] [PubMed]

38. Maier, F.; Lewis, C.J.; Horstkoetter, N.; Eggers, C.; Kalbe, E.; Maarouf, M.; Timmermann, L. Patients' expectations of deep brain stimulation, and subjective perceived outcome related to clinical measures in Parkinson's disease: A mixed-method approach. *J. Neurol. Neurosurg. Psychiatry* **2013**, *84*, 1273–1281. [CrossRef] [PubMed]

39. Montel, S.R.; Bungener, C. What relation is there between deep brain stimulation and coping strategies in Parkinson's disease? *Mov. Disord. Off. J. Mov. Disord. Soc.* **2008**, *23*, 1780–1784. [CrossRef] [PubMed]

40. Montel, S.R.; Bungener, C. Coping and quality of life of patients with Parkinson disease who have undergone deep brain stimulation of the subthalamic nucleus. *Surg. Neurol.* **2009**, *72*, 105–110, discussion 110–111. [CrossRef] [PubMed]

41. Soulas, T.; Sultan, S.; Gurruchaga, J.; Palfi, S.; Fénelon, G. Depression and coping as predictors of change after deep brain stimulation in Parkinson's disease. *World Neurosurg.* **2011**, *75*, 525–532. [CrossRef] [PubMed]

42. Moss-Morris, R.; Weinman, J.; Petrie, K.; Horne, R.; Cameron, L.; Buick, D. The revised illness perception questionnaire (IPQ-R). *Psychol. Health* **2002**, *17*, 1–16. [CrossRef]

43. Carver, C.S. You want to measure coping but your protocol's too long: Consider the brief COPE. *Int. J. Behav. Med.* **1997**, *4*, 92–100. [CrossRef]

44. Wolf, E.J.; Harrington, K.M.; Clark, S.L.; Miller, M.W. Sample size requirements for structural equation models: An evaluation of power, bias, and solution propriety. *Educ. Psychol. Meas.* **2013**, *73*, 913–934. [CrossRef]

45. Lee, S.-Y.; Song, X.-Y. Evaluation of the bayesian and maximum likelihood approaches in analyzing structural equation models with small sample sizes. *Multivar. Behav. Res.* **2004**, *39*, 653–686. [CrossRef]

46. Spiegelhalter, A.R.; Abrams, K.R.; Myles, J.P. *Bayesian Approaches to Clinical Trials and Health-Care Evaluation*; John Wiley Sons: Chichester, UK, 2004.

47. Cohen, J. *Statistical Power Analysis for the Behavioral Sciences*, 2nd ed.; Lawrence Erlbaum Associates: Hillsdale, NJ, USA, 1988.

48. Gilbert, F. Deep brain stimulation: Inducing self-estrangement. *Neuroethics* **2018**, *11*, 157–165. [CrossRef]

49. Gilbert, F.; Goddard, E.; Viaña, J.N.M.; Carter, A.; Horne, M. I miss being me: Phenomenological effects of deep brain stimulation. *AJOB Neurosci.* **2017**, *8*, 96–109. [CrossRef]

50. Evans, D.; Norman, P. Illness representations, coping and psychological adjustment to Parkinson's disease. *Psychol. Health* **2009**, *24*, 1181–1196. [CrossRef] [PubMed]

51. Schüpbach, W.M.M.; Chastan, N.; Welter, M.L.; Houeto, J.L.; Mesnage, V.; Bonnet, A.M.; Agid, Y. Stimulation of the subthalamic nucleus in Parkinson's disease: A 5 year follow up. *J. Neurol. Neurosurg. Psychiatry* **2005**, *76*, 1640–1644. [CrossRef] [PubMed]

52. Hurt, C.S.; Burn, D.J.; Hindle, J.; Samuel, M.; Wilson, K.; Brown, R.G. Thinking positively about chronic illness: An exploration of optimism, illness perceptions and well-being in patients with Parkinson's disease. *Br. J. Health Psychol.* **2014**, *19*, 363–379. [CrossRef]

53. Gilbert, F.; Cook, M.; O'Brien, T.; Illes, J. Embodiment and estrangement: Results from a first-in-human "Intelligent BCI" trial. *Sci. Eng. Ethics* **2019**, *25*, 83–96. [CrossRef] [PubMed]

5

A Decade of Progress in Deep Brain Stimulation of the Subcallosal Cingulate for the Treatment of Depression

Sharafuddin Khairuddin [1,†]**, Fung Yin Ngo** [1,†]**, Wei Ling Lim** [1,2]**, Luca Aquili** [3]**, Naveed Ahmed Khan** [4]**, Man-Lung Fung** [1]**, Ying-Shing Chan** [1]**, Yasin Temel** [5] **and Lee Wei Lim** [1,2,*]

[1] Neuromodulation Laboratory, School of Biomedical Sciences, Li Ka Shing Faculty of Medicine, The University of Hong Kong, L4 Laboratory Block, 21 Sassoon Road, Hong Kong, China; sharaf@hku.hk (S.K.); fyngo1@connect.hku.hk (F.Y.N.); weilingl@sunway.edu.my (W.L.L.); fungml@hku.hk (M.-L.F.); yschan@hku.hk (Y.-S.C.)

[2] Department of Biological Sciences, School of Science and Technology, Sunway University, Bandar Sunway 47500, Malaysia

[3] School of Psychological and Clinical Sciences, Charles Darwin University, NT0815 Darwin, Australia; luca.aquili@cdu.edu.au

[4] Department of Biology, Chemistry and Environmental Sciences, College of Arts and Sciences, American University of Sharjah, Sharjah 26666, UAE; naveed5438@gmail.com

[5] Departments of Neuroscience and Neurosurgery, Maastricht University, 6229ER Maastricht, The Netherlands; y.temel@maastrichtuniversity.nl

* Correspondence: drlimleewei@gmail.com

† These authors have joint first authorship.

Abstract: Major depression contributes significantly to the global disability burden. Since the first clinical study of deep brain stimulation (DBS), over 446 patients with depression have now undergone this neuromodulation therapy, and 29 animal studies have investigated the efficacy of subgenual cingulate DBS for depression. In this review, we aim to provide a comprehensive overview of the progress of DBS of the subcallosal cingulate in humans and the medial prefrontal cortex, its rodent homolog. For preclinical animal studies, we discuss the various antidepressant-like behaviors induced by medial prefrontal cortex DBS and examine the possible mechanisms including neuroplasticity-dependent/independent cellular and molecular changes. Interestingly, the response rate of subcallosal cingulate Deep brain stimulation marks a milestone in the treatment of depression. DBS achieved response and remission rates of 64–76% and 37–63%, respectively, from clinical studies monitoring patients from 6–24 months. Although some studies showed its stimulation efficacy was limited, it still holds great promise as a therapy for patients with treatment-resistant depression. Overall, further research is still needed, including more credible clinical research, preclinical mechanistic studies, precise selection of patients, and customized electrical stimulation paradigms.

Keywords: deep brain stimulation; treatment-resistant depression; major depressive disorder; subcallosal cingulate; medial prefrontal cortex

1. Introduction

Major depressive disorder (MDD) contributes significantly to the global disability burden and social burden [1,2]. In the US from 2005 to 2010, the economic burden of patients with major depressive disorder increased by 21.5% to $210.5 billion [3]. The main symptoms of MDD include severe sadness, anxiety, cognitive deterioration, and suicidal thoughts [4]. Although its etiology is uncertain, genetic predisposition, developmental deficits, hormonal imbalance, and a stressful lifestyle may increase the risk for MDD [5–10].

Prior to the discovery of antidepressant medication, surgical ablation was used to effectively treat MDD in the US and Europe [11]. Pharmacological antidepressants first appeared in the late 20th century and these first-generation drugs became the first line treatment for depression [12]. However, newer generations of antidepressants were barely more effective than first-generation tricyclic antidepressants [13] and this has led to the emergence of treatment resistance. Treatment-resistant depression (TRD) is the failure to respond to the three different classes of treatment: antidepressants, psychotherapy, or electroconvulsive therapy given at a sufficient dose and time [14,15]. Approximately 20% to 30% of patients are refractory to pharmacotherapy and nearly 60% respond inadequately [16,17], which can result in worse clinical responses, leading to additional social burdens [18]. As the pathogenesis of MDD involves multiple structures, a broad-acting safe therapy needs to be developed [19,20].

With much progress in surgical techniques and advances in cardiac pacemakers, electrical stimulation has matured to become an adjustable stimulatory regimen [21]. Deep brain stimulation (DBS) is a procedure whereby deep brain structures are stimulated via precisely implanted electrodes. It was first used to alleviate movement disorders in patients with Parkinson's disease [22]. With advances in our understanding of the limbic circuitry, the focus has shifted to the antidepressant-like effects of DBS [23]. Some recent clinical studies have shown that DBS holds great promise in treating patients with TRD, and mechanistic studies in animals are currently in progress.

The use of DBS as a treatment for TRD was first proposed in a study by Kruger et al. on the differences in regional cerebral blood flow (rCBF) between remitted patients and bipolar depression (BD) patients [24]. They observed that rCBF in Brodmann Area 25 (BA25) was higher in remitted and BD patients compared to control patients and this was also seen in healthy patients with self-rated high negative affect [25]. Furthermore, Kruger et al. noted that mood provocation did not change the rCBF to this region in BD patients compared to MDD patients, indicating that dysfunction in the region was specific to depression [24]. Mayberg et al., who are pioneers of DBS as a treatment for depression, subsequently targeted BA25 after detecting metabolic abnormalities within the region that were consistent with those found in patients with TRD [19]. This landmark paper led to further developments in the application of DBS of this region as a treatment for depression.

Indeed, several research groups have used DBS to treat depression by targeting different brain regions in the limbic system. Jimenez et al. applied DBS to the inferior thalamic peduncle, whereas Schlaepfer et al. applied DBS in the nucleus accumbens core [26,27] and successfully performed DBS on the medial forebrain bundle [28]. With rapid developments in DBS as a treatment for TRD, research is now focusing on the subcallosal cingulate (SCC). This review aims to examine and consolidate clinical and preclinical research on the use of DBS as a treatment for depression, targeting the subcallosal cingulate in humans and the ventromedial prefrontal cortex, the anatomical correlate in rodents.

2. Outline of the Review

The online PubMed database was searched for research articles in English using a Boolean operation with keywords including "deep brain stimulation" AND "depression" AND "subcallosal cingulate" OR "rodent" AND "medial prefrontal cortex". Relevant articles cited in the reference lists of the identified publications were also included. PubMed was utilized due to its extensive collection of indexed peer-reviewed journals. This review highlights the development of DBS as a treatment for TRD and discusses the findings and limitations of preclinical and clinical studies published in the recent decade. The neuroplasticity-dependent and -independent aspects of the molecular and cellular changes due to DBS are also discussed. Lastly, some potential approaches that may improve the precision, safety, and efficacy of DBS are proposed.

3. The Development of Deep Brain Stimulation as a Treatment for Depression

Deep brain stimulation involves the stereotactic implantation of thin electrodes in deep brain structures that are used to deliver electrical stimulation generated by a subcutaneous pulse generator [29,30]. Stimulation is generally applied at either a low/moderate frequency (5–90 Hz) or high frequency (100–400 Hz). Since the inception of DBS, a number of studies have demonstrated that this modality has the ability to treat pain, obsessive-compulsive disorder, and Parkinson's disease [16,21,31]. Its efficacy has been verified in Parkinson's disease patients, in which high frequency stimulation (HFS) of specific brain region(s) in the basal ganglia was able to stop tremors [21,32]. The use of DBS has been given FDA approval for the management of obsessive-compulsive disorder since 2007, but it is only provided under a humanitarian device exemption [33,34].

The following sections summarize the clinical studies on deep brain stimulation in the subcallosal cingulate for treating patients with treatment-resistant depression and preclinical studies of deep brain stimulation in the medial prefrontal cortex (mPFC) of rodents.

4. Clinical and Preclinical Studies of SCC DBS for the Treatment of Depression

Clinical studies of depression utilize rating scales of depression that assess changes in depressive symptoms in patients. Some scales are completed by the researcher such as the Hamilton Depression Rating Scale (HDRS) and the Montgomery-Åsberg Depression Rating Scale (MADRS). These rating scales should allow more consistent assessment between patients, but can lack consensus in their interpretation among researchers, which could lead to misdiagnosis [35]. Another weakness of rating scales conducted in this manner is that the accuracy of the results is dependent on the communication skills of the patient, which might be hampered by the disease itself. Other scales are completed by patients such as the Beck Anxiety Inventory (BAI), Beck Depression Inventory (BDI), and Quick Inventory of Depressive Symptomatology (QIDS). These rating scales should allow for a more accurate reporting of depressive symptoms, although the number and/or depth of questions may vary across different tests.

4.1. Progress in the Development of SCC-DBS

Different papers have referred to the SCC and similar regions under different names, e.g., the subcallosal cingulate gyrus (SCG), the subgenual cingulate, as well as Brodmann areas. Different historical names allow for different historical context. The subgenual cortex is used more interchangeably with the term Brodmann Area 25, named after Korbinian Brodmann. The subgenual cortex is located in the cingulate region as a narrow band in the caudal portion of the subcallosal area adjacent to the paraterminal gyrus. By comparison, the SCG is comprised of Brodmann areas 25, 24, and 32 [36]; SCG circuits; and limbic structures. The SCG is pivotal in mood, learning, reward, and memory [37] and has been implicated as an aberrant region in MDD. As the SCC can be effectively targeted by antidepressants, this makes the SCG a potential target of DBS against TRD [38,39]. Tables 1 and 2 list 39 clinical studies on the treatment efficacy of SCC-DBS for TRD.

Table 1. A list of clinical studies on deep brain stimulation of the human subcallosal cingulate.

Authors	Main Inclusion Criteria	No. of Patients	Stimulation Target & DBS Design	Stimulation Parameters	Clinical Evaluation	Major Outcomes	Adverse Effects
Sankar et al. 2020 [40]	TRD MDE; Current MDE ≥ 12 months; HRSD-17 score ≥ 20; Non-responsive (NR) ≥ 4 antidepressant therapies; HRSD-17 score ≥ 20.	27	Target SCG	Implantation Bilateral Stimulation Monopolar Frequency 130 Hz Amplitude 3–6 V Pulse Width 90 µs	Volumetric analysis, Whole brain grey and white matter analysis	Left and average SCG volume significantly higher in responders compared to non-responders. Right and average amygdala volume significantly higher in responders compared to non-responders. Left, right, and average thalamus volume significantly higher in responders compared to non-responders. Brain grey matter volume significantly lower in responders compared to non-responders. Ratio of grey to white matter volume significantly higher in responders compared to non-responders.	N.A.
Riva-Posse et al. (2019) [41]	TRD MDE; Current MDE ≥ 12 months; HRSD-17 score ≥ 20; Non-responsive (NR) ≥ 4 antidepressant therapies; HRSD-17 score ≥ 20; GAF < 50.	9	Target SCC Study Design Intraoperative Sessions: 6 min session of 3 min stimulation ON and 3 min stimulation OFF. Number of sessions: 12 trials (one at each of the eight available contacts. Four per hemisphere, plus four sham trials). Sham-controlled, double-blinded trials (one case w/single blind trial)	Implantation Bilateral Stimulation Monopolar Frequency 130 Hz Amplitude 6 mA Pulse Width 90 µs	ECG, EDA, MRI Volume of Tissue Activated, Structural Connectivity Analysis	Autonomic changes with SCC-DBS correspond to salient behavioral responses. Distant effects of SCC-DBS in the midcingulate cortex. Increase in heart rate was only seen with left SCC-DBS. No significant relationship with skin conductance. These findings aid in the optimal selection of contacts and parameters in SCC-DBS surgery.	N.A.
Eitan et al. (2018) [42]	Both sexes, 21–70 years; Non-psychotic MDD; First MDE onset before 45 years old with current MDE ≥ 12 months; NR ≥ 4 antidepressant therapies; MADRS ≥ 22; GAF < 50; MMSE > 24; No changes in current antidepressant treatments ≥ 4 wks prior to study.	9	Target BA25 Study Design Double-blind, randomized. Two groups: High- OR low-frequency DBS for 12 months from 1 month after electrode implantation.	Implantation Bilateral Stimulation Monopolar Frequency 20 Hz or 130 Hz Amplitude 4–8 mA Pulse Width 91 µs	MADRS, HRSD-17, QIDS-SR, Q-LES-Q, GAF, HAM-A, CGI, PGI, CANTAB battery.	Four out of nine patients responded ◊ at the end of DBS (≥40% reduction in MADRS from baseline). The effect of DBS at 6–12 months was higher than DBS at 1–6 months. High-frequency DBS showed higher efficacy than low-frequency DBS. Non-responders crossed over after first 6 months of DBS.	Severe One patient overdosed on medication (dothiepin and valium).

Table 1. *Cont.*

Authors	Main Inclusion Criteria	No. of Patients	Stimulation Target & DBS Design	Stimulation Parameters	Clinical Evaluation	Major Outcomes	Adverse Effects
Merkl et al. (2018) [43]	Diagnosed MDD and disease lasted for >2 years; HAMD-24 score ≥ 20; ATHF Score ≥ 3; TRD: NR ≥ 2 antidepressant therapies; Failed to respond to antidepressants and ECT; No changes in current antidepressant treatments ≥6 wks prior to study.	8	Target SCG; Study Design: Randomized; Two groups: sham-DBS (delayed onset) OR non-delayed onset group for the first 8 weeks in a blinded manner. Open-label DBS afterwards for up to 28 months.	Implantation: Bilateral; Stimulation: Monopolar; Frequency: 130 Hz; Amplitude: 5–7 V; Pulse Width: 90 µs	HAMD-24, BDI, MADRS.	Three out of eight patients responded ** after 6 months DBS; three out of seven with the same criteria after 12 months. Two out of six responded ** at the end of DBS, follow-up at 28 months. Two out of six patients reached remission □ at the end of DBS, follow-up at 28 months. This study showed a delayed response in patients; no significant antidepressant effects between sham and active stimulation compared to baseline.	Non-severe: Headache; Pain; Scalp tingling; Dizziness; Light hypomania; Inconvenient movement; Severe: NIL
Howell et al. (2018) [44]	Both sexes aged 18–70 years; current MDE ≥ 12 months; NR ≥ 4 antidepressant therapies; HRSD-17 score ≥ 20; GAF score ≤ 50.	6	Target SCC (Cingulum Bundle and Forceps Minor)	Implantation: Bilateral; Stimulation: Monopolar; Frequency: 130 Hz; Amplitude: 4 V; Pulse Width: 90 µs	HDRS-17, MRI Field-cable modeling (non-VTA-based analysis)	All of the subjects responded. Left and right cingulum bundles as well as forceps minor are the most likely therapeutic targets. Right cingulum bundle activation beyond a threshold may protract recovery. Uncinate fasciculus and frontal pole were activated to a lesser extent, may not be necessary for anti-depressive effect of SCC-DBS. Time to a stable response (TSR) was 8–189 days, 1-year HDRS-17 was 2–11. Field cable modeling was more accurate than volume of activated tissue at approximating axonal activation. Overstimulation of CB-DBS can be detrimental to the recovery process.	N.A.
Waters et al. (2018) [45]	Both sexes aged 18–70 years; current MDE ≥ 12 months; NR ≥ 4 antidepressant therapies; HRSD-17 score ≥ 20; GAF score ≤ 50.	4	Target SCC; Study Design: Single-blinded, Session: 3 min	Implantation: Bilateral; Stimulation: Monopolar; Frequency: 130 Hz; Amplitude: 3–5 V; Pulse Width: 90 µs	HDRS-17, EEG	Symptom severity scores decreased. three out of four patients in remission (HDRS-17 ≤ 7). Test-retest reliability across four repeated measures over 14 months met or exceeded standards for valid test construction in three out of four patients for cortical-evoked responses studied.	N.A.

Table 1. *Cont.*

Authors	Main Inclusion Criteria	No. of Patients	Stimulation Target & DBS Design	Stimulation Parameters	Clinical Evaluation	Major Outcomes	Adverse Effects
Smart et al. (2018) [46]	TRD patients enrolled from two separate clinical trials for Deep Brain Stimulation. Trial 1 Both sexes aged 18–70 years; Diagnosis of a Major Depressive Episode or Bipolar Type II—current episode depressed. Current episode duration of at least 1 year, Non-responsive (NR) ≥ 4 antidepressant therapies. Trial 2 Both sexes aged 25–70 years; Current depressive episode of at least 2 years duration OR a history of more than four lifetime depressive episodes, Non-responsive (NR) ≥ 4 antidepressant therapies.	14	Target SCC Study Design Double-blinded. Intraoperative behavioral testing: Frequency: 130 Hz Pulse width: 90 μs Current: 6 mA Eight patients continued SCC local field potential.	Implantation Bilateral Stimulation Monopolar Frequency 130 Hz Amplitude 6–8 mA for St. Jude Medical devices, 3.5–5 V for Medtronic devices Pulse Width 90 μs	HDRS-17, MRI, LFP.	11 of 14 patients met the criteria for DBS antidepressant response by 6 months. Of the three 6 month non-responders, one responded after the 6 month study endpoint but without a contact change (Patient 2), one responded after a contact switch in the left hemisphere (Patient 7), and one remained a non-responder (Patient 6). Mean baseline HDRS-17 of 23.8 and SD of 2.8; HDRS-17 of 9.6 and SD of 4.5 at month 6; 19.9 weeks for stable response with SD of 20 weeks. Precision on the left may be more important than precision on the right, which is supported by theta decreases.	N.A.
Choi et al. (2018) [47]	Both sexes aged 18–70 years; current MDE ≥ 12 months; NR ≥ 4 antidepressant therapies; HRSD-17 score ≥ 20; GAF score ≤ 50.	15	Target SCC Study Design Patients went through SCC-DBS, followed by MRI scans.	Implantation Bilateral Stimulation Monopolar Frequency 130 Hz Amplitude 6 mA Pulse Width 90 μs	HDRS-17, MRI, DWI, Volume of Tissue Activated	Significant differences in the pathway activation changes over time between remitters and non-remitters. Non-remitters had significantly larger net changes in their pathway activation connection in both the near and long term relative to the initial plan.	N.A.
Conen et al. (2018) [48]	TRD (unipolar); NR ≥ 4 antidepressant therapies; MADRS Score ≥ 22.	7	Targets SCC followed by Ventral Anterior Capsule, nucleus accumbens (separately, unless patient in remission, and later combined, for non-responding patients). Study Design DBS was applied sequentially for 3 months per region, for a total period ranging from 16–45 months.	N.A.	MADRS, HAM-D 17, GAF.	Remitters had higher regional cerebral blood flow in the baseline prefrontal cortex and subsequent tests when compared to non-remitters and non-responders. Chronic DBS increased prefrontal cortex regional cerebral blood flow. Remitted patients had higher prefrontal cerebral blood flow at baseline.	N.A.

Table 1. *Cont.*

Authors	Main Inclusion Criteria	No. of Patients	Stimulation Target & DBS Design	Stimulation Parameters	Clinical Evaluation	Major Outcomes	Adverse Effects
Holtzheimer et al. (2017) [15]	Both sexes aged 21–70 years; Unipolar, non-psychotic MDD; First MDE onset before 45 years old with current MDE ≥ 12 months; NR ≥ 4 antidepressant therapies, MADRS Score ≥ 22; GAF < 50; MMSE > 24; No changes in current antidepressant treatments ≥ 4 wks prior to study.	60 (DBS) 30 (Sham)	Target SCC Study Design DBS or sham stimulation 2 weeks after implantation for 6 months in randomized and double-blind manner. Two groups: DBS or sham then both groups received open-label stimulation for 6 months or 2 years.	Implantation Bilateral Stimulation Monopolar Frequency 130 Hz Amplitude 4–8 mA Pulse Width 91 μs	MADRS, GAF HRSD-17, 30-item Inventory of Depressive Symptomatology, QIDS-SR, WSAS, PGI, CGI, QOL, HAM-A.	Insignificant difference in response * between sham and DBS at the end of the 6-month double-blind phase. 38 patients responded * and 20 remitted □ after 6 month DBS. In 2 years of open-label active DBS, 48% achieved antidepressant response and 25% achieved remission—clinically meaningful long-term outcomes.	Severe Eight of 40 events reported related to device or surgery: six infections (in five patients), one skin erosion over the extension wires, and one postoperative seizure.
McInerney et al. (2017) [14]	Current MDE ≥ 12 months; HRSD-17 Score ≥ 20; NR ≥ 4 antidepressant therapies.	20	Target SCC Study Design DBS for 12 months open-label	Implantation Bilateral Stimulation Monopolar Frequency 130 Hz Amplitude 3.5–5 V Pulse Width 90 μs	Wisconsin Card Sorting Task (WCST), Hopkins Verbal Learning Test, Controlled Oral Word Association Test (COWA), Finger Tap Test, Stroop Test, HRSD-17.	Significant reduction in HRSD-17 from baseline to experimental follow-up. Baseline scores differed significantly between responders and non-responders. 11 patients responded ** and nine were non-responders. WCST Test results indicated that the total errors were predictive of responsiveness to DBS. No significant deterioration in cognition and psychomotor speed. Improvements in verbal memory and verbal fluency.	N.A.
Riva-Posse et al. (2018) [49]	Both sexes aged 18–70 years; current MDE ≥ 12 months; NR ≥ 4 antidepressant therapies; HRSD-17 score ≥ 20; GAF score ≤ 50.	11	Target SCC Study Design DBS from 4 weeks after surgery and lasted for 6 months, open-label. Stimulation contacts were changed in non-responders and they were stimulated for 6 more months.	Implantation Bilateral Stimulation Monopolar Frequency 130 Hz Amplitude 6–8 mA Pulse Width 91 μs	HRSD-17	Eight out of 11 responded ** and six remitted □□ after 6 month DBS. Nine responded ** and six remitted □□ after 12 month DBS. Two did not respond throughout the study. Tractography-based surgery reduced variability in the effects of stimulation on patient-specific brain circuitry.	N.A.
Tsolaki et al. (2017) [50]	TRD	2	Target SCC	Implantation Bilateral Stimulation Monopolar Frequency 130 Hz Amplitude 8 mA Pulse Width 91 μs	MRI, DTI, CT, FSL Probabilistic tractography, Volume of Tissue Activated, MADRS.	One patient was a responder (81% change in MADRS score). Responder's contacts were closer to the Tractography-guided optimized target (TOT), unlike the non-responder.	N.A.

Table 1. *Cont.*

Authors	Main Inclusion Criteria	No. of Patients	Stimulation Target & DBS Design	Stimulation Parameters	Clinical Evaluation	Major Outcomes	Adverse Effects
Accolla et al. (2016) [51]	MDD; NR to treatments; Currently in a depressive episode as in DSM-IV Axis I disorders; HAMD-24 score of ≥ 20.	5	Target BA25. Study Design Double-blind. Each homologous electrode pair was activated separately on 5 consecutive days, then antidepressant effects was assessed 24 h later. Open-label DBS for up to 24 months. Pre- and post-DBS MRI images were taken.	Implantation N.A. Stimulation Monopolar Frequency 130 Hz Amplitude 5 V Pulse Width 90 µs	HAMD-24, BDI.	Four out of five patients did not show sustained response ** to DBS (also ≥50% reduction in DBI). One patient responded ** to DBS of the bilateral posterior gyrus rectus instead of the intended target (BA25).	N.A.
Richieri et al. (2016) [52]	Diagnosed MDD; Severe cognitive defects and relapsed after ECT.	1	Target BA25 Study Design DBS at Day 5 after electrode implantation.	Implantation Bilateral Stimulation Bipolar Frequency 130 Hz Amplitude 4.2 V Pulse Width 90 µs	QIDS SR-16	Remitted (QIDS SR-16 3/48) at 1 month after DBS and maintained at the end of DBS.	Seizure
Hilimire et al. (2015) [53]	Both sexes aged 18–70 years; Current MDE ≥ 12 months, Non-responsive (NR) ≥ 4 antidepressant therapies, HRSD-17 score ≥ 20, GAF score ≤ 50.	7	Target SCC Study Design DBS for 6 months, open-label. Behavioral testing and electrophysiological recording (i) before electrode implantation, (ii) after 1 month DBS and (iii) after 6 month DBS.	Implantation Bilateral Stimulation Monopolar Frequency 130 Hz Amplitude 4–8 mA Pulse Width 91 µs	HDRS-17, Emotional self-referential task, EEG recording.	Reduced proportion of negative self-descriptive words compared to baseline after 1 month and 6 month DBS. Significant reduction in P1 amplitude compared to baseline (for negative word self-description) after 1 month and 6 month DBS, and P3 amplitudes at 6 month DBS only. Reduced depression severity.	N.A.
Martin-Blanco et al. (2015) [54]	Both sexes aged 18–70 years; current MDE ≥ 12 months; NR ≥ 4 antidepressant therapies; HRSD-17 score ≥ 20; GAF score ≤ 50.	7	Target SCG Study Design Chronic DBS for 9 months on average for clinical stabilization. A PET scan was acquired (i) during active stimulation and (ii) after 48 h of inactive stimulation.	Implantation Bilateral Stimulation Monopolar Frequency 135 Hz Amplitude 3.5–5 V Pulse Width 120–210 µs	HAMD-17, PET	Decreased metabolism in BA24, BA6, caudate putamen after 48 h DBS. This study suggests metabolic changes spread after longer periods of no stimulation. No clinical changes were detected according to HAMD-17.	N.A.

Table 1. *Cont.*

Authors	Main Inclusion Criteria	No. of Patients	Stimulation Target & DBS Design	Stimulation Parameters	Clinical Evaluation	Major Outcomes	Adverse Effects
Puigdemont et al. (2015) [55]	Severe TRD; Both sexes aged 18–70 years; current MDE ≥ 12 months; NR ≥ 4 antidepressant therapies; HRSD-17 score ≥ 20; GAF score ≤ 50.	5	Target SCG. Study Design. Randomized, Double-blind. After stable clinical remission to DBS, patients were allocated to two groups, one with (i) 3 month DBS-ON, then (ii) 3 month sham stimulation (ON-OFF arm) or OFF-ON arm and the other, vice-versa.	Implantation. Bilateral Stimulation. Monopolar. Frequency 130–135 Hz. Amplitude 3.5–5 V. Pulse Width 120–240 µs	Volume of Tissue Activated, HRSD-17	Active stimulation: four of five patients were remitted patients. Sham stimulation: Only two patients remained in remission, another two relapsed, and one showed a progressive worsening without reaching relapse criteria.	N.A.
Serra-Blasco et al. (2015) [56]	Treatment-Resistant Depression (TRD) Group. Resistant to pharmacological treatment; min. stage IV of Thase-Rush scale; HDRS score ≥ 18. First Episode MDD (FE MDD) Group. HDRS score ≥ 14; Newly diagnosed MDD.	16	Target SCG. Study Design. DBS began at 48 h postoperative and ended when each patient had stabilized response for at least three consecutive visits, tests conducted before surgery, and 12 months after DBS treatment.	Implantation. Bilateral Stimulation. Monopolar. Frequency 135 Hz. Amplitude 3.5–5 V. Pulse Width 120–210 µs	Rey Auditory Verbal Learning Test, Trail Making Tests-A and -B, Wechsler Adult Intelligence Scale III, Tower of London Test, HDRS-17.	FE MDD and TRD saw significant improvements over time in memory. No significant difference was observed in both groups on executive functioning, language, and processing speed. DBS was well tolerated and had no adverse effect on neuropsychological and cognitive function.	N.A.
Choi et al. (2015) [57]	Both sexes aged 18–70 years; current MDE ≥ 12 months; NR ≥ 4 antidepressant therapies; HDRS-17 score ≥ 20; GAF score ≤ 50.	9	Target SCC. Intraoperative Sessions: 6 min session of 3 min stimulation ON, and 3 min stimulation OFF. Number of sessions: 12 trials (one at each of the eight available contacts; four per hemisphere, plus four sham trials). Study Design. Sham-controlled, Double-blind trials (one case w/single blind trial).	Acute Implantation. Bilateral Stimulation. Monopolar. Frequency 130 Hz. Amplitude 6 mA. Pulse Width 90 µs	MRI with FSL analysis, Volume of Tissue Activated.	Behavioral switch was apparent to patients within the first minute of the initiation of stimulation and effects were sustained while stimulation remained on. Three common white matter bundles were affected by stimulation: (i) the uncinate fasciculus, (ii) the forceps minor, and (iii) the left cingulum bundle. Seven of nine patients with left hemispheric contact had a response to treatment at 6 months.	
Sun et al. (2015) [58]	NR ≥ 4 antidepressant therapies, Mean HRSD-17 score of 25 (3).	20	Target SCC. Session: 100 min, w/15 min break. EEG recording sessions/day. Session 1: DBS On. Session 2: DBS Random (On/Off). Session 3: DBS (Off)	Implantation. Bilateral Stimulation. Monopolar. Frequency 130 Hz. Amplitude 2–7.25 mA OR 2–6 V. Pulse Width 90 µs	EEG, HDRS-17.	Suppression of gamma oscillations by DBS during working memory performance and the treatment efficacy of DBS for TRD may be associated with the improved GABAergic neurotransmission, previously shown to be deficient in MDD. The present study also suggests that modifying treatment parameters to achieve suppression of gamma oscillations and increased theta-gamma coupling may lead to optimized DBS efficacy for TRD.	N.A.

Table 1. *Cont.*

Authors	No. of Patients	Main Inclusion Criteria	Stimulation Target & DBS Design	Stimulation Parameters	Clinical Evaluation	Major Outcomes	Adverse Effects
Perez-Caballero et al. (2014) [59]	8	18–70 years old with MDE; Resistant to pharmacological treatment and at most, a partial response to ECT; HAMD-17 Score ≥ 18.	Target SCG Study Design All patients received chronic DBS within 48 h after implantation. Four patients took NSAIDs for up to 30 days postoperative, four patients did not.	Implantation Quadrupolar Stimulation 135 Hz Amplitude 3.5–5 V Pulse Width 120–210 μs	HDRS-17	At week 1 after surgery, all patients without NSAID prescription responded ** and two remitted □□□, three patients with NSAID responded **, and two remitted □□□. At week 4 after surgery, three patients without NSAID remitted □□□, no patients with NSAID responded **	N.A.
Merkl et al. (2013) [60]	6	MDD; NR to treatments; Currently in a depressive episode as in DSM-IV Axis I disorder; HAMD-24 score of ≥ 20; HDRS-24 score ≥ 24.	Target SCG Study Design DBS on 11–19 days after electrode implantation, 24 h acute stimulation followed by sham stimulation for each of the three electrode pairs. Up to 6 months of chronic stimulation.	Implantation Bilateral Stimulation Monopolar Frequency 130 Hz Amplitude 2.5–10 V Pulse Width 90 μs	HAMD-24, MADRS BDI, TMT-A, TMT-B, CVLI, TAP, Boston Naming Test, Stroop Test, Word Fluency Test.	Non-significant reduction in HAMD-24, BDI, and MADRS scores for acute DBS and sham stimulation. 0/4 contact pair locations showed significant BDI and MADRS improvements. Contact pair 3/7 for Patient 4 saw a 77% reduction in HAMD-24 score and 62% reduction of MADRS score. Reduced HDRS-24, BDI, and MADRS scores at the end of chronic stimulation. Two out of six remissions □ at the end of chronic stimulation.	Mild Headache; Pain; Scalp tingling; Dizziness; Sore throat; Hardware-related; Severe NIL
Ramasubbu et al. (2013) [61]	4	Aged between 20–60 years; Diagnosed MDD; HAMD-17 score ≥ 20; NR ≥ 4 antidepressant therapies. (Enrolled patients were among the most treatment resistant).	Target SCC Study Design Double-blind DBS optimization. Open-label continuous DBS for 6 months after optimization period. Varied parameters for each patient during optimization.	Implantation Bilateral Stimulation Monopolar Frequency 0/5/20/50/130/185 Hz Amplitude 0–10.5 V Pulse Width 0/90/150/ 270/450 μs	HAMD-17, MADRS, HAM-A, CGI.	Postoperative optimization: All four patients showed maximal response at longer pulse widths; three patients experienced a 50% reduction in HAMD-17 score. Longer pulse widths were correlated to short-term improvement. Longer pulse width also induced insomnia, confusion, and drowsiness; improved by turning off stimulation. Chronic stimulation: two patients responded ** at the end of open-label DBS, with longer pulse width. Electrode targets suggested to be individualized, as opposed to standard as in movement disorders, owing to the complexity of cortical gyral anatomy	Mild Anxiety; Drowsiness; Confusion; Insomnia.

62   Deep Brain Stimulation for Neurological Disorders

Table 1. *Cont.*

Authors	Main Inclusion Criteria	No. of Patients	Stimulation Target & DBS Design	Stimulation Parameters	Clinical Evaluation	Major Outcomes	Adverse Effects
Torres et al. (2013) [62]	Type I bipolar depression; Poor response to ECT and pharmacotherapy.	1	Target SCC Study Design DBS from 15 days after implantation and follow-up for 9 months.	Implantation N.A. Stimulation Monopolar Frequency 130 Hz Amplitude 6 mA Pulse Width 91 µs	HDRS-17, BDI, MADRS, GAF, Young Mania Scale.	Scores improved across tests. Psychotic symptoms disappeared. Manic episodes reduced.	N.A.
Broadway et al. (2012) [63]	Both sexes aged 18–70 years; current MDE ≥ 12 months; NR ≥ 4 antidepressant therapies; HRSD-17 score ≥ 20; GAF score ≤ 50.	12	Target SCC Study Design DBS for up to 24 weeks.	Implantation N.A. Stimulation Monopolar Frequency 130 Hz Amplitude 6–8 mA Pulse Width 90 µs	HRSD-17, Frontal and posterior Theta cordance.	Reduced HDRS-17 scores between baseline and the end of DBS among all patients. Six patients had significantly reduced HRSD-17 scores ** at the end of DBS. Increased frontal theta cordance between baseline and week 4 in responders correlated with their decreased depressive state at later time points.	N.A.
Hamani et al. (2012) [64]	TRD; NR to respond to pharmacotherapy, psychotherapy, transcranial magnetic stimulation, ECT, vagus nerve stimulation. Relapsed after receiving 6 month SCC-DBS.	1	Target SCC Study Design Administered tranylcypromine before surgery. DBS for 6 months.	Implantation Bilateral Stimulation Monopolar Frequency 130 Hz Amplitude 2.5 V Pulse Width 90 µs	HAMD-17	Before relapse: SCC-DBS reduced HAMD-17 score from 22 to 9 after 4 month DBS. After relapse: MAOI supplementation restored the therapeutic effect of DBS; HAMD-17 score lowered from 22 to 16 (after 2 weeks), to 8 (after 2 months) and to 9 (after 4 months).	N.A.
Holtzheimer et al. (2012) [65]	Both sexes aged 18–70 years; current MDE ≥ 12 months; NR ≥ 4 antidepressant therapies; HRSD-17 score ≥ 20; GAF score ≤ 50.	17	Target SCC Study Design Intraoperative testing of electrode location for 12 or 17 patients. Stimulation: (i) 4 weeks of sham stimulation, followed by (ii) 24 weeks of open label DBS for 24 weeks, followed by (iii) single-blind discontinuation for 1 week and open label stimulation for up to 2 years.	Implantation Bilateral Stimulation Monopolar Frequency 130 Hz Amplitude 4–8 mA Pulse Width 91 µs	HRSD-17, BDI-II, GAF.	Reduced depression and increased function. 11 patients responded ** and seven further remitted □□ after 2 year DBS. Efficacy was similar for patients with MDD and those with BP. A modest sham stimulation effect was found, likely due to a decrease in depression after the surgical intervention, but prior to entering the sham phase.	Anxiety; Worsened depression; Nausea; Headache; Infection; Suicide attempts.

Table 1. *Cont.*

Authors	Main Inclusion Criteria	No. of Patients	Stimulation Target & DBS Design	Stimulation Parameters	Clinical Evaluation	Major Outcomes	Adverse Effects
Lozano et al. (2012) [66]	Both sexes aged 30–60 years; First MDE before 35 years; HRSD-17 score ≥ 20; GAF < 50.	21	Target SCG; Study Design DBS for 12 months, open label.	Implantation Bilateral; Stimulation N.A.; Frequency 110–140 Hz; Amplitude 3.5–7 mA; Pulse Width 65–182 μs	HRSD-17, CGI-S.	Improved global functioning and less severe depression. 13 patients responded **, based on HRSD-17 scores.	Gastrointestinal problems; Skin problem; Suicide; Spasms; Weight gain; Insomnia.
Puigdemont et al. (2012) [67]	18–70 years old with MDE; Resistant to pharmacological treatment and at most, a partial response to ECT; HAMD-17 Score ≥ 18.	8	Target SCG; Study Design Intraoperative feedback was provided during surgery for electrode placement. DBS began at 48 h postoperative and ended when each patient had stabilized their response for at least three consecutive visits.	Implantation Bilateral; Stimulation Monopolar; Frequency 135 Hz; Amplitude 3.5–5 V; Pulse Width 90 μs	HAMD-17, MADRS, CGI.	Seven patients responded ** and three remitted □□ after 6 month DBS. Five patients responded ** and four remitted □□ after 12 month DBS. Three out of four remitted patients after 12 month DBS had remitted after 3 month DBS.	Suicide ideation; Neck pain; Recurrence; Depression; Cephalalgia.
Kennedy et al. (2011) [18]	Current MDE ≥ 12 months; HRSD-17 score ≥ 20; NR ≥ 4 antidepressant therapies.	20	Target SCG; DBS patients were monitored for 3–6 years.	Implantation Bilateral; Stimulation Monopolar; Frequency 124.7 Hz (average); Amplitude 4.3 V (average); Pulse Width 70.6 μs	HAMD-17 36-item Short-Form Healthy Survey Questionnaire.	64.3% patients responded ** at the last follow-up visit. 35% patients remitted □□ at the last follow-up visit. Scores at the last visit tended towards maintenance of therapeutic scores at 3 years.	Depression; Suicidal thoughts; Suicide (All determined to be unrelated to DBS).
Guinjoan et al. (2010) [68]	Chronic TRD; Family history of affective disorders; Poor response to antidepressants, ECT, and psychotherapy.	1	Target BA25; Study Design Positioning was aided by intraoperative feedback. Bilateral DBS was conducted for 12 months. Followed by unilateral-left, then right DBS, for 6 months.	Implantation Bilateral; Stimulation Monopolar; Frequency 130 Hz; Amplitude 3.5–5 V; Pulse Width 90 μs	HAMD-17, BDI.	Patient's condition plateaued after 6 month bilateral DBS. Left unilateral DBS led to rapid worsening in mood. Right unilateral DBS reversed the symptoms and the patient made significant improvements over bilateral stimulation. Patient remitted at 18 months.	Orthostatic hypotension.

Table 1. *Cont.*

Authors	Main Inclusion Criteria	No. of Patients	Stimulation Target & DBS Design	Stimulation Parameters	Clinical Evaluation	Major Outcomes	Adverse Effects
Holtzheimer and Mayberg (2010) [69]	Showed signs and symptoms of MDD; Had suicidal ideation in current MDE; Did not improve in symptoms with pharmacotherapy, psychotherapy, and ECT HAM-D score was 25	1	Target SCC Study Design Positioning of electrodes was aided by intraoperative feedback 24 weeks of open-label DBS and chronic stimulation beyond the assessment	Implantation Bilateral Stimulation Monopolar Frequency 130 Hz Amplitude 6 mA Pulse Width 91 µs	HAMD-17	HAMD-17 score lowered to 9 at the end of DBS follow-up. Sustained antidepressant response up to 2 years after surgery	N.A.
Hamani et al. (2009) [70]	Diagnosed MDD; current MDE ≥ 12 months; HAMD-17 score >20; GAF ≤ 50; NR ≥ 4 antidepressant therapies.	20	Target SCG Study Design DBS began at 2 weeks after surgery and lasted for 12 months	Implantation Bilateral Stimulation Monopolar Frequency 130 Hz Amplitude 3-5 V Pulse Width 90 µs	HAMD-17	11 responded ** at the end of 6 month DBS follow-up. Electrodes in responders were positioned ventrally relative to the landmarks of the medial prefrontal lobe.	N.A.
Puigdemont et al. (2009) [71]	Suffered from MDD, with several MDE accompanied by psychotic symptoms; Responded poorly to pharmacotherapy and ECT; Relapse following SCG-DBS with different features; Psychotic as opposed to depressive from previous episodes.	1	Target SCG Study Design DBS for 4 months, then switched off because of relapse and administered ECT for 3 weeks Resumed DBS until 12 months from the beginning of DBS.	Implantation Bilateral Stimulation Monopolar Frequency 135 Hz Amplitude 3.6 V Pulse Width 90 µs	HAMD-17	Sustained response without the need of ECT before relapse. Maintained remission in DBS after ECT until the end of follow-up.	N.A.

Table 1. *Cont.*

Authors	Main Inclusion Criteria	No. of Patients	Stimulation Target & DBS Design	Stimulation Parameters	Clinical Evaluation	Major Outcomes	Adverse Effects
Lozano et al. (2008) [72]	Current MDE ≥ 12 months; HRSD-17 score ≥ 20; NR ≥ 4 antidepressant therapies.	20	Target SCG Study Design Blinded-DBS in between and after surgery, monitored for up to 1 year.	Implantation Bilateral Stimulation Monopolar Frequency 130 Hz Amplitude 3.5–5 V Pulse Width 90 µs	HRSD-17, Beck Anxiety Inventory, BDI, CGI-S, PET scans, Neuropsychological tests.	Mean HRSD-17 score lower than baseline at all time points. 12 patients responded ** to DBS, 7 remitted □□ after 6 month DBS. 11 patients responded ** to DBS, 7 were nearly remitted or remitted □□ after 12 month DBS. Eight responses maintained from 6 month to 12 month DBS. PET Scans: decreases in orbital, medial prefrontal cortex, and insula. Increases in lateral prefrontal cortex, parietal, anterior, and posterior cingulate by 6 months; increases in metabolic activity in regions adjacent to SCG.	Seven patients without adverse effects. Wound Infection; Headache; Pain; Seizure; Worsened mood; Irritability.
McNeely et al. (2008) [73]	Current MDE ≥ 12 months, HRSD-17 score ≥ 20, Non-responsive (NR) ≥ 4 antidepressant therapies,	6	Target BA25 Continuous DBS for 12 months.	Implantation Bilateral Stimulation Monopolar Frequency 130 Hz Amplitude 3–4.5 V Pulse Width 60 µs	HRSD-17 Object alternation Test Iowa gambling task Visual delayed recall memory Verbal delayed memory Verbal list learning Stroop color-word	6 months: four responded at the end of DBS ** General Neuropsychological Performance: Manual Motor Skills: Improved for dominant and non-dominant hand by 12 months. Verbal learning: Restored impairments in two patients at the end of 12 months. No significant correlations between change in mood and neuropsychological function at 6 and 12 months.	N.A.
Neimat et al. (2008) [74]	Family history of severe MDD. Failed to respond to antidepressants, adjuncts, and ECT. Relapsed after ablative cingulotomy	1	Target BA25 Study Design Started DBS on the day after electrode implantation and lasted for 30 months	Implantation Bilateral Stimulation Monopolar Frequency 130 Hz Amplitude 4.5 V Pulse Width 60 µs	HAMD-17	HAMD-17 score decreased from 19 before surgery to 8 at 6 months after DBS. Sustained remission until the end of DBS study (scored 7)	N.A.

Table 1. *Cont.*

Authors	Main Inclusion Criteria	No. of Patients	Stimulation Target & DBS Design	Stimulation Parameters	Clinical Evaluation	Major Outcomes	Adverse Effects
Mayberg et al. (2005) [19]	Current MDE ≥ 12 months, HRSD-17 score ≥ 20, Non-responsive (NR) ≥ 4 antidepressant therapies.	6	Target BA25 Study Design 1–5 min on-off stimulation in acute DBS for 5 days postoperative. Chronic DBS for 6 months after pulse generator was implanted and optimized for 4 wks	Implantation Bilateral Stimulation Monopolar Acute: Frequency 10–130 Hz Amplitude 0.0–9.0V Pulse Width 30–250 μs Chronic: Frequency 130 Hz Amplitude 4 V Pulse Width 60 μs	HDRS-17, MADRS, CGI, Positive and Negative Affective Scale.	Acute effects: Sudden feeling of calmness Chronic effects: five patients responded ** after 2 month DBS. Response maintained in four patients at the end of 6 month DBS. Three patients achieved remission □□ or near remission at the end of 6 month DBS.	Mild Lightheadedness; Psychomotor slowing; Skin infection; Skin erosion.

* ≥40% reduction in MADRS and average GAF in months 4–6 not worse than baseline; ** ≥50% reduction in HRSD-17 (HAMD-17) score from baseline; *** ≥40% reduction in HRSD-17 score from baseline; ◊ ≥40% reduction in MADRS compared to mean baseline; □ HAMD-24 scores or MADRS scores ≤ 10 after DBS; □□ HRSD score < 8. □□□ HRSD score ≤ 8; Abbreviations: ATHF = Anti-depressant Treatment History Form, BA25 = Brodmann Area 25, BDI/-II = Beck Depression Inventory/-II, CGI, PGI, CANTAB = Clinician and Patient Global Impression of Severity and Improvement (CGI; PGI) and cognitive function (CANTAB); CVLT = California verbal learning test, DBS = deep brain stimulation, DWI = Diffusion-weighted imaging, ECG = electrocardiogram, ECT = electroconvulsive therapy, EDA = electrodermal activity, EEG = electroencephalography, GAF = Global assessment function, HAM-A = Hamilton Anxiety Rating Scale, HRSD-17/HDRS-17 = Hamilton Rating Scale for Depression/ Hamilton Depression Rating Scale, (f)MRI = (functional) magnetic resonance imaging; MADRS/MARDS = Montgomery-Åsberg Depression Rating Scale, MAOI = monoamine oxidase inhibitors, MDD = major depressive disorder, MDE = major depressive episodes, MMSE = Mini-Mental State Examination, NSAID = non-steroidal anti-inflammatory drug, NR = non-responsive, PET = positron emission tomography, QIDS/-SR = Quick Inventory of Depressive Symptomatology/-self report, Q-LES-Q = Quality of Life and Satisfaction Questionnaire, SCC = subcallosal cingulate, SCG = subcallosal cingulate gyrus, SCR = skin conductance response, QOL = Quality of Life Enjoyment and Satisfaction Questionnaire, TRD = treatment-resistant depression, WSAS = Work and Social Adjustment Scale.

Table 2. Summary of response and remission rates from clinical studies.

Authors	≤ 6 months		6–12 months		12–24 months		≥ 24 months	
	Response (%)	Remission (%)	Response (%)	Remission (%)	Response (%)	Remission (%)	Response (%)	Remission (%)
Sankar et al. 2020 [40]	NA	NA	NA	NA	NA	NA	NA	NA
Riva Posse et al. (2019) [41]	NA	NA	NA	NA	NA	NA	NA	NA
Eitan et al. (2018) [42]	NA	NA	NA	NA	44.4	NA	NA	NA
Merkl et al. (2018) [43]	37.5	12.5	43	14.2	33	33	33	NA
Howell et al. (2018) [44]	-	-	33.3	66.7	-	-	-	-
Waters et al. (2018) [45]	NA	NA	NA	NA	NA	NA	NA	NA
Smart et al. (2018) [46]	-	-	78.5	-	-	-	-	-
Choi et al. (2018) [47]	NA	NA	NA	NA	NA	NA	NA	NA
Conen et al. (2018) [48]	-	-	28.6	42.9	-	-	-	-
Holtzheimer et al. (2017) [15]	22 20 (sham)	10 7 (sham)	28 30 (sham)	12 7 (sham)	54 52 (sham)	17 20 (sham)	48 44 (sham)	25 12 (sham)
McInerney et al. (2017) [14]	-	-	55	-	-	-	-	-
Riva-Posse et al. (2018) [49]	72.7	54.5	81.8	54.5	-	-	-	-
Tsolaki et al. 2017 [50]	50	-	-	-	-	-	-	-
Accolla et al. (2016) [51]	-	-	-	-	79	20	-	-
Richieri et al. (2016) [52]	100 (Case Study)	-	-	-	-	-	-	-
Hilimire et al. (2015) [53]	NA	NA	NA	NA	NA	NA	NA	NA
Martin-Blanco et al. (2015) [54]	NA	NA	NA	NA	NA	NA	NA	NA
Puigdemont et al. (2015) [55]	-	80	-	-	-	-	-	-
Serra-Blasco et al. (2015) [56]	-	-	-	-	75 (F.E.) 87 (TRD)	-	-	-
Choi et al. 2015 [57]	NA	NA	NA	NA	NA	NA	NA	NA
Sun et al. 2015 [58]	NA	NA	NA	NA	NA	NA	NA	NA
Perez-Caballero et al. (2014) [59]	50	-	-	-	-	-	-	-
Merkl et al. (2013) [60]	-	-	-	30	-	-	-	-
Ramasubbu et al. (2013) [61]	50	-	-	-	-	-	-	-
Torres et al. (2013) [62]	100 (2 Case Studies)	-	100 (2 Case Studies)	-	100 (2 Case Studies)	-	100 (2 Case Studies)	-
Broadway et al. (2012) [63]	50	-	-	-	-	-	-	-
Hamani et al. (2012) [64]	-	100 (Case Study)	100 (Case Study)	-	-	-	-	-
Holtzheimer et al. (2012) [65]	18	41	36	36	58	92	-	-
Lozano et al. (2012) [66]	57	-	48	-	62	-	-	-
Puigdemont et al. (2012) [67]	37.5	37.5	87.5	37.5	62.5	50	-	-
Kennedy et al. (2011) [18]	-	-	62.5	-	46.2	-	75	-
Guinjoan et al. (2010) [68]	100 (Case Study)	-	100 (Case Study)	-	100 (Case Study)	-	-	100 (Case Study)
Holtzheimer and Mayberg (2010) [69]	100 (Case Study)	-	100 (Case Study)	-	100 (Case Study)	-	100 (Case Study)	-
Hamani et al. (2009) [70]	-	-	55	-	-	-	-	-
Puigdemont et al. (2009) [71]	100 (Case Study)	-	100 (Case Study)	-	-	-	-	-
Lozano et al. (2008) [72]	35	10	60	35	-	-	-	-
McNeely et al. (2008) [73]	66	NA	-	-	-	-	-	-
Neimat et al. (2008) [74]	100 (Case Study)	NA	-	-	-	-	100 (Case Study)	-
Mayberg et al. (2005) [19]	66	50	-	-	-	-	-	-
Average	63.8%	43.9%	66.5%	36.5%	69.3%	42.4%	76%	62.5%
Range	18–100	10–100	28.6–100	12–66.7	33–100	17–92	33–100	12–100

The first evidence-based clinical study on SCC-DBS was published by Mayberg et al. in 2005 [19]. Among six patients with an average of 5.6 years of major depressive episode (MDE), four responded to the treatment, but three remitted or nearly remitted during the stimulation, even without changing medications. The authors found that the metabolic activity in the SCC normalized from a hyperactive state and was accompanied by reduced local blood flow as detected by Positron Emission Tomography (PET) [19]. In a study from 2003 to 2006 by Lozano et al. on chronic DBS in 20 patients with an average of 6.9 years of current MDE, 11 patients responded, but seven remitted [72], which was similar to the response and remission rates of Mayberg et al. In a 3.5-year follow-up study, the response rate was consistent across time points, but the remission rate increased from 18.8% to 42.9% at the last visit [18]. Both studies reported changes in structures distal to SCC after DBS, which explains the persistent response throughout the DBS treatments [18,72].

In a case report by Neimat et al., a 55-year-old female TRD patient who relapsed after a subgenual cingulotomy, achieved sustained remission for up to 30 months with SCC-DBS treatment [74]. In a case reported by Guinjoan et al. in 2010, a 60-year-old male TRD patient responded to unilateral SCC-DBS in the right hemisphere, but unilateral stimulation in the left hemisphere worsened his mood. This is in line with the asymmetrical response to antidepressants in the SCC region. However, the authors noted a further study was needed with more patients to validate the effects of unilateral stimulation on mood enhancement [68].

Similarly, in a preliminary study in 2012 by Puigdemont et al. on eight patients with an average of 6.3 years of current MDE, they found that five patients responded at the end of the 12-month DBS, but three out of four final remitters remitted after 3 months of DBS [67]. Their cognitive functions were not exacerbated and their memory functions were actually improved in cognitive assessments in 2015 [56]. Concurrently, a clinical study conducted in three different medical centers also reported similar efficacies of SCC-DBS, suggesting that DBS has reliable stimulation effects. Among 21 patients with an average of 5 years of current MDE, 13 responded to the treatment and the rest performed better than at baseline by the end of the study, although one patient committing suicide by medication overdose [66].

4.2. Remission Rates

Some previous studies reported higher initial response and/or remission rates compared to more recent studies [19,67,72]. In the study by Perez-Caballero et al., they suggested that electrode insertion-induced inflammation could affect response and remission rates. Four of the eight recruited patients took non-steroidal anti-inflammatory drugs (NSAIDs), which resulted in a diminished antidepressant response toward DBS, whereas the other four not taking NSAIDs gradually responded and remitted. The authors also analyzed the role of inflammation in the early DBS response in rats [59], which is discussed in a later section of this review. A later study in 2015 by Puigdemont et al. reported that remission was maintained in four out of five remitted patients in the 3-month active stimulation group, whereas only two patients remitted in the sham stimulation group. They concluded that continuous active stimulation was important in maintaining the therapeutic effect [55]. This was supported by an earlier case of a 27-year-old patient on DBS for 2 years whose symptoms worsened due to battery depletion, but improved again upon battery replacement [69].

Table 2 reflects the different response and remission rates, at 6-month intervals, across the duration of the studies in Table 1. This reporting allows for a cursory longitudinal tracking in understanding how response and remission may change with time. Among the reviewed studies on DBS, the response rate ranged from 18% to 87.5% and remission rate ranged from 10% to 92% (excluding all case studies) across the different time points (see Table 2), which were comparable to earlier clinical studies [19,72]. However, large-scale controlled trials are needed to further validate the efficacy of DBS in patients with TRD. Some predictive markers discovered in these studies could facilitate the selection of more responsive patients and increase the safety of DBS. A noteworthy study by Holtzheimer and Mayberg demonstrated some changes in the response and remission rates with DBS [69]. The authors noted that several months after a response and/or remission in their depressive symptoms, worsening of symptoms was temporarily observed at 16 weeks. They attributed the temporary worsening of symptoms to the difficulty of some patients reintegrating into society. In an earlier study by Lozano et al. in 2008, they also observed a similar occurrence at 4 months. These findings highlight the complexity of treating neuropsychiatric diseases, as the recovery periods are not always consistent and can be affected by different factors.

4.3. Significant Challenges in the Development of SCC-DBS

A larger study that aimed to recruit 201 patients was conducted by Holtzheimer et al. in 2017 to further validate the therapeutic effects of DBS [15]. A futility analysis conducted after 90 patients had been recruited showed no significant differences between the DBS and sham groups, leading to the early termination of the study. During a 6-month double-blind trial, no significant differences were found in the response of the DBS group compared to the sham group. However, among 77 patients that received subsequent open-label DBS for up to 2 years, 38 responded and 20 remitted. Holtzheimer et al. offered several explanations for the observed result. First, the patients selected for the study had an average current episode duration of around 12 years, whereas most studies recruited patients with an average current depressive episode of about 3–5 years. Holtzheimer also posited the possibility of suboptimal contact during the first 12 months, further affecting the results. This landmark paper was initially thought to be the death knell for DBS as a treatment for TRD. However, a summit of key academics within the field determined that DBS protocols required further modification and patient recruitment needed refining to better assess the therapeutic effects of DBS for TRD [75]. Considering that multiple other studies showed the efficacy and effectiveness of DBS for TRD, the conference considered several possibilities for the discrepancies in the findings, some conclusions were that DBS was initiated too early before optimal targeting was secured, a lack of specificity and standardization in the improvement of symptoms, high placebo effects typically seen in the treatment of psychiatric disorders, and study design. The heterogeneity of the symptoms of the disease was also emphasized, which suggested that different circuitry might be involved in different individuals. The key conclusions from the summit included that patient selection should be better and more refined, study designs should be either fast to fail or fast to succeed, registries should be established for better subject tracking, and longitudinal data should be collected. The paper stressed that the complexities of the disease were real and better experimental designs were needed to truly reflect the effects of DBS as a treatment for TRD for a better response and remission rate and to allow the elucidation of the mechanistic role of DBS.

4.4. Adverse Effects

The safety of SCC-DBS was subsequently assessed following the initial results of the efficacy of DBS in treating TRD. In 2008, McNeely et al. conducted a trial on six patients with an average of 5.6 years of current MDE. They found that mood was significantly improved during the 1-year DBS treatment without serious cognitive deterioration [73]. Moreines et al. found that DBS treatment in both unipolar and bipolar TRD patients with at least 2 years of current MDE improved executive functions and stabilized their memory [76]. Similarly, SCC-DBS for 6 months followed by depression treatment in patients with MDD, who had increased negative emotional processing and/or reduced positive emotions, resulted in reduced negative emotional bias [53]. Martín-Blanco et al. reported that a 52-year-old female had a seizure after 5 weeks of DBS. As severe MDD may predispose patients to seizures, the authors recommended that patients should be evaluated for seizures before administering DBS and parameters might need to be adjusted to within safe ranges [52]. In a study in 2017 by McInerney et al. on 20 unipolar TRD patients with an average of 6.9 years of MDE, they reported that 11 patients responded at the end of the 12-month DBS without further deterioration of cognitive functions. They also found a correlation between verbal fluency and mood improvement, which could be predictive of the DBS response [14]. The side effects reported in this review range from mild symptoms, such as headaches, dizziness and gastrointestinal irritation [43,66], to more severe effects including suicidal ideation and device malfunction [15,67]. This reporting should not discourage the development of therapies. Indeed, many treatments including serotonin-selective reuptake inhibitors have severe side effects, including increased fractures and suicidal ideations [77,78]. In the study of therapies, it is important to report these side effects and to note that these therapies are administered by a professional, whose role is to detect and modulate the therapies accordingly.

4.5. Stimulation Parameters

Several studies have attempted to optimize the parameters of DBS for treating mood disorders. As previously mentioned, Eitan et al. reported that high-frequency stimulation (HFS) was more effective at lowering MADRS scores compared with low frequency stimulation [42]. Indeed, the most commonly used stimulation frequency was in the high frequency range of 130–135 Hz, although some studies have tested frequencies between 5 and 185 Hz [19,61] (see Table 1). The pulse width used in DBS also varied greatly across studies. In a study by Ramasubbu et al., they found that a long pulse width of 180–270 µs was effective [61]. However, this study also reported that DBS with a long pulse width caused patients to experience stimulation-induced insomnia, anxiety, confusion, and drowsiness. Previous studies by Lozano et al. and Holtzheimer et al. demonstrated that shorter pulse widths of 30–60 µs led to clinical improvements in depression symptoms without these side effects [66,72]. Indeed, Ramasubbu et al. suggested that longer pulse widths with lower amplitudes and shorter pulse widths with higher amplitudes could produce comparable therapeutic benefits. The amplitude of the stimulating current used in DBS to elicit a therapeutic response also tended to vary across studies. The amplitude is the first parameter to be adjusted when patients do not respond to the treatment. Among 38 clinical studies, the overall current range was 2–8 mA and voltage range was 2.5–10.5 V. The variability in the amplitude underscores the personalized nature of DBS, which requires specific adjustments to achieve individual therapeutic effects.

4.6. Electrode Implantation

Several clinical DBS studies have also tried to improve the accuracy of electrode implantation in order to precisely target regions of interest. The pioneering work by Mayberg et al. used PET scans of pathological glucose metabolism to guide the electrode implantation. Riva-Posse et al. used individualized tractography maps based on a group connectome blueprint of past responders to DBS to identify optimal target regions for electrode implantation [49]. Riva-Posse et al. used a four-bundle white matter blueprint, which resulted in good clinical outcomes in eight out of 11 patients, which suggests that the use of this method could improve the precision of implantation. Similarly, Tsolaki et al. investigated the use of FMRIB Software Library (FSL) probabilistic tractography in SCC-DBS [50]. Several studies have used other methods to try to specify the optimal stimulation points. Choi et al. investigated the best contact positions that elicited the best response during intraoperative testing [57]. They used diffusion-directed magnetic resonance imaging and patient-specific tractography maps to guide the implantation. They also used fiber tract probabilistic tractography to determine the putative fiber tract activation in patients, which was used to guide the electrode implantation for the best response, rather than the salient response. Contacts in the left hemisphere were found to produce the best consistent intraoperative response to DBS in seven out of nine patients at 6 months. Smart et al. validated this result in their study using local field potentials following unilateral HFS-DBS [46]. They found that left-sided stimulation evoked broadband effects, compared with right sided stimulation, which evoked only beta and gamma bands. Additionally, a decrease in theta bands was consistently accompanied by behavioral improvements. They concluded that the precision of electrodes in the left-hemisphere was more important and instructive than in the right hemisphere. In contrast, Guinjoan et al. and Howell et al. found that right hemisphere targets were critical for behavioral improvements [44,68]. Guinjoan et al. showed that right unilateral DBS could reverse and remit a patient's worsening mood induced by left unilateral DBS. Howell et al. showed that right cingulate bundle activation beyond a threshold could protract the recovery. Further research is needed to elucidate the differences in these studies.

4.7. Other Responses to DBS

With regard to other potential responses to DBS, recent studies have attempted to characterize non-behavioral evoked responses. Conen et al. identified higher rCBF in patients at baseline and during DBS therapy compared to non-remitters and non-responders [48]. Riva-Posse et al. observed autonomic changes in responders undergoing DBS [41]. In a study by Smart et al., assessing the efficacy of DBS, they found consistent changes in left theta local field potentials, which could provide another consistent parameter to monitor. Based on this finding, they proceeded to adjust the contacts for one non-responder, who was able to achieve a response by the end of the study. In a study by Sankar et al. on responders and non-responders who had previously undergone SCG-DBS, they found that both groups had significant volume differences in the left and average SCG; in the right and average amygdala; and in the left, right, and average thalamus (Sankar et al. 2020). Additionally, non-responders had significantly greater grey matter volume compared to responders and a greater grey to white matter ratio. This important information provides yet more criteria for assessing if a patient might respond to DBS. Expanding the breadth of data obtained during clinical trials has the potential to advise clinicians on the efficacy of DBS, and to help predict non-responders and adjust the stimulation parameters. This will improve patient welfare and allows for a more accurate examination of the mechanisms of DBS in improving depressive-like symptoms.

Furthermore, it would be prudent to use preclinical results to advise clinical cases. In a previous preclinical study, Hamani et al. reported that DBS supplemented with tranylcypromine increased the antidepressant-like response in animals by 20%–30% compared to either treatment alone. They later reported on a patient who relapsed after 4 years of remission following DBS treatment [64]. Based on their previous work, they administered tranylcypromine before the DBS treatment, which allowed the patient to enter remission again.

5. Preclinical Studies of Electrical Stimulation in the Medial Prefrontal Cortex in Rodents

Following the success of a number of preliminary clinical studies, several preclinical studies were conducted to investigate the antidepressant-like effects of DBS [79]. The mPFC in rats is widely regarded to be homologous to the SCC in humans. The mPFC together with the amygdala, hippocampus, and hypothalamus controls the stress response, autonomic functions, and cognition in rats [80–83]. Using PET imaging, glucose metabolism was observed to normalize in the mPFC from a hyperactive state following DBS, which was similarly observed in the SCC after 1 h of DBS [84]. However, the homology between subdivisions of mPFC and SCC is still under debate. The vmPFC can be further subdivided into the infralimbic (IL) and prelimbic (PrL) regions. Although there are overlaps, the IL and PrL innervate different regions to different extents, including the lateral hypothalamus, dorsal raphe nucleus, and amygdala, among efferent regions [85–87]. The PrL has been shown to innervate to important limbic regions associated with SCC projections [87]. Meanwhile, the infralimbic cortex (IL) is believed to be structurally homologous based on comparisons involving tractography analysis [88–90]. Some assert that the whole ventromedial prefrontal cortex (vmPFC) is homologous to the SCC [91,92]. Others assert that the vmPFC is functionally distinct from the dorsal medial prefrontal cortex [70,91]. Nevertheless, the vmPFC is generally regarded as homologous to BA25, although a thorough understanding of specific correlations remains to be seen. Table 3 lists 29 preclinical studies on the effects of vmPFC-DBS on animal behaviors.

5.1. vmPFC Stimulation

Hamani et al. published the first preclinical study of vmPFC-DBS in rats in 2010. They used the forced swim test (FST), which models "helplessness" in animals including anxiolytic-like and anti-anhedonic-like behavior. They found DBS reduced the immobility score in FST, indicating antidepressant-like effects. The authors attributed the behavioral changes to serotonergic function in the dorsal raphe nucleus (DRN) as lesions in this structure abolished the behavioral effects in FST [91]. Another animal study in 2012 found the optimal stimulation frequency and amplitude of vmPFC-DBS was 130 Hz and 200 μA that produced anti-anhedonic-like effects and produced a charge density similar to DBS in humans [93]. They found a lesion in the DRN abolished the higher sucrose consumption due to DBS, even with a normal hippocampal brain-derived neurotrophic factor (BDNF) profile. They postulated that an interaction between BDNF and neurochemical substances potentiated the antidepressant-like response [92]. The anti-anhedonic-like effects of DBS were also supported in studies by Rea et al. and Edemann-Callesen et al. They conducted an intracranial, self-stimulation paradigm in Flinders sensitive line and Flinders resistant line rats to assess reward-seeking behaviors, which demonstrated that the anti-anhedonic-like effect of vmPFC-DBS was independent of the dopaminergic reward system [94,95]. Bruchim-Samuel et al. reported that modulation of the ventral tegmental area could prolong the behavioral changes. They found that intermittent acute patterned stimulation administered to the ventral tegmental area of Flinders sensitive line rats resulted in antidepressant-like and anti-anhedonic-like behaviors [96]. Strikingly, a study by Bregman et al. in 2018 found that the antidepressant-like effect of DBS was serotonin transporter-independent. This could be of benefit to some patients with a mutated serotonin transporter-promoter gene (5-HTTLPR), which underlies the poor response to conventional selective serotonin re-uptake inhibitors that target serotonin transporters [97].

Beside changes in neurochemical and neurotrophin profiles, neuroplasticity changes induced by DBS have also been investigated. For instance, Bambico et al. reported increased hippocampal neurogenesis and BDNF levels after vmPFC-DBS, which led to anti-anhedonic-like behaviors, but was not sufficient for an overall antidepressant-like effect [98]. Correspondingly, Liu et al. found a correlation between vmPFC-HFS and hippocampal neurogenesis and improvements in short- and long-term memory in middle-aged rats. This suggests that DBS has therapeutic potential in age-dependent memory deficits [99].

5.2. Other Brain Targets

As preclinical studies have progressed, several brain targets of DBS have been established. Hamani et al. in 2014 demonstrated that DBS in the nucleus accumbens induced a similar antidepressant-like effect to DBS in the vmPFC, even though the stimulations modulated different circuits. This may contribute to more customized stimulation targeting based on the patient's symptoms [100]. Bregman et al. reported that the HFS of the medial forebrain bundle induced antidepressant-like behaviors in the FST [101]. Interestingly, this antidepressant effect was not mediated by increases in either serotonin or dopamine release in the nucleus accumbens. Lim et al. in 2015 emphasized that only HFS of the vmPFC led to anti-anhedonic-like effects and these pronounced antidepressant-like effects were induced by modulating the activity of serotonergic neurons in the DRN [102]. However, the authors did not investigate the effects of different stimulation parameters on depressive-like behaviors in various DBS targets. The study by Etiévant et al. supported the modulation of DRN by DBS and added that glial integrity was a prerequisite to the antidepressant-like outcome [103]. In another study, mice subjected to chronic social defeat stress were administered 7 days of 5-h vmPFC-DBS, which resulted in increased social interactive behavior accompanied by DRN modulation [104]. Interestingly, a recent study demonstrated that the potentiation of the anxiolytic response to vmPFC stimulation was associated with exposure to an enriched environment. This indicates that an enriched living environment can facilitate the beneficial effects of DBS intervention [105]. Creed et al. conducted DBS on the entopeduncular and the subthalamic nuclei to compare antidepressant-like effects [106]. Chronic Subthalamic nucleus DBS was reported to impair performance in the learned helplessness task, with no significant effects in anxiety tests. These results were associated with decreased hippocampal BDNF and TrkB mRNA. Interestingly, entopeduncular nucleus DBS did not increase depressive-like behavior in the learned helplessness task, indicating a superior target over the subthalamic nucleus for the treatment of depressive-like behaviors. Meng et al. reported reductions in depressive-like behaviors in animals stimulated in the lateral habenula; this observation was associated with elevations in dopamine, norepinephrine, and serotonin in both blood serum and in the hippocampus [107].

5.3. vmPFC-Linked Modulation of Other Structures

Other structures have been found to be modulated by vmPFC-DBS. For example, Lim et al. reported that activation of the medial subthalamic nucleus contributed to antidepressant-like behavior [108]. In a rat model of post-traumatic stress disorder, IL-DBS reduced firing in the basolateral amygdala, which attenuated fear and produced a slight anxiolytic-like effect [109]. A recent study showed that DBS resulted in elevated spontaneous firing of noradrenergic locus coeruleus neurons and strengthened the coherence between the prefrontal cortex and locus coeruleus. The latter was protective against stress and was responsible for the antidepressant-like effect seen in FST [110]. On the other hand, Insel et al. reported that there was reduced communication between IL and ventral hippocampus in rats after 10 days of 8-h IL-DBS and such coherence was higher in depressed subjects [111]. Jiménez-Sánchez et al. in 2016 reported two studies on acute IL-DBS in naive and olfactory bulbectomized rat models. In naive animals, IL-DBS induced antidepressant-like behaviors and increased prefrontal glutamate efflux, which activated the α-amino-3-hydroxy-5-methyl-4-isoxazolepropionic acid receptor (AMPAR) to modulate DRN output [81]. In olfactory bulbectomized rats, similar changes were noted in the prefrontal serotonergic and glutamatergic output with the activation of AMPAR and antidepressant-like behaviors [33].

5.4. Synergism with Other Treatments

Antidepressant-like effects in different DBS paradigms are leading to some advancements in the field. One such investigation by Laver et al. in 2014 examined the use of augmentation agents such as buspirone, risperidone, and pindolol to enhance DBS efficacy. However, these agents did not increase the antidepressant response of the rats receiving DBS treatment, when compared to those co-administered monoamine oxidase inhibitors in previous studies [64,112]. It is possible that a response may become evident in clinical trials. Perez-Caballero et al. in 2014 reported an interesting early response to stimulation, in which sham-treated rats had reduced immobility and increased swimming in FST at weeks 1 and 2, but not at week 6 post treatment. They reasoned that this was caused by insertion-induced inflammation as pretreatment by indomethacin reduced the expression of pro-inflammatory mediators (TNF-α, COX1, COX2) and reversed the antidepressant-like behaviors in sham-treated animals [59]. Rummel et al. in 2016 reported that chronic continuous HFS did not have more benefits than chronic intermittent stimulation in treatment-resistant rats with congenitally learned helplessness [113].

5.5. Other Biological Parameters Modulated

Similar to the research direction of clinical studies, preclinical studies have also attempted to characterize other biological parameters of DBS, including more precise electrode implantation. Lehto et al. characterized real-time fMRI responses in the brain following DBS, and found strong connectivity between the vmPFC and amygdala, which validated vmPFC as a target region [114]. Perez-Cabalerro et al. used PET scans to study the immediate effects of electrode implantation. They found that metabolism was decreased locally (vmPFC), but was increased in ventral regions, including dorsal and ventral hippocampus, piriform and insular cortex, nucleus accumbens, ventral tegmental area, ventral pallidum, hypothalamus, and the preoptic area [115]. This was in agreement with other studies on the effect of DBS on depressive-like behavior, but it is noteworthy to see these effects simply via electrode insertion.

Table 3. A list of preclinical studies on deep brain stimulation of the medial prefrontal cortex in rodents.

Authors	Target	Animal	Animal Models & DBS Design	Stimulation Parameters	Behavioral Tests	Outcomes
Jia et al. (2019) [116]	vmPFC	Sprague-Dawley rats, male.	CUS animal model. Open field test and forced swim test before DBS.	Unipolar High Frequency Frequency: 130 Hz Amplitude: 100 µA Pulse Width: 90 µs Low Frequency Frequency: 20 Hz Amplitude: 400 µA Pulse Width: 0.2 µs	Sucrose preference test	CUS rats had a lowered sucrose preference compared to control rats.
					Open field test	No significant difference in locomotion was recorded between CUS and control groups.
					Forced swim test	Both High- and Low-Frequency Stimulation reduced immobility compared to sham rats.
Papp et al. (2019) [117]	vmPFC	Wistar-Kyoto rats, male (DBS) Wistar rats, male [Venlafaxine(VFX)-treated]	CMS animal model. Two, 2-h DBS sessions were conducted, one on the preceding evening and the other on the following morning before each sucrose intake test and the NORT T1 session.	Frequency: 130 Hz Amplitude: 250 µA Pulse width: 90 µs	Sucrose intake test	During the first 2 wks of CMS, sucrose intake decreased >50% across groups. VFX treatment restored sucrose intake levels.
					Novel object recognition test	Wistar Kyoto rats: DBS rescued novel object recognition test across all groups. Wistar rats: VFX rescued novel object recognition test in CMS animals administered with D2 antagonist, but not in D2-administered CMS animals. VFX also did not rescue groups administered with D3 antagonist.
Bhaskar et al. (2018) [105]	vmPFC	Wistar rats, male.	Naïve animal model. DBS for 15 min prior to and throughout behavioral testing.	Bipolar Frequency: 100 Hz Amplitude: 200 µA Pulse Width: 100 µs	Home-cage emergence test	Enriched environment potentiated the efficacy of HFS on reduced escape latency time in the Naïve animal model.

Table 3. *Cont.*

Authors	Target	Animal	Animal Models & DBS Design	Stimulation Parameters	Behavioral Tests	Outcomes
					Elevated plus maze	HFS with an enriched environment reduced the anxiety index and increased head dips.
					Novel object recognition test	No significant difference.
Bregman et al. (2018) [97]	vmPFC	SERT homozygous knockout and wildtype mice, male.	Serotonin transporter (SERT) knockout model. DBS for 4 h before forced swim test and open field test.	Bilateral Monopolar Frequency: 130 Hz Amplitude: 100 μA Pulse Width: 90 μs	Forced swim test	Both wild-type and knockout-DBS mice had reduced immobility time compared to sham.
					Open field test	Knockout-DBS mice had lower locomotion counts than sham and wild-type mice.
Lehto et al. (2018) [114]	IL	Sprague-Dawley rats, male.	Naïve animal model. All stimulation paradigms consisted of three blocks of 60 s of rest and 18 s of stimulation, ending with an additional rest period, giving a total paradigm of 4 min 54 s.	Monopolar Frequency: 20/35/70/100/130/160/200 Hz tested in randomized order. Amplitude: 1.4–1.7 mA distributed equally among the three electrode channels Pulse Width: 180 μs	N.A.	fMRI conducted to characterize changes in the brain following DBS. IL-DBS at varying stimulation parameters significantly triggered the amygdala. Orientation selective stimulation was able to recruit neuronal pathways of distinct orientations relative to the position of the electrode.
Papp et al. (2018) [118]	vmPFC	Wistar rats, male.	CMS animal model. Two, 2-h DBS sessions were conducted, one on the previous evening and one the next morning 15 min before each behavioral test.	Bipolar Frequency: 130 Hz, Amplitude: 250 μA, Pulse Width: 90 μs	Sucrose intake test	DBS increased sucrose intake across all treatment groups, except for imipramine-treated animals.
					Elevated plus maze	DBS increased the anxiolytic open arm entries in all treatment groups.

Table 3. *Cont.*

Authors	Target	Animal	Animal Models & DBS Design	Stimulation Parameters	Behavioral Tests	Outcomes
					Novel object recognition test	DBS rescued the abolished novel object recognition in CMS sham-treated animals, across all treatment groups.
					Paw-pressure test	Ibuprofen, tramadol, and morphine significantly increased the paw withdrawal threshold in naïve animals relative to respective vehicle alone, demonstrating a clear analgesic effect.
					Open field test	No analgesics altered the motor activity of rats.
Perez-Caballero et al. (2018) [115]	IL	Wistar rats, male.	Six independent sets of animals using naïve (unoperated controls) and DBS-off animals.	N.A.	Modified forced swim test	Electrode implantation induced a significant reduction in the immobility scores of vehicle-treated animals. Ibuprofen abolished the antidepressant-like effect of electrode implantation in the modified forced swim test, increasing the DBS-off animal's immobility. Neither morphine nor tramadol counteracted the antidepressant-like effect of DBS-off animals.

Table 3. *Cont.*

Authors	Target	Animal	Animal Models & DBS Design	Stimulation Parameters	Behavioral Tests	Outcomes
					Novelty suppressed feeding test	Electrode implantation reduced latency to feed compared to naïve animals. Ibuprofen increased latency to feed relative to VEH-treated animals. Neither morphine nor tramadol reduced the latency to feed in electrode-implanted animals.
Torres-Sanchez et al. (2018) [110]	vmPFC	Wistar rats, male.	Naïve animal model. DBS for (i) 4 h at 24 h after surgery, then (ii) 2 h at 48 h after surgery	Bipolar Monophasic Frequency: 130 Hz Amplitude: 100 µA Pulse Width: 90 µs	Forced swim test	Reduced immobility time and increased climbing compared to control.
Volle et al. (2018) [119]	vmPFC	Sprague-Dawley rats, male.	Stimulation was delivered 1 week after surgery for either (i) a single day (acute stimulation; 8 h/day) or (ii) 12 days (chronic stimulation daily for 8 h/day) using a portable stimulator (ANS model 3510) to different groups of rats	Frequency: 130 Hz Amplitude: 200 µA Pulse Width: 90 µs	N.A.	Both treatments increase serotonin (5-HT) release, although fluoxetine resulted in a higher sustained concentration, even upon chronic treatment. Chronic DBS resulted in lowered 5HT release by Day 12. DBS reduced raphe SERT expression. DBS induced changes in 5-HT1B receptor expression, whereas fluoxetine induced changes in 5-HT1A receptors expression in the prefrontal cortex. Research highlighted different effects of both treatments on the serotonergic system.

Table 3. *Cont.*

Authors	Target	Animal	Animal Models & DBS Design	Stimulation Parameters	Behavioral Tests	Outcomes
Reznikov et al. (2017) [109]	IL	Sprague-Dawley rats, male.	Posttraumatic stress disorder animal model. 3-day fear conditioning DBS from 1 week after extinction recall to the end of experiment, 8 h/day, or 2 h before and 4 h after behavioral tests.	Frequency: 130 Hz Amplitude: 100 µA Pulse Width: 90 µs	Extinction recall test	Higher freezing scores in DBS-weak extinction than DBS-strong extinction.
					Open field test	No significant difference between groups.
					Novelty suppressed feeding test	Reduced latency to feeding in DBS-weak extinction, but not strong extinction.
					Elevated plus maze	No significant difference observed between groups.
Bruchim-Samuel et al. (2016) [96]	vmPFC VTA	Flinders Sensitive Line rats, male. Sprague-Dawley rats, male. (Control)	Flinders Sensitive Line model. DBS for 15 min/day, for 10 days.	Bilateral, Monopolar vmPFC Stimulation Frequency: 20 Hz Amplitude: 400 µA Pulse Width: 200 µs VTA Stimulation (control) Frequency: 10 Hz Amplitude: 300 µA Pulse Width: 200 µs	Sweetened condensed milk intake test	No significant difference between vmPFC groups. Significant difference between VTA groups for Flinders Sensitive Line rats.
					Novelty Exploration Test	No significant difference between vmPFC groups. Significant difference between VTA groups for Flinders sensitive line rats.
					Forced swim test	Decreased immobility for vmPFC-stimulated rats after DBS for 10 days, half relapsed at day 28. VTA-stimulated Sprague-Dawley rats had persistently reduced immobility until the end of the experiment.
Jiménez-Sánchez et al. (2016) [33]	IL	Wistar rats, male.	Olfactory bulbectomized model animal model. DBS 1 h daily stimulation, beginning 2 days after electrode implantation before behavioral testing.	Bipolar Biphasic Frequency: 130 Hz Amplitude: 200 µA Pulse Width: 90 µs	Social interaction test	Increased duration of active contact.

Table 3. *Cont.*

Authors	Target	Animal	Animal Models & DBS Design	Stimulation Parameters	Behavioral Tests	Outcomes
					Sucrose preference test	Increased percentage of sucrose consumption in total liquid consumption.
					Forced swim test	Reduced immobility and increased climbing but not swimming.
					Hyperemotionality test	Reduced total behavioral scores when compared to olfactory bulbectomized sham rats.
Jiménez-Sánchez et al. (2016) [81]	IL PrL	Wistar rats, male.	Naïve animal model. DBS for 1 h daily before behavioral testing.	Bipolar Biphasic Frequency: 130 Hz Amplitude: 200 µA Pulse Width: 90 µs	Forced swim test	Reduced immobility and increased climbing in IL-DBS No significant behavioral changes in PrL-DBS.
					Open field test	Insignificant locomotor changes in IL-DBS.
					Novelty suppressed feeding test	Decreased latency to feed in IL-DBS.
Rummel et al. (2016) [113]	vmPFC	Flinders Sensitive Line rats, male. Congenitally learned helplessness rats, Male.	Experiment 1 Chronic intermittent DBS 1 week after surgery in Flinders sensitive line rats, 30 min each morning and extra 30-min stimulation on afternoons before the day of behavioral test. Experiment 2 Chronic continuous DBS 1 week after surgery for 16 days. Experiment 3 Chronic intermittent DBS in congenitally learned helplessness rats, procedures followed that in experiment 1.	Chronic intermittent DBS Frequency: 130 Hz Amplitude: 300 µA Pulse Width: 100 µs Chronic continuous DBS Frequency: 130 Hz Amplitude: 150 µA Pulse Width: 100 µs	Sucrose consumption test	Chronic intermittent DBS increased sucrose intake in Flinders sensitive line rats but not in congenitally learned helplessness rats. Chronic continuous DBS did not affect sucrose intake in Flinders sensitive line rats and congenitally learned helplessness rats.

Table 3. *Cont.*

Authors	Target	Animal	Animal Models & DBS Design	Stimulation Parameters	Behavioral Tests	Outcomes
					Forced swim test	Chronic intermittent DBS and chronic continuous DBS increased latency to immobility in Flinders sensitive line rats but not congenitally learned helplessness rats.
					Learned helplessness paradigm	Chronic intermittent DBS and chronic continuous DBS decreased helplessness in Flinders sensitive line rats but not cLH rats.
					Sucrose intake test	No significant difference observed.
					Novelty exploration test	No significant difference observed.
Bambico et al. (2015) [98]	vmPFC	Fisher rats, Male.	CUS animal model CUS for ~4 weeks until anhedonia inferred by SPI scores, then performed implantation DBS for 3 weeks after implantation, 8 h per day, 7 days per week	Frequency: 130 Hz Amplitude: 100 μA Pulse Width: 90 μs	Novelty-suppressed feeding test	Reduced latency to feeding in CUS-DBS animals compared to CUS-sham animals.

Table 3. *Cont.*

Authors	Target	Animal	Animal Models & DBS Design	Stimulation Parameters	Behavioral Tests	Outcomes
Edemann-Callesen et al. (2015) [94]	vmPFC; Medial forebrain bundle.	Flinders sensitive line rats, male. Sprague-Dawley rats, male.	Naïve animal model DBS was applied in an Intra-cranial self-stimulation protocol.	Bilateral, Monopolar Frequency: 20–200 Hz Amplitude: 170–560 μA Pulse Width: 100 μs	Open field test	No significant difference observed.
					Elevated plus maze test	More time in open arms in CUS-DBS animals compared to CUS-sham animals.
					Forced swim test	Reduced immobility time in CUS-DBS animals compared to CUS-sham animals.
					Intra-cranial self-stimulation	For Flinders Sensitive Line rats, vmPFC-DBS did not affect the reward-seeking behavior compared to medial forebrain bundle DBS.
Etiévant et al. (2015) [103]	IL	Sprague-Dawley rats, male.	Naïve animal model. DBS for 4 h after forced swim pre-test and 2 h before forced swim test.	Bipolar Unilateral Frequency: 130 Hz Amplitude: 150 μA Pulse Width: 60 μs	Forced swim test	Reduced immobility duration in IL-DBS compared to control.
Insel et al. (2015) [111]	IL	Sprague-Dawley rats, male.	Naïve animal model. DBS for 8 h per day, for 10 days.	Monopolar Bilateral Frequency: 130 Hz Amplitude: 100 μA Pulse Width: 90 μs	Spontaneous behavior recording	Coherence between ventral hippocampus and IL was reduced after 10-day DBS compared to sham in 2–4 Hz brain activity range, but was not reduced after only 1 day of treatment. Coherence was not affected by fluoxetine, indicating that IL-DBS observations were independent of the serotonergic pathways.

Table 3. *Cont.*

Authors	Target	Animal	Animal Models & DBS Design	Stimulation Parameters	Behavioral Tests	Outcomes
Lim et al. (2015) [102]	vmPFC	Sprague-Dawley rats, male.	Experiment 1 Naïve animal model. Experiment 2 CUS animal model. CUS for 3 weeks, each stressor lasted for 10-14 h DBS for 15 min before home-cage emergence test, before and during open field test.	Bipolar Biphasic Experiment 1 Frequency:10/100 Hz Amplitude: 100 μA Pulse Width: 100 μs Experiment 2 Frequency: 100 Hz Amplitude: 100μA Pulse Width: 100μs	Home-cage emergence test	HFS reduced escape latency time in Naïve and CUS animal model.
					Open-field test	Insignificant effect in Naïve animals for both HFS and LFS. Increased time spent in the central zone for HFS-CUS.
					Food-intake test	HFS increased food intake in naïve animals. No significance difference observed in CUS animals.
					Sucrose-intake test	Insignificant in Naïve animals for both HFS and LFS. Increased sucrose intake in HFS-CUS.
					Forced swim test	Insignificant in Naïve for both HFS and LFS. Reduced immobility duration in HFS-CUS.
Lim et al. (2015) [108]	PrL	Sprague-Dawley rats, male.	Naïve animal model. DBS for 15 min before and during sucrose intake test (same for forced swim test) and before sacrifice for 1 h.	Bipolar Biphasic Frequency: 100 Hz Amplitude: 100 μA Pulse Width: 100 μs	Sucrose intake test	Increased sucrose consumption.
					Forced swim test	Reduced immobility.
Liu et al. (2015) [99]	vmPFC	Sprague-Dawley rats, male. 4 months old and 12 months old.	Acute DBS Naïve animal model. DBS for 30 min before the behavioral tests. Chronic DBS Naïve animal model. DBS for 1 h daily including days of behavioral tests.	Bipolar Biphasic Acute DBS Frequency: 10/100 Hz Amplitude: 50/100/200/400 μA Pulse Width: 100 μs Chronic DBS Frequency: 100 Hz Amplitude: 100 μA Pulse Width: 100 μs	Novel object recognition test	Acute HFS at 200 μA produced higher novel object exploration than familiar object in short-term memory test. Chronic HFS increased novel object exploration in short- and long-term memory than familiar object, as well as the durations.

Table 3. *Cont.*

Authors	Target	Animal	Animal Models & DBS Design	Stimulation Parameters	Behavioral Tests	Outcomes
					Morris water maze	Shorter latency to reach platform on day 1 and 2 in chronic HFS compared to sham. More time spent in the target quadrant and less in the opposite quadrant in chronic HFS compared to sham.
Hamani et al. (2014) [100]	vmPFC	Sprague-Dawley rats, male.	Naïve animal model. DBS for 4 h after FST on day 1, 2 h before swimming on day 2. DBS 1 week after forced swim test, 4 h on day 1, 2 h on day 2, then assessed in open field test	Monopolar Frequency: 130 Hz Amplitude: 100 µA Pulse Width: 90 µs	Forced swim test	Reduced immobility and increased climbing frequency between groups.
					Open field test	No significant difference in locomotion observed.
Laver et al. (2014) [112]	vmPFC	Sprague-Dawley rats, male.	Naïve animal model. Serotonin reuptake inhibitors/vehicle were injected i.p. 1 h and 5 h after forced swim test on day 1 and 1 h before forced swim test on day 2. DBS for 4 h on day 1 of forced swim pre-test and 2 h before forced swim test on day 2.	Monopolar Bilateral Frequency: 130 Hz Amplitude: 100 µA Pulse Width: 90 µs	Forced swim test	DBS-saline, DBS-buspirone, DBS-Risperidone, DBS-pindolol-treated animals had higher swimming and lower observed immobility frequencies.
					Open field test	No significant difference observed
Perez-Caballero et al. (2013) [45]	IL	Wistar rats, male.	CUS animal model. Electrode implantation after week 4 of CUS, then CUS resumed. DBS for 4 h after forced swim pre-test and 2 h before forced swim test. Some animals received pre-treatment with indomethacin or ibuprofen.	Bipolar Monophasic Frequency: 130 Hz Amplitude: 100 µA Pulse Width: 90 µs	Forced swim test	Reduced immobility and increased swimming in DBS-off-IL and DBS-on-IL compared to sham- and naïve-animals. Increased immobility and reduced swimming in DBS-off-IL animals treated with NSAIDs.

Table 3. *Cont.*

Authors	Target	Animal	Animal Models & DBS Design	Stimulation Parameters	Behavioral Tests	Outcomes
Rea et al. (2014) [95]	vmPFC	Flinders sensitive line rats, male. Flinders resistant line rats, male. (Control)	DBS for 30 min each morning for 2 weeks. Extra DBS for 30 min in the afternoon before the day of behavioral tests and during behavioral tests.	Monopolar Frequency: 130 Hz Amplitude: 300 μA Pulse Width: 100 μs	Open field test	No significant difference.
					Forced swim test	DBS reduced immobility in both groups of rats.
					Sucrose consumption test	DBS increased sucrose consumption in both groups of rats.
Veerakumar et al. (2014) [104]	vmPFC	C57BL/6 mice, male.	Chronic social defeat stress animal model. DBS for 5 h/day, for 7 days.	Bipolar Unilateral Frequency: 160 Hz Amplitude: 150 μA Pulse Width: 60 μs	Social interaction test	Before DBS, defeat-susceptible mice showed lower interaction times. Defeated animals with DBS spent longer in the interaction zone than sham and similar to non-stressed animals. DBS increased the total distance traveled.
Hamani et al. (2012) [92]	vmPFC	Wistar rats, male.	CUS animal model. DBS for 8 h/day, for 2 weeks	Monopolar Frequency: 130 Hz Amplitude: 200 μA Pulse Width: 90 μs	Sucrose preference test	Higher preference observed in CUS-treated DBS animals when compared to CUS-sham animals. Higher sucrose consumption in CUS-treated DBS than CUS-sham alone.
Hamani et al. (2010) [93]	vmPFC, IL, PrL	Sprague-Dawley rats, male	Naïve animal model DBS for 4 h after FST on day 1, 2 h before swimming on day 2	Frequency: 20 Hz/130 Hz Amplitude: 100/200/300/400 μA Pulse Width: 90 μs	Forced swim test	Parameters of 130 Hz, 90 μs, 200 μA reduced immobility the most in vmPFC-DBS, also at 100 μA and 300 μA. PrL stimulation at 130 Hz, 90 μs, 200 μA reduced immobility, but IL stimulation was insignificant.

Table 3. *Cont.*

Authors	Target	Animal	Animal Models & DBS Design	Stimulation Parameters	Behavioral Tests	Outcomes
Hamani et al. (2010) [91]	vmPFC	Sprague-Dawley rats, male	Naïve animal model, with serotonergic depletion, or norepinephrine lesion. DBS for Forced Swim Test Day 1: 4 h after forced swim test Day 2: 2 h before forced swim test DBS for open field test, novelty suppressed feeding test, and learned helplessness. Pre-test Day 1: 4 h Pre-test Day 2: 2 h	Monopolar Frequency: 130 Hz Amplitude: 100 µA Pulse Width: 90 µs	Forced swim test	DBS reduced immobility and increased swimming counts in naïve animals. DBS in animals with ibotenic acid injection had lower immobility and higher swimming counts than control. Rats with DBS without serotonergic depletion exhibited lower immobility than DBS animals with serotonergic depletion. Rats with DBS without norepinephrine lesion had lower immobility than control, similar reduction in immobility was shown in animals with DBS and norepinephrine lesion.
					Open field test	No significant difference.
					Novelty suppressed feeding test	DBS reduced latency to feed compared to control.
					Learned helplessness paradigm	Insignificant difference in escape latency between DBS and control.

Table 3. *Cont.*

Authors	Target	Animal	Animal Models & DBS Design	Stimulation Parameters	Behavioral Tests	Outcomes
			Animals predisposed to helplessness. DBS for 2 h before baseline assessment, 2 h before footshock at 2 days after baseline test, and DBS for 2 h before sucrose consumption test on the next day	Monopolar Frequency: 130 Hz Amplitude: 100 µA Pulse Width: 90 µs	Sucrose consumption test	DBS reduced the sucrose drinking time in animals after footshock, but this was insignificant.

Abbreviations: Cg, cingulate cortex; CUS, chronic unpredictable stress; EPM, elevated plus maze; FST, forced swim test; HFS, high-frequency stimulation; IL, infralimbic cortex; LFS, low-frequency stimulation; MWM, Morris water maze test; NORT, novel object recognition test; NSFT, novelty-suppressed feeding test; OBX, olfactory bulbectomy; OFT, open field test; PrL, prelimbic cortex; SD, Sprague-Dawley; SPI, sucrose preference index; vmPFC, ventromedial prefrontal cortex.

Preclinical studies have progressed from studying the behavioral effects of DBS to understanding the accompanying cellular and molecular changes, be they local or distal nodes in the neurocircuitry. However, issues concerning the rodent homologs of SCC and the effect of stimulation in the subdivisions of vmPFC have yet to be resolved and are discussed in the later part of the review.

6. Potential Mechanisms of Stimulation-Induced Antidepressant-Like Activities

Several preclinical studies reported that DBS modulates neuronal activities in different brain regions, leading to antidepressant-like behaviors (Figure 1A). The network-wide cellular and molecular changes caused by vmPFC-DBS can be classified into neuroplasticity-dependent and -independent changes (Figure 1B). Neuroplasticity-dependent effects included neurogenesis, increased synaptic plasticity, enhanced neurotrophin signaling, and potential activation of glial cell-mediated changes, whereas neuroplasticity-independent effects included changes in serotonergic (5-HT) and glutamatergic neurotransmission patterns, either locally or in distal structures. Other changes outside the scope of this review might also be relevant.

Figure 1. (**A**) Changes in local and distal neuronal activity after electrical stimulation of the ventromedial prefrontal cortex. (**B**) Neuroplasticity-dependent and -independent changes in different structures following vmPFC-DBS. Abbreviations: AH, anterior hypothalamus; AMPAR, α-amino-3-hydroxy-5-methyl-4-isoxazolepropionic acid receptor; BDNF, brain-derived neurotrophic factor; BLA, basolateral amygdaloid nucleus; Cg1,2, cingulate gyrus area 1, 2; CM, centromedial thalamic nucleus; DG, dentate gyrus; DMH, dorsomedial hypothalamus; DRD, dorsal raphe nucleus, dorsal part; DRVL, dorsal raphe nucleus, ventrolateral part; IntMC, interposed cerebellar nucleus, magnocelluar part; LA, lateral amygdaloid nucleus; LEnt, lateral entorhinal cortex; LHb, lateral habenula; MD, mediodorsal thalamic nucleus; mPFC, medial prefrontal cortex; OrbF, orbitofrontal cortex; PaMP, paraventricular hypothalamic nucleus, medial parvicellular; Pir, piriform cortex; PrL, prelimbic cortex; TeA, temporal association area; and 5-HT, serotonin.

Neuroplasticity-Dependent Effects of Electrical Stimulation

(i) Neurogenesis is a Long-Term Cellular Change Brought About by Electrical Stimulation

Post-mortem studies, pharmacological analyses, and electroconvulsive therapy reports have led to the neurogenic hypothesis of the pathogenesis of depression, whereby atrophy and apoptosis of hippocampal neurons correlated with depression and neurogenesis induce antidepressant-like effects [120,121]. As CA1 and subiculum in the hippocampus project substantially to the IL and the latter feeds back to the hippocampus via the relay nucleus reuniens in the thalamus [102,122], vmPFC-DBS induces a corollary of hippocampal neuromodulation that may mediate the antidepressant-like outcome. Etiévant et al. found that there was increased neurogenesis in the dentate gyrus of the dorsal and ventral hippocampus in rodents after 1-h IL-DBS, as detected by positive BrdU cells, and this was accompanied by reduced immobility in FST [103]. Similarly, Liu et al. reported proliferation of neuronal progenitors after chronic vmPFC-DBS, as demonstrated by increased positive BrdU and Dcx cell counts, as well as upregulated expressions of genes related to neurogenesis (NeuN, Syn, Dcx, Nes) and neuronal differentiation and protective functions (Angpt2, S100a4). These results were correlated with enhanced memory function, which may serve as another indication of vmPFC-DBS [99]. Bambico et al. confirmed that new cells with mature neuronal phenotype were found in the hippocampus after vmPFC-DBS, as detected by BrdU and NeuN co-expression. They also reported that temozolomide-induced reduction of these cells led to a longer latency to feed in a novelty-suppressed feeding test, but did not significantly change immobility in FST. This prompted the authors to further examine the anxiolytic-like and anti-anhedonic-like effects of vmPFC-DBS. In contrast, Winter et al. showed that 1 h of vmPFC-DBS with established DBS parameters in rodents did not increase the percentage of BrdU and Dcx double-stained cells in the dentate gyrus compared to the control [123]. Although research on the interaction between neurogenesis and substrates such as serotonin is ongoing, BDNF may be required to exert this antidepressant-like effect [98]. Neurogenesis is a widely investigated mechanism of DBS and these results indicate positive effects in the hippocampal region.

(ii) Synaptic Plasticity is Altered More Rapidly by Electrical Stimulation than by Neurogenesis

Disruption in synaptic functions and signaling are implicated in the pathophysiology of MDD, considering their importance in neurotransmission and ultimately, in cell survival [20]. Chronic stress, a risk factor of MDD, was shown to cause retraction of dendrites in the medial prefrontal cortex [124] and CA3 of the hippocampus [125] in rodents. In the latter, the long-term potentiation (LTP) of synapses was compromised, affecting long-term memory formation [126]. Regarding the changes in synaptic plasticity caused by vmPFC-DBS, Liu et al. reported denser secondary dendritic spines in the dentate gyrus, as demonstrated by upregulated Syn expression correlated with Nes and Dcx. The authors also reported a slight (1.2 fold) increase in hippocampal BDNF gene expression, a regulator of synaptic plasticity [99]. More recently, Bezchlibnyk et al. found that 1 h of IL-DBS resulted in longer dendritic length and branch points localized in the basal and apical regions of hippocampal CA1 neurons, respectively. These results indicated that the acute stimulation stressed the indispensable connections between the hippocampus and vmPFC, which may have implications in MDD and its treatment [127].

Chakravarty et al. found that 5 days of 6-h vmPFC-DBS daily in 9-week-old C57Bl/6 mice resulted in a larger hippocampal volume and increased hippocampal synaptic density, as indicated by upregulated synaptophysin expression, a presynaptic marker [128]. Similarly, Veerakumar et al. found that chronic vmPFC-DBS in transgenic mice increased dendrite length and complexity of the 5-HT DRN neurons and upregulated the expression of postsynaptic markers synaptophysin and PSD-95 [104]. Moreover, Etiévant et al. reported synaptogenesis in the DRN, as indicated by higher expressions of PSD-95 and synapsin. This may explain the prolonged DRN neuronal activation during and after vmPFC-DBS, leading to an antidepressant-like effect [103]. According to earlier reviews, dendritic spines can respond swiftly and provide surfaces for synapse formation [126,129]. Given the more dynamic properties of synapses compared to neurogenesis, synaptic plasticity may serve as an early indicator of vmPFC-DBS efficacy. More preclinical studies characterizing the dynamics of synaptic plasticity under vmPFC-DBS are anticipated.

(iii) Neurotrophin Signaling Underlies the Antidepressant-Like Effect of Electrical Stimulation

The neurotrophin BDNF is important in synaptic regulation, neuronal survival, and differentiation of new neuron terminals in the adult brain [130–132]. Preclinical studies reported that depressive-like rats subjected to chronic unpredictable stress [92,98] or olfactory bulbectomy [33] had lower BDNF levels, whereas DBS increased BDNF levels, thus preventing the development of depressive-like behaviors. Extracellularly, pro-BDNF is cleaved by tissue plasminogen activator/plasmin to form mature BDNF. The high-affinity tropomyosin-related kinase B (TrkB) receptor is activated by BDNF [133], leading to downstream phosphorylation of kinases, including protein kinase B (Akt) and extracellular signal-regulated kinases (ERK), which are important mediators of anti-apoptosis and proliferation, respectively [134]. Moreover, BDNF-TrkB triggers Serine 133 phosphorylation of transcription factor cAMP response element binding (CREB), leading to the formation of the dimer. The phosphorylated CREB dimer forms a larger transcriptional complex and alters multiple gene expressions including BDNF itself [135]. Encouragingly, Jiménez-Sánchez et al. showed that IL-DBS administered to olfactory bulbectomized rats activated these signaling pathways, as demonstrated by lowered Akt/pAkt, ERK/pERK, and CREB/pCREB ratios during 1 h of stimulation that increased again after stopping the stimulation, which was similar to the expression pattern of BDNF [33]. Further molecular studies are needed to characterize the action of vmPFC-DBS toward different targets in this signaling cascade.

(iv) Potential Involvement of Glial Cells in Mediating the Outcome of Electrical Stimulation

Glial cells may be involved in the pathogenesis of depression, as revealed by post-mortem studies of MDD patients, which found lower densities in the prefrontal cortex and amygdala, but increased levels in the hippocampal hilus [136–138]. The latter may be activated as a result of neuronal injury and decreasing neuronal populations [139,140]. Glial cells metabolically support neurons and regulate glutamate synthesis and thus, regulate synaptic plasticity. They may be modulated by DBS to potentiate the therapeutic effects [136]. This mechanism was supported in a study by Etiévant et al., which found that glial lesion by L-alpha-aminoadipic acid injection diminished antidepressant-like behaviors, hippocampal neurogenesis, and LTP induced by IL-DBS [103]. These findings led to the hypothesis that the neuronal-glial relationship is a determinant of the antidepressant-like efficacy of DBS, but this requires further study. Perez-Caballero et al. also studied the effects of electrode implantation and analgesic supplements [115]. They found that implantation with non-NSAID analgesic treatments, like tramadol and morphine, did not ameliorate the anti-depressant effects of the electrode implantation. This observation was accompanied by an increase in glial marker GFAP-positive cells. This finding suggests that the supplementation of non-NSAIDs postoperatively could improve the comfort of patients.

Neuroplasticity-Independent Effects of Electrical Stimulation

Besides modulating neuroplasticity-dependent mechanisms, DBS may manipulate some neuroplasticity-independent pathways to induce antidepressant-like effects. In a chronic mild stress model, depressive-like behaviors developed without significant deterioration of hippocampal neurogenesis or neuronal survival [141]. There are two likely inter-related neurotransmission systems that potentiate DBS efficacy, namely serotonergic and glutamatergic systems.

(i) An Alternative Action of the Serotonergic System by Electrical Stimulation

Results from preclinical studies have established an important role of the vmPFC-DRN axis and downstream 5-HT neurotransmission in the treatment of depression. Hamani et al. first reported that 5-HT neurotransmission was augmented by DBS, as shown by a four-fold increase in hippocampal

5-HT after 1 h of vmPFC-DBS [91]. The authors also suggested a relationship between the integral 5-HT system and DBS efficacy, as 5-HT depletion induced by DRN lesions with 5,7-dihydroxytryptamine injection diminished the antidepressant-like effects of vmPFC-DBS [91,92]. Similarly, a study by Perez-Caballero et al. showed that the administration of para-chlorophenylalanine ester impeded 5-HT biosynthesis and diminished the antidepressant-like behaviors in early DBS among IL sham-treated animals [59]. Interestingly, Volle et al. showed that DBS and fluoxetine could rescue the 5-HT system via different mechanisms [119]. Both treatments increased the amount of 5-HT at the end of the chronic treatments, but chronic fluoxetine treatment was associated with decreased expression of 5-HT$_{1A}$ in the prefrontal cortex and the hippocampus, whereas chronic DBS increased 5-HT$_{1B}$ expression in the prefrontal cortex, globus pallidus, substantia nigra, and raphe nuclei.

A study by Veerakumar et al. in a transgenic mouse model of chronic social defeat stress revealed normalization of 5-HT neuron excitability in DRN after vmPFC-DBS [104]. Moreover, Jiménez-Sánchez et al. found increased prefrontal 5-HT efflux after 1 h of IL-DBS in olfactory bulbectomized rats [33] and in naive rats [81]. Etiévant et al. also found spontaneous DRN 5-HT neuron activity increased with IL-DBS [103]. Strikingly, an electrophysiological study performed by Srejic et al. showed that IL-DBS decreased the firing rate of DRN neurons, including serotonergic subtypes via the activation of GABAergic interneurons and possibly by the inhibition of excitatory glutamatergic neurons that modulate the firing of 5-HT [142]. Hence, the positive response to DBS could be enhanced by more selective targeting of the neuronal population by pharmacological adjuncts or coupling with optogenetic techniques. A study by Bregman et al. in 2018 using a serotonin transporter knockout mouse model found that DBS increased hippocampal 5-HT concentration, despite mice responding poorly to fluoxetine, a conventional selective serotonin reuptake inhibitor that acts on serotonin transporter [97]. These findings revealed a novel antidepressant-like activity of DBS involving the 5-HT system primarily in the DRN [79].

(ii) Glutamatergic Neurotransmission is a Promising Target of Electrical Stimulation

Jiménez-Sánchez et al. showed that there was enhanced prefrontal glutamatergic efflux together with changes in the local 5-HT profile [33,81]. The administration of AMPAR agonist and antagonist and subsequent FST showed that the increased glutamate led to antidepressant-like behaviors in animals [81]. The authors also found increased synthesis of the GluA1 subunit of AMPAR and postulated that their postsynaptic membrane insertion may explain the antidepressant-like outcome after 1 h of IL-DBS [33]. The activated glutamate output from the medial prefrontal cortex and frontal cortex enhanced 5-HT neuronal firing in the DRN [143], resulting in the antidepressant-like effect. However, Etiévant et al. argued that their activation was attributed to increased synaptogenesis in the DRN as previously described [103]. Nevertheless, Lim et al. hypothesized that a glutamatergic projection from the vmPFC to the medial subthalamic nucleus [144] may account for the antidepressant-like effects of vmPFC-DBS, as seen by increased c-Fos-immunoreactive cells in the medial subthalamic nucleus, increased sucrose consumption, and reduced immobility duration in FST [108]. With the emergence of glutamate-targeting pharmacotherapy [81], the ability to modulate glutamatergic transmission of DBS would add to the therapeutic novelty.

7. Concerns and Limitations of the Electrical Stimulation Studies

The small sample sizes in several clinical studies might compromise the credibility of the DBS efficacy, even in studies with similar recruited DBS subjects or consistent outcomes [18,56]. Most of the clinical studies were open-label, which means the responses could be prone to the placebo effect, despite the early response characterized by Perez-Caballero [59]. Efficacy of DBS treatment could be overestimated, unless countered by long stimulation, randomization, and blinding [18,145], such as double-blinded and sham-controlled studies [55]. A major criterion in preclinical studies is that they should mimic clinical studies. As it is unfeasible to stimulate animals for 24 h a day as in clinical designs [128], the scheduling of the stimulations and behavioral assessments will thus be relevant to the validity of the outcomes. Stimulation during behavioral tests will be most similar to clinical studies, but this may interfere with the physiological functions of the animals [79]. Besides, DBS is normally carried out in animals for relatively short periods and the effects might not correlate well with chronic stimulation [33]. Some preclinical studies were conducted in naive animal models and would not be compatible with clinical trials as TRD patients will be recruited exclusively in clinical settings [33,93]. Moreover, carry-over effects and lesion effects may interfere with the results in both settings. Carry-over effects refer to behavioral or neurochemical changes after DBS ceases. This needs to be counteracted by a washout period to allow the subjects to resume their baseline physiological states before the next stimulation [79]. Lesion effects occur where responses are observed after electrode implantation [19,60,72]. This needs to be differentiated from true responses observed in preclinical studies by sham-treatment [67], otherwise, the therapeutic effect will be over-estimated. Generally speaking, care must be taken in the design of experiments and data analysis of preclinical studies to increase their translational value to clinical studies.

8. Prospective Approaches to Enhance Deep Brain Stimulation Safety and Efficacy

Clinical response to SCC-DBS and various predictors can facilitate precise patient selection and customize the stimulation targets, thereby yielding maximal therapeutic outcomes with minimal adverse effects. For example, a lower baseline frontal theta cordance and incremental increase in the early stage of DBS indicates a clinical response [63]. Efforts have been made toward a more standardized approach to localize SCG in DBS responders [70]. Recently, real-time recording of the local field potential at the site of electrode implantation coupled with electroencephalogram have revealed network-wide clinical changes in DBS, which may improve the surgical precision [146]. Tractography-guided localization of electrodes, being more customized and precise, can improve the response rate [49]. A rechargeable DBS system should also be considered for long-term stimulation to reduce the need for surgery to replace batteries [17]. Lastly, given the high cost and invasiveness of DBS, more stringent regulation and evidence from randomized controlled studies are necessary to justify the benefits in TRD patients [147,148].

9. Conclusions

Major depressive disorder is a debilitating psychiatric condition, which is affected by treatment resistance. Although safety concerns were raised on the risks of ablative treatment, it paved the way for deep brain stimulation as an adjustable therapy against depression. This review summarized the efficacies of deep brain stimulation in the subcallosal cingulate, one of the most extensively studied targets of stimulation, and in the ventromedial prefrontal cortex, which is the rodent homolog. Research on DBS initially focused on symptomatic relief. As the decades have progressed, studies have started to branch out and utilize modern technology to improve targeting of brain regions and to investigate a broader list of symptoms in patients. This has allowed us to better understand the impact of DBS on underreported parameters, such as heart rate, skin conductance, and brain waveforms. Additionally, preclinical research has expanded our understanding of the molecular factors modulated by stimulation. Besides the local effects, DBS has been shown to modulate distal structures, which can involve numerous projections to and from the stimulated targets, and can contribute to the antidepressant effects. This review also described some of the neuroplasticity-dependent and -independent changes brought about by DBS. Progress in different areas of research has helped lay the groundwork for the next wave of DBS research investigating more targeted and more effective applications of DBS for treating MDD. Last but not least, with further customization, more precise approaches, and more stringent regulation, it is anticipated that deep brain stimulation has great promise to treat severe, refractory depressive disorders in the near future.

Author Contributions: Methodology, Investigation, Formal Analysis, Data Curation, Visualization, & Writing-Original Draft Preparation, Review & Editing: S.K., F.Y.N. and L.W.L.; Conceptualization, Supervision, Project Administration, Resources, & Funding Acquisition: L.W.L.; Validation: S.K., L.A., W.L.L. & L.W.L.;

Manuscript Intellectual Inputs: W.L.L., L.A., N.A.K., M.-L.F., Y.-S.C. and Y.T. All authors have read and agreed to the published version of the manuscript.

References

1. Collaborators. GBD 2017 Disease and Injury Incidence and Prevalence. Global, regional, and national incidence, prevalence, and years lived with disability for 354 diseases and injuries for 195 countries and territories, 1990–2017: A systematic analysis for the Global Burden of Disease Study 2017. *Lancet* **2018**, *392*, 1789–1858.
2. Ferrari, A.J.; Charlson, F.J.; Norman, R.E.; Patten, S.B.; Freedman, G.; Murray, C.J.; Vos, T.; Whiteford, H.A. Burden of depressive disorders by country, sex, age, and year: Findings from the global burden of disease study 2010. *PloS Med.* **2013**, *10*, e1001547. [CrossRef] [PubMed]
3. Greenberg, P.E.; Fournier, A.-A.; Sisitsky, T.; Pike, C.T.; Kessler, R.C. The economic burden of adults with major depressive disorder in the United States (2005 and 2010). *J. Clin. Psychiatry* **2015**, *76*, 155–162. [CrossRef] [PubMed]
4. American Psychiatric Association. *Diagnostic and Statistical Manual of Mental Disorders*, 5th ed.; American Psychiatric Association Publishing: Washington, DC, USA, 2013.
5. Kendler, K.S.; Walters, E.E.; Neale, M.C.; Kessler, R.C.; Heath, A.C.; Eaves, L.J. The Structure of the Genetic and Environmental Risk Factors for Six Major Psychiatric Disorders in Women: Phobia, Generalized Anxiety Disorder, Panic Disorder, Bulimia, Major Depression, and Alcoholism. *Arch. Gen. Psychiatry* **1995**, *52*, 374–383. [CrossRef] [PubMed]
6. Kendler, K.S.; Gardner, C.O.; Lichtenstein, P. A developmental twin study of symptoms of anxiety and depression: Evidence for genetic innovation and attenuation. *Psychol. Med.* **2008**, *38*, 1567–1575. [CrossRef]
7. Rudolph, M.; Rosanowski, F.; Eysholdt, U.; Kummer, P. Anxiety and depression in mothers of speech impaired children. *Int. J. Pediatric Otorhinolaryngol.* **2003**, *67*, 1337–1341. [CrossRef]
8. Montero-Pedrazuela, A.; Venero, C.; Lavado-Autric, R.; Fernández-Lamo, I.; García-Verdugo, J.M.; Bernal, J.; Guadaño-Ferraz, A. Modulation of adult hippocampal neurogenesis by thyroid hormones: Implications in depressive-like behavior. *Mol. Psychiatry* **2006**, *11*, 361–371. [CrossRef]
9. Monteagudo, P.T.; Falcão, A.A.; Verreschi, I.T.N.; Zanella, M.-T. The imbalance of sex-hormones related to depressive symptoms in obese men. *Aging Male* **2016**, *19*, 20–26. [CrossRef]
10. Rohr, U.D. The impact of testosterone imbalance on depression and women's health. *Maturitas* **2002**, *41*, 25–46. [CrossRef]
11. Malhi, G.S.; Bridges, P.K.; Malizia, A.L. Neurosurgery for mental disorders (NMD) A clinical worldwide perspective: Past, present and future. *Int. J. Psychiatry Clin. Pract.* **1997**, *1*, 119–129. [CrossRef]
12. López-Muñoz, F.; Alamo, C. Monoaminergic Neurotransmission: The History of the Discovery of Antidepressants from 1950s Until Today. *Curr. Pharm. Des.* **2009**, *15*, 1563–1586. [CrossRef]
13. Baghai, T.C.; Blier, P.; Baldwin, D.S.; Bauer, M.; Goodwin, G.M.; Fountoulakis, K.N.; Kasper, S.; Leonard, B.E.; Malt, U.F.; Stein, D.; et al. General and comparative efficacy and effectiveness of antidepressants in the acute treatment of depressive disorders: A report by the WPA section of pharmacopsychiatry. *Eur. Arch. Psychiatry Clin. Neurosci.* **2011**, *261*, 207–245. [CrossRef]
14. McInerney, S.J.; McNeely, H.E.; Geraci, J.; Giacobbe, P.; Rizvi, S.J.; Ceniti, A.K.; Cyriac, A.; Mayberg, H.S.; Lozano, A.M.; Kennedy, S.H. Neurocognitive Predictors of Response in Treatment Resistant Depression to Subcallosal Cingulate Gyrus Deep Brain Stimulation. *Front. Hum. Neurosci.* **2017**, *11*, 74. [CrossRef] [PubMed]
15. Holtzheimer, P.E.; Husain, M.M.; Lisanby, S.H.; Taylor, S.F.; Whitworth, L.A.; McClintock, S.; Slavin, K.V.; Berman, J.; McKhann, G.M.; Patil, P.G.; et al. Subcallosal cingulate deep brain stimulation for treatment-resistant depression: A multisite, randomised, sham-controlled trial. *Lancet Psychiatry* **2017**, *4*, 839–849. [CrossRef]
16. Temel, Y.; Hescham, S.A.; Jahanshahi, A.; Janssen, M.L.; Tan, S.K.; van Overbeeke, J.J.; Ackermans, L.; Oosterloo, M.; Duits, A.; Leentjens, A.F.; et al. Neuromodulation in psychiatric disorders. *Int. Rev. Neurobiol.* **2012**, *107*, 283–314. [PubMed]
17. Morishita, T.; Fayad, S.M.; Higuchi, M.-a.; Nestor, K.A.; Foote, K.D. Deep Brain Stimulation for Treatment-resistant Depression: Systematic Review of Clinical Outcomes. *Neurotherapeutics* **2014**, *11*, 475–484. [CrossRef]

18. Kennedy, S.H.; Giacobbe, P.; Rizvi, S.J.; Placenza, F.M.; Nishikawa, Y.; Mayberg, H.S.; Lozano, A.M. Deep Brain Stimulation for Treatment-Resistant Depression: Follow-Up After 3 to 6 Years. *Am. J. Psychiatry* **2011**, *168*, 502–510. [CrossRef] [PubMed]

19. Mayberg, H.S.; Lozano, A.M.; Voon, V.; McNeely, H.E.; Seminowicz, D.; Hamani, C.; Schwalb, J.M.; Kennedy, S.H. Deep Brain Stimulation for Treatment-Resistant Depression. *Neuron* **2005**, *45*, 651–660. [CrossRef]

20. Duman, R.S.; Aghajanian, G.K.; Sanacora, G.; Krystal, J.H. Synaptic plasticity and depression: New insights from stress and rapid-acting antidepressants. *Nat. Med.* **2016**, *22*, 238–249. [CrossRef]

21. Gardner, J. A history of deep brain stimulation: Technological innovation and the role of clinical assessment tools. *Soc. Stud. Sci.* **2013**, *43*, 707–728. [CrossRef]

22. Benabid, A.L.; Pollak, P.; Louveau, A.; Henry, S.; de Rougemont, J. Combined (thalamotomy and stimulation) stereotactic surgery of the VIM thalamic nucleus for bilateral Parkinson disease. *Appl. Neurophysiol.* **1987**, *50*, 344–346. [CrossRef] [PubMed]

23. Faria, M.A. Violence, mental illness, and the brain—A brief history of psychosurgery: Part 2—From the limbic system and cingulotomy to deep brain stimulation. *Surg. Neurol. Int.* **2013**, *4*, 75. [CrossRef] [PubMed]

24. Krüger, S.; Seminowicz, D.; Goldapple, K.; Kennedy, S.H.; Mayberg, H.S. State and trait influences on mood regulation in bipolar disorder: Blood flow differences with an acute mood challenge. *Biol. Psychiatry* **2003**, *54*, 1274–1283. [CrossRef]

25. Zald, D.H.; Mattson, D.L.; Pardo, J.V. Brain activity in ventromedial prefrontal cortex correlates with individual differences in negative affect. *Proc. Natl. Acad. Sci. USA* **2002**, *99*, 2450–2454. [CrossRef]

26. Jimenez, F.; Velasco, F.; Salin-Pascual, R.; Hernandez, J.A.; Velasco, M.; Criales, J.L.; Nicolini, H. A patient with a resistant major depression disorder treated with deep brain stimulation in the inferior thalamic peduncle. *Neurosurgery* **2005**, *57*, 585–593. [CrossRef]

27. Schlaepfer, T.E.; Cohen, M.X.; Frick, C.; Kosel, M.; Brodesser, D.; Axmacher, N.; Joe, A.Y.; Kreft, M.; Lenartz, D.; Sturm, V. Deep brain stimulation to reward circuitry alleviates anhedonia in refractory major depression. *Neuropsychopharmacology* **2008**, *33*, 368–377. [CrossRef]

28. Schlaepfer, T.E.; Bewernick, B.H.; Kayser, S.; Madler, B.; Coenen, V.A. Rapid effects of deep brain stimulation for treatment-resistant major depression. *Biol. Psychiatry* **2013**, *73*, 1204–1212. [CrossRef]

29. Kringelbach, M.L.; Aziz, T.Z. Deep brain stimulation: Avoiding the errors of psychosurgery. *JAMA* **2009**, *301*, 1705–1707. [CrossRef]

30. Holtzheimer, P.E.; Mayberg, H.S. Neuromodulation for treatment-resistant depression. *F1000 Med. Rep.* **2012**, *4*, 22. [CrossRef]

31. Philip, M.L.; Richard, H.T.; Jeffrey, V.R.; Paul, B.F. Brain Neuromodulation Techniques: A Review. *Neuroscientist* **2016**, *22*, 406–421.

32. Blomstedt, P.; Hariz, M.I. Deep brain stimulation for movement disorders before DBS for movement disorders. *Parkinsonism Relat. Disord.* **2010**, *16*, 429–433. [CrossRef] [PubMed]

33. Jiménez-Sánchez, L.; Linge, R.; Campa, L.; Valdizán, E.M.; Pazos, Á.; Díaz, Á.; Adell, A. Behavioral, neurochemical and molecular changes after acute deep brain stimulation of the infralimbic prefrontal cortex. *Neuropharmacology* **2016**, *108*, 91–102. [CrossRef] [PubMed]

34. Greenberg, B.D.; Gabriels, L.A.; Malone, D.A.; Friehs, G.M.; Okun, M.S.; Shapira, N.A.; Foote, K.D.; Cosyns, P.R.; Kubu, C.S.; Malloy, P.F.; et al. Deep brain stimulation of the ventral internal capsule/ventral striatum for obsessive-compulsive disorder: Worldwide experience. *Mol. Psychiatry* **2010**, *15*, 64–79.

35. Kriston, L.; von Wolff, A. Not as golden as standards should be: Interpretation of the Hamilton Rating Scale for Depression. *J. Affect. Disord.* **2011**, *128*, 175–177. [CrossRef]

36. Hamani, C.; Mayberg, H.; Stone, S.; Laxton, A.; Haber, S.; Lozano, A.M. The subcallosal cingulate gyrus in the context of major depression. *Biol. Psychiatry* **2011**, *69*, 301–308. [CrossRef]

37. Andrade, P.; Noblesse, L.H.M.; Temel, Y.; Ackermans, L.; Lim, L.W.; Steinbusch, H.W.M.; Visser-Vandewalle, V. Neurostimulatory and ablative treatment options in major depressive disorder: A systematic review. *Acta Neurochir.* **2010**, *152*, 565–577. [CrossRef]

38. Fitzgerald, P.B.; Laird, A.R.; Maller, J.; Daskalakis, Z.J. A meta-analytic study of changes in brain activation in depression. *Hum. Brain Mapp.* **2008**, *29*, 683–695. [CrossRef]

39. Mayberg, S.H.; Brannan, K.S.; Mahurin, K.R.; Jerabek, A.P.; Brickman, S.J.; Tekell, L.J.; Silva, A.J.; McGinnis, G.S.; Glass, C.T.; Martin, T.C.; et al. Cingulate function in depression: A potential predictor of treatment response. *NeuroReport* **1997**, *8*, 1057–1061. [CrossRef]

40. Sankar, T.; Chakravarty, M.M.; Jawa, N.; Li, S.X.; Giacobbe, P.; Kennedy, S.H.; Rizvi, S.J.; Mayberg, H.S.; Hamani, C.; Lozano, A.M. Neuroanatomical predictors of response to subcallosal cingulate deep brain stimulation for treatment-resistant depression. *J. Psychiatry Neurosci.* **2020**, *45*, 45–54. [CrossRef]

41. Riva-Posse, P.; Inman, C.S.; Choi, K.S.; Crowell, A.L.; Gross, R.E.; Hamann, S.; Mayberg, H.S. Autonomic arousal elicited by subcallosal cingulate stimulation is explained by white matter connectivity. *Brain Stimul.* **2019**, *12*, 743–751. [CrossRef]

42. Eitan, R.; Fontaine, D.; Benoit, M.; Giordana, C.; Darmon, N.; Israel, Z.; Linesky, E.; Arkadir, D.; Ben-Naim, S.; Iserlles, M.; et al. One year double blind study of high vs low frequency subcallosal cingulate stimulation for depression. *J. Psychiatr. Res.* **2018**, *96*, 124–134. [CrossRef]

43. Merkl, A.; Aust, S.; Schneider, G.-H.; Visser-Vandewalle, V.; Horn, A.; Kühn, A.A.; Kuhn, J.; Bajbouj, M. Deep brain stimulation of the subcallosal cingulate gyrus in patients with treatment-resistant depression: A double-blinded randomized controlled study and long-term follow-up in eight patients. *J. Affect. Disord.* **2018**, *227*, 521–529. [CrossRef]

44. Howell, B.; Choi, K.S.; Gunalan, K.; Rajendra, J.; Mayberg, H.S.; McIntyre, C.C. Quantifying the axonal pathways directly stimulated in therapeutic subcallosal cingulate deep brain stimulation. *Hum. Brain Mapp.* **2019**, *40*, 889–903. [CrossRef]

45. Waters, A.C.; Veerakumar, A.; Choi, K.S.; Howell, B.; Tiruvadi, V.; Bijanki, K.R.; Crowell, A.; Riva-Posse, P.; Mayberg, H.S. Test-retest reliability of a stimulation-locked evoked response to deep brain stimulation in subcallosal cingulate for treatment resistant depression. *Hum. Brain Mapp.* **2018**, *39*, 4844–4856. [CrossRef]

46. Smart, O.; Choi, K.S.; Riva-Posse, P.; Tiruvadi, V.; Rajendra, J.; Waters, A.C.; Crowell, A.L.; Edwards, J.; Gross, R.E.; Mayberg, H.S. Initial Unilateral Exposure to Deep Brain Stimulation in Treatment-Resistant Depression Patients Alters Spectral Power in the Subcallosal Cingulate. *Front. Comput. Neurosci.* **2018**, *12*. [CrossRef]

47. Choi, K.S.; Noecker, A.M.; Riva-Posse, P.; Rajendra, J.K.; Gross, R.E.; Mayberg, H.S.; McIntyre, C.C. Impact of brain shift on subcallosal cingulate deep brain stimulation. *Brain Stimul.* **2018**, *11*, 445–453. [CrossRef]

48. Conen, S.; Matthews, J.C.; Patel, N.K.; Anton-Rodriguez, J.; Talbot, P.S. Acute and chronic changes in brain activity with deep brain stimulation for refractory depression. *J. Psychopharmacol.* **2018**, *32*, 430–440. [CrossRef]

49. Riva-Posse, P.; Choi, K.S.; Holtzheimer, P.E.; Crowell, A.L.; Garlow, S.J.; Rajendra, J.K.; McIntyre, C.C.; Gross, R.E.; Mayberg, H.S. A connectomic approach for subcallosal cingulate deep brain stimulation surgery: Prospective targeting in treatment-resistant depression. *Mol. Psychiatry* **2017**. [CrossRef]

50. Tsolaki, E.; Espinoza, R.; Pouratian, N. Using probabilistic tractography to target the subcallosal cingulate cortex in patients with treatment resistant depression. *Psychiatry Res. Neuroimaging* **2017**, *261*, 72–74. [CrossRef]

51. Accolla, E.A.; Aust, S.; Merkl, A.; Schneider, G.-H.; Kühn, A.A.; Bajbouj, M.; Draganski, B. Deep brain stimulation of the posterior gyrus rectus region for treatment resistant depression. *J. Affect. Disord.* **2016**, *194*, 33–37. [CrossRef]

52. Richieri, R.; Borius, P.Y.; Lagrange, G.; Faget-Agius, C.; Guedj, E.; Mc Gonigal, A.; Régis, J.M.; Lançon, C.; Bartolomei, F. Unmasking Partial Seizure after Deep Brain Stimulation for Treatment-Resistant Depression: A Case Report. *Brain Stimul.* **2016**, *9*, 636–638. [CrossRef]

53. Hilimire, M.R.; Mayberg, H.S.; Holtzheimer, P.E.; Broadway, J.M.; Parks, N.A.; DeVylder, J.E.; Corballis, P.M. Effects of Subcallosal Cingulate Deep Brain Stimulation on Negative Self-Bias in Patients with Treatment-Resistant Depression. *Brain Stimul.* **2015**, *8*, 185–191. [CrossRef]

54. Martin-Blanco, A.; Serra-Blasco, M.; Perez-Egea, R.; de Diego-Adelino, J.; Carceller-Sindreu, M.; Puigdemont, D.; Molet, J.; Alvarez, E.; Perez, V.; Portella, M.J. Immediate cerebral metabolic changes induced by discontinuation of deep brain stimulation of subcallosal cingulate gyrus in treatment-resistant depression. *J. Affect. Disord.* **2015**, *173*, 159–162. [CrossRef]

55. Puigdemont, D.; Portella, M.J.; Pérez-Egea, R.; Molet, J.; Gironell, A.; de Diego-Adeliño, J.; Martín, A.; Rodríguez, R.; Àlvarez, E.; Artigas, F.; et al. A randomized double-blind crossover trial of deep brain stimulation of the subcallosal cingulate gyrus in patients with treatment-resistant depression: A pilot study of relapse prevention. *J. Psychiatry Neurosci. Jpn.* **2015**, *40*, 224–231. [CrossRef]

56. Serra-Blasco, M.; de Vita, S.; Rodriguez, M.R.; de Diego-Adelino, J.; Puigdemont, D.; Martin-Blanco, A.; Perez-Egea, R.; Molet, J.; Alvarez, E.; Perez, V.; et al. Cognitive functioning after deep brain stimulation in

subcallosal cingulate gyrus for treatment-resistant depression: An exploratory study. *Psychiatry Res.* **2015**, *225*, 341–346. [CrossRef]

57. Choi, K.S.; Riva-Posse, P.; Gross, R.E.; Mayberg, H.S. Mapping the "Depression Switch" During Intraoperative Testing of Subcallosal Cingulate Deep Brain Stimulation. *JAMA Neurol.* **2015**, *72*, 1252–1260. [CrossRef]

58. Sun, Y.; Giacobbe, P.; Tang, C.W.; Barr, M.S.; Rajji, T.; Kennedy, S.H.; Fitzgerald, P.B.; Lozano, A.M.; Wong, W.; Daskalakis, Z.J. Deep Brain Stimulation Modulates Gamma Oscillations and Theta-Gamma Coupling in Treatment Resistant Depression. *Brain Stimul.* **2015**, *8*, 1033–1042. [CrossRef]

59. Perez-Caballero, L.; Pérez-Egea, R.; Romero-Grimaldi, C.; Puigdemont, D.; Molet, J.; Caso, J.R.; Mico, J.A.; Pérez, V.; Leza, J.C.; Berrocoso, E. Early responses to deep brain stimulation in depression are modulated by anti-inflammatory drugs. *Mol. Psychiatry* **2013**, *19*, 607. [CrossRef]

60. Merkl, A.; Schneider, G.-H.; Schönecker, T.; Aust, S.; Kühl, K.-P.; Kupsch, A.; Kühn, A.A.; Bajbouj, M. Antidepressant effects after short-term and chronic stimulation of the subgenual cingulate gyrus in treatment-resistant depression. *Exp. Neurol.* **2013**, *249*, 160–168. [CrossRef]

61. Ramasubbu, R.; Anderson, S.; Haffenden, A.; Chavda, S.; Kiss, Z.H. Double-blind optimization of subcallosal cingulate deep brain stimulation for treatment-resistant depression: A pilot study. *J. Psychiatry Neurosci.* **2013**, *38*, 325–332. [CrossRef] [PubMed]

62. Torres, C.V.; Ezquiaga, E.; Navas, M.; Sola, R.G. Deep brain stimulation of the subcallosal cingulate for medication-resistant type I bipolar depression: Case report. *Bipolar. Disord.* **2013**, *15*, 719–721. [CrossRef] [PubMed]

63. Broadway, J.M.; Holtzheimer, P.E.; Hilimire, M.R.; Parks, N.A.; DeVylder, J.E.; Mayberg, H.S.; Corballis, P.M. Frontal Theta Cordance Predicts 6-Month Antidepressant Response to Subcallosal Cingulate Deep Brain Stimulation for Treatment-Resistant Depression: A Pilot Study. *Neuropsychopharmacology* **2012**, *37*, 1764–1772. [CrossRef] [PubMed]

64. Hamani, C.; Giacobbe, P.; Diwan, M.; Balbino, E.S.; Tong, J.; Bridgman, A.; Lipsman, N.; Lozano, A.M.; Kennedy, S.H.; Nobrega, J.N. Monoamine oxidase inhibitors potentiate the effects of deep brain stimulation. *Am. J. Psychiatry* **2012**, *169*, 1320–1321. [CrossRef] [PubMed]

65. Holtzheimer, P.E.; Kelley, M.E.; Gross, R.E.; Filkowski, M.M.; Garlow, S.J.; Barrocas, A.; Wint, D.; Craighead, M.C.; Kozarsky, J.; Chismar, R.; et al. Subcallosal Cingulate Deep Brain Stimulation for Treatment-Resistant Unipolar and Bipolar Depression. *Arch. Gen. Psychiatry* **2012**, *69*, 150–158. [CrossRef] [PubMed]

66. Lozano, A.M.; Giacobbe, P.; Hamani, C.; Rizvi, S.J.; Kennedy, S.H.; Kolivakis, T.T.; Debonnel, G.; Sadikot, A.F.; Lam, R.W.; Howard, A.K.; et al. A multicenter pilot study of subcallosal cingulate area deep brain stimulation for treatment-resistant depression. *J. Neurosurg.* **2011**, *116*, 315–322. [CrossRef] [PubMed]

67. Puigdemont, D.; Pérez-Egea, R.; Portella, M.J.; Molet, J.; de Diego-Adeliño, J.; Gironell, A.; Radua, J.; Gómez-Anson, B.; Rodríguez, R.; Serra, M.; et al. Deep brain stimulation of the subcallosal cingulate gyrus: Further evidence in treatment-resistant major depression. *Int. J. Neuropsychopharmacol.* **2012**, *15*, 121–133. [CrossRef]

68. Guinjoan, S.M.; Mayberg, H.S.; Costanzo, E.Y.; Fahrer, R.D.; Tenca, E.; Antico, J.; Cerquetti, D.; Smyth, E.; Leiguarda, R.C.; Nemeroff, C.B. Asymmetrical contribution of brain structures to treatment-resistant depression as illustrated by effects of right subgenual cingulum stimulation. *J. Neuropsychiatry Clin. Neurosci.* **2010**, *22*, 265–277. [CrossRef] [PubMed]

69. Holtzheimer, P.E., 3rd; Mayberg, H.S. Deep brain stimulation for treatment-resistant depression. *Am. J. Psychiatry* **2010**, *167*, 1437–1444. [CrossRef]

70. Hamani, C.; Mayberg, H.; Snyder, B.; Giacobbe, P.; Kennedy, S.; Lozano, A.M. Deep brain stimulation of the subcallosal cingulate gyrus for depression: Anatomical location of active contacts in clinical responders and a suggested guideline for targeting. *J. Neurosurg.* **2009**, *111*, 1209. [CrossRef]

71. Puigdemont, D.; Portella, M.J.; Pérez-Egea, R.; de Diego-Adeliño, J.; Gironell, A.; Molet, J.; Duran-Sindreu, S.; Álvarez, E.; Pérez, V. Depressive Relapse After Initial Response to Subcallosal Cingulate Gyrus-Deep Brain Stimulation in a Patient with a Treatment-Resistant Depression: Electroconvulsive Therapy as a Feasible Strategy. *Biol. Psychiatry* **2009**, *66*, e11–e12. [CrossRef]

72. Lozano, A.M.; Mayberg, H.S.; Giacobbe, P.; Hamani, C.; Craddock, R.C.; Kennedy, S.H. Subcallosal Cingulate Gyrus Deep Brain Stimulation for Treatment-Resistant Depression. *Biol. Psychiatry* **2008**, *64*, 461–467. [CrossRef] [PubMed]

73. McNeely, E.H.; Mayberg, S.H.; Lozano, M.A.; Kennedy, H.S. Neuropsychological Impact of Cg25 Deep Brain Stimulation for Treatment-Resistant Depression: Preliminary Results Over 12 Months. *J. Nerv. Ment. Dis.* **2008**, *196*, 405–410. [CrossRef] [PubMed]

74. Neimat, J.S.; Hamani, C.; Giacobbe, P.; Merskey, H.; Kennedy, S.H.; Mayberg, H.S.; Lozano, A.M. Neural stimulation successfully treats depression in patients with prior ablative cingulotomy. *Am. J. Psychiatry* **2008**, *165*, 687. [CrossRef] [PubMed]

75. Bari, A.A.; Mikell, C.B.; Abosch, A.; Ben-Haim, S.; Buchanan, R.J.; Burton, A.W.; Carcieri, S.; Cosgrove, G.R.; D'Haese, P.-F.; Daskalakis, Z.J.; et al. Charting the road forward in psychiatric neurosurgery: Proceedings of the 2016 American Society for Stereotactic and Functional Neurosurgery workshop on neuromodulation for psychiatric disorders. *J. Neurol. Neurosurg. Psychiatry* **2018**, *89*, 886–896. [CrossRef]

76. Moreines, J.L.; McClintock, S.M.; Kelley, M.E.; Holtzheimer, P.E.; Mayberg, H.S. Neuropsychological function before and after subcallosal cingulate deep brain stimulation in patients with treatment-resistant depression. *Depress. Anxiety* **2014**, *31*, 690–698. [CrossRef]

77. Nyandege, A.N.; Slattum, P.W.; Harpe, S.E. Risk of Fracture and the Concomitant Use of Bisphosphonates With Osteoporosis-Inducing Medications. *Ann. Pharmacother.* **2015**, *49*, 437–447. [CrossRef]

78. Cox, G.R.; Callahan, P.; Churchill, R.; Hunot, V.; Merry, S.N.; Parker, A.G.; Hetrick, S.E. Psychological therapies versus antidepressant medication, alone and in combination for depression in children and adolescents. *Cochrane Database Syst. Rev.* **2014**, *11*, CD008324. [CrossRef]

79. Hamani, C.; Nobrega, J.N. Preclinical Studies Modeling Deep Brain Stimulation for Depression. *Biol. Psychiatry* **2012**, *72*, 916–923. [CrossRef]

80. Vertes, R.P. Interactions among the medial prefrontal cortex, hippocampus and midline thalamus in emotional and cognitive processing in the rat. *Neuroscience* **2006**, *142*, 1–20. [CrossRef]

81. Jiménez-Sánchez, L.; Castañé, A.; Pérez-Caballero, L.; Grifoll-Escoda, M.; López-Gil, X.; Campa, L.; Galofré, M.; Berrocoso, E.; Adell, A. Activation of AMPA Receptors Mediates the Antidepressant Action of Deep Brain Stimulation of the Infralimbic Prefrontal Cortex. *Cereb. Cortex* **2016**, *26*, 2778–2789. [CrossRef]

82. Ferry, A.T.; Öngür, D.; An, X.; Price, J.L. Prefrontal cortical projections to the striatum in macaque monkeys: Evidence for an organization related to prefrontal networks. *J. Comp. Neurol.* **2000**, *425*, 447–470. [CrossRef]

83. McFarland, N.R.; Haber, S.N. Thalamic Relay Nuclei of the Basal Ganglia Form Both Reciprocal and Nonreciprocal Cortical Connections, Linking Multiple Frontal Cortical Areas. *J. Neurosci.* **2002**, *22*, 8117–8132. [CrossRef]

84. Parthoens, J.; Verhaeghe, J.; Stroobants, S.; Staelens, S. Deep Brain Stimulation of the Prelimbic Medial Prefrontal Cortex: Quantification of the Effect on Glucose Metabolism in the Rat Brain Using [18 F] FDG MicroPET. *Mol. Imaging Biol.* **2014**, *16*, 838–845. [CrossRef]

85. Hajós, M.; Richards, C.D.; Székely, A.D.; Sharp, T. An electrophysiological and neuroanatomical study of the medial prefrontal cortical projection to the midbrain raphe nuclei in the rat. *Neuroscience* **1998**, *87*, 95–108. [CrossRef]

86. Wood, M.; Adil, O.; Wallace, T.; Fourman, S.; Wilson, S.P.; Herman, J.P.; Myers, B. Infralimbic prefrontal cortex structural and functional connectivity with the limbic forebrain: A combined viral genetic and optogenetic analysis. *Brain Struct. Funct.* **2019**, *224*, 73–97. [CrossRef] [PubMed]

87. Sesack, S.R.; Deutch, A.Y.; Roth, R.H.; Bunney, B.S. Topographical organization of the efferent projections of the medial prefrontal cortex in the rat: An anterograde tract-tracing study with Phaseolus vulgaris leucoagglutinin. *J. Comp. Neurol.* **1989**, *290*, 213–242. [CrossRef] [PubMed]

88. Chandler, L.J.; Gass, J.T. The plasticity of extinction: Contribution of the prefrontal cortex in treating addiction though inhibitory learning. *Front. Psychiatry* **2013**, *4*. [CrossRef]

89. Uylings, H.B.; van Eden, C.G. Qualitative and quantitative comparison of the prefrontal cortex in rat and in primates, including humans. *Prog. Brain Res.* **1990**, *85*, 31–62. [PubMed]

90. Lim, L.W.; Tan, S.K.; Groenewegen, H.J.; Temel, Y. Electrical brain stimulation in depression: Which target(s)? *Biol. Psychiatry* **2011**, *69*, e5–e6, author reply e7–e8. [CrossRef] [PubMed]

91. Hamani, C.; Diwan, M.; Macedo, C.E.; Brandao, M.L.; Shumake, J.; Gonzalez-Lima, F.; Raymond, R.; Lozano, A.M.; Fletcher, P.J.; Nobrega, J.N. Antidepressant-like effects of medial prefrontal cortex deep brain stimulation in rats. *Biol. Psychiatry* **2010**, *67*, 117–124. [CrossRef]

92. Hamani, C.; Machado, D.C.; Hipólide, D.C.; Dubiela, F.P.; Suchecki, D.; Macedo, C.E.; Tescarollo, F.; Martins, U.; Covolan, L.; Nobrega, J.N. Deep Brain Stimulation Reverses Anhedonic-Like Behavior in a

Chronic Model of Depression: Role of Serotonin and Brain Derived Neurotrophic Factor. *Biol. Psychiatry* **2012**, *71*, 30–35. [CrossRef] [PubMed]

93. Hamani, C.; Diwan, M.; Isabella, S.; Lozano, A.M.; Nobrega, J.N. Effects of different stimulation parameters on the antidepressant-like response of medial prefrontal cortex deep brain stimulation in rats. *J. Psychiatr. Res.* **2010**, *44*, 683–687. [CrossRef] [PubMed]

94. Edemann-Callesen, H.; Voget, M.; Empl, L.; Vogel, M.; Wieske, F.; Rummel, J.; Heinz, A.; Mathé, A.A.; Hadar, R.; Winter, C. Medial Forebrain Bundle Deep Brain Stimulation has Symptom-specific Anti-depressant Effects in Rats and as Opposed to Ventromedial Prefrontal Cortex Stimulation Interacts With the Reward System. *Brain Stimul.* **2015**, *8*, 714–723. [CrossRef] [PubMed]

95. Rea, E.; Rummel, J.; Schmidt, T.T.; Hadar, R.; Heinz, A.; Mathé, A.A.; Winter, C. Anti-Anhedonic Effect of Deep Brain Stimulation of the Prefrontal Cortex and the Dopaminergic Reward System in a Genetic Rat Model of Depression: An Intracranial Self-Stimulation Paradigm Study. *Brain Stimul.* **2014**, *7*, 21–28. [CrossRef] [PubMed]

96. Bruchim-Samuel, M.; Lax, E.; Gazit, T.; Friedman, A.; Ahdoot, H.; Bairachnaya, M.; Pinhasov, A.; Yadid, G. Electrical stimulation of the vmPFC serves as a remote control to affect VTA activity and improve depressive-like behavior. *Exp. Neurol.* **2016**, *283*, 255–263. [CrossRef] [PubMed]

97. Bregman, T.; Nona, C.; Volle, J.; Diwan, M.; Raymond, R.; Fletcher, P.J.; Nobrega, J.N.; Hamani, C. Deep brain stimulation induces antidepressant-like effects in serotonin transporter knockout mice. *Brain Stimul.* **2018**, *11*, 423–425. [CrossRef]

98. Bambico, F.R.; Bregman, T.; Diwan, M.; Li, J.; Darvish-Ghane, S.; Li, Z.; Laver, B.; Amorim, B.O.; Covolan, L.; Nobrega, J.N.; et al. Neuroplasticity-dependent and -independent mechanisms of chronic deep brain stimulation in stressed rats. *Transl. Psychiatry* **2015**, *5*, e674. [CrossRef]

99. Liu, A.; Jain, N.; Vyas, A.; Lim, L.W. Ventromedial prefrontal cortex stimulation enhances memory and hippocampal neurogenesis in the middle-aged rats. *eLife* **2015**, *4*, e04803. [CrossRef]

100. Hamani, C.; Amorim, B.O.; Wheeler, A.L.; Diwan, M.; Driesslein, K.; Covolan, L.; Butson, C.R.; Nobrega, J.N. Deep brain stimulation in rats: Different targets induce similar antidepressant-like effects but influence different circuits. *Neurobiol. Dis.* **2014**, *71*, 205–214. [CrossRef]

101. Bregman, T.; Reznikov, R.; Diwan, M.; Raymond, R.; Butson, C.R.; Nobrega, J.N.; Hamani, C. Antidepressant-like Effects of Medial Forebrain Bundle Deep Brain Stimulation in Rats are not Associated With Accumbens Dopamine Release. *Brain Stimul.* **2015**, *8*, 708–713. [CrossRef]

102. Lim, L.W.; Prickaerts, J.; Huguet, G.; Kadar, E.; Hartung, H.; Sharp, T.; Temel, Y. Electrical stimulation alleviates depressive-like behaviors of rats: Investigation of brain targets and potential mechanisms. *Transl. Psychiatry* **2015**, *5*, e535. [CrossRef] [PubMed]

103. Etiévant, A.; Oosterhof, C.; Bétry, C.; Abrial, E.; Novo-Perez, M.; Rovera, R.; Scarna, H.; Devader, C.; Mazella, J.; Wegener, G.; et al. Astroglial Control of the Antidepressant-Like Effects of Prefrontal Cortex Deep Brain Stimulation. *EBioMedicine* **2015**, *2*, 898–908. [CrossRef] [PubMed]

104. Veerakumar, A.; Challis, C.; Gupta, P.; Da, J.; Upadhyay, A.; Beck, S.G.; Berton, O. Antidepressant-like effects of cortical deep brain stimulation coincide with pro-neuroplastic adaptations of serotonin systems. *Biol. Psychiatry* **2014**, *76*, 203–212. [CrossRef] [PubMed]

105. Bhaskar, Y.; Lim, L.W.; Mitra, R. Enriched Environment Facilitates Anxiolytic Efficacy Driven by Deep-Brain Stimulation of Medial Prefrontal Cortex. *Front. Behav. Neurosci.* **2018**, *12*, 204. [CrossRef] [PubMed]

106. Creed, M.C.; Hamani, C.; Nobrega, J.N. Effects of repeated deep brain stimulation on depressive- and anxiety-like behavior in rats: Comparing entopeduncular and subthalamic nuclei. *Brain Stimul.* **2013**, *6*, 506–514. [CrossRef]

107. Meng, H.; Wang, Y.; Huang, M.; Lin, W.; Wang, S.; Zhang, B. Chronic deep brain stimulation of the lateral habenula nucleus in a rat model of depression. *Brain Res.* **2011**, *1422*, 32–38. [CrossRef]

108. Lim, L.W.; Janssen, M.L.F.; Kocabicak, E.; Temel, Y. The antidepressant effects of ventromedial prefrontal cortex stimulation is associated with neural activation in the medial part of the subthalamic nucleus. *Behav. Brain Res.* **2015**, *279*, 17–21. [CrossRef]

109. Reznikov, R.; Bambico, F.R.; Diwan, M.; Raymond, R.J.; Nashed, M.G.; Nobrega, J.N.; Hamani, C. Prefrontal Cortex Deep Brain Stimulation Improves Fear and Anxiety-Like Behavior and Reduces Basolateral Amygdala Activity in a Preclinical Model of Posttraumatic Stress Disorder. *Neuropsychopharmacology* **2017**, *43*, 1099–1106. [CrossRef]

110. Torres-Sanchez, S.; Perez-Caballero, L.; Mico, J.A.; Celada, P.; Berrocoso, E. Effect of Deep Brain Stimulation of the ventromedial prefrontal cortex on the noradrenergic system in rats. *Brain Stimul.* **2018**, *11*, 222–230. [CrossRef]

111. Insel, N.; Pilkiw, M.; Nobrega, J.N.; Hutchison, W.D.; Takehara-Nishiuchi, K.; Hamani, C. Chronic deep brain stimulation of the rat ventral medial prefrontal cortex disrupts hippocampal–prefrontal coherence. *Exp. Neurol.* **2015**, *269*, 1–7. [CrossRef]

112. Laver, B.; Diwan, M.; Nobrega, J.N.; Hamani, C. Augmentative therapies do not potentiate the antidepressant-like effects of deep brain stimulation in rats. *J. Affect. Disord.* **2014**, *161*, 87–90. [CrossRef]

113. Rummel, J.; Voget, M.; Hadar, R.; Ewing, S.; Sohr, R.; Klein, J.; Sartorius, A.; Heinz, A.; Mathé, A.A.; Vollmayr, B.; et al. Testing different paradigms to optimize antidepressant deep brain stimulation in different rat models of depression. *J. Psychiatr. Res.* **2016**, *81*, 36–45. [CrossRef] [PubMed]

114. Lehto, L.J.; Filip, P.; Laakso, H.; Sierra, A.; Slopsema, J.P.; Johnson, M.D.; Eberly, L.E.; Low, W.C.; Grohn, O.; Tanila, H.; et al. Tuning Neuromodulation Effects by Orientation Selective Deep Brain Stimulation in the Rat Medial Frontal Cortex. *Front. Neurosci.* **2018**, *12*, 899. [CrossRef] [PubMed]

115. Perez-Caballero, L.; Soto-Montenegro, M.L.; Hidalgo-Figueroa, M.; Mico, J.A.; Desco, M.; Berrocoso, E. Deep brain stimulation electrode insertion and depression: Patterns of activity and modulation by analgesics. *Brain Stimul.* **2018**, *11*, 1348–1355. [CrossRef] [PubMed]

116. Jia, L.; Sun, Z.; Shi, D.; Wang, M.; Jia, J.; He, Y.; Xue, F.; Ren, Y.; Yang, J.; Ma, X. Effects of different patterns of electric stimulation of the ventromedial prefrontal cortex on hippocampal–prefrontal coherence in a rat model of depression. *Behav. Brain Res.* **2019**, *356*, 179–188. [CrossRef]

117. Papp, M.; Gruca, P.; Lason, M.; Niemczyk, M.; Willner, P. The role of prefrontal cortex dopamine D2 and D3 receptors in the mechanism of action of venlafaxine and deep brain stimulation in animal models of treatment-responsive and treatment-resistant depression. *J. Psychopharmacol.* **2019**, *33*, 748–756. [CrossRef]

118. Papp, M.; Gruca, P.; Lason, M.; Tota-Glowczyk, K.; Niemczyk, M.; Litwa, E.; Willner, P. Rapid antidepressant effects of deep brain stimulation of the pre-frontal cortex in an animal model of treatment-resistant depression. *J. Psychopharmacol* **2018**, *32*, 1133–1140. [CrossRef]

119. Volle, J.; Bregman, T.; Scott, B.; Diwan, M.; Raymond, R.; Fletcher, P.J.; Nobrega, J.N.; Hamani, C. Deep brain stimulation and fluoxetine exert different long-term changes in the serotonergic system. *Neuropharmacology* **2018**, *135*, 63–72. [CrossRef]

120. Santarelli, L.; Saxe, M.; Gross, C.; Surget, A.; Battaglia, F.; Dulawa, S.; Weisstaub, N.; Lee, J.; Duman, R.; Arancio, O.; et al. Requirement of Hippocampal Neurogenesis for the Behavioral Effects of Antidepressants. *Science* **2003**, *301*, 805. [CrossRef]

121. Pittenger, C.; Duman, R.S. Stress, depression, and neuroplasticity: A convergence of mechanisms. *Neuropsychopharmacology* **2008**, *33*, 88–109. [CrossRef]

122. Vertes, R.P.; Hoover, W.B.; Szigeti-Buck, K.; Leranth, C. Nucleus reuniens of the midline thalamus: Link between the medial prefrontal cortex and the hippocampus. *Brain Res. Bull.* **2007**, *71*, 601–609. [CrossRef]

123. Winter, C.; Bregman, T.; Voget, M.; Raymond, R.; Hadar, R.; Nobrega, J.N.; Hamani, C. Acute high frequency stimulation of the prefrontal cortex or nucleus accumbens does not increase hippocampal neurogenesis in rats. *J. Psychiatr. Res.* **2015**, *68*, 27–29. [CrossRef] [PubMed]

124. Cook, S.C.; Wellman, C.L. Chronic stress alters dendritic morphology in rat medial prefrontal cortex. *J. Neurobiol.* **2004**, *60*, 236–248. [CrossRef] [PubMed]

125. Magariños, A.M.; McEwen, B.S.; Flügge, G.; Fuchs, E. Chronic psychosocial stress causes apical dendritic atrophy of hippocampal CA3 pyramidal neurons in subordinate tree shrews. *J. Neurosci. Off. J. Soc. Neurosci.* **1996**, *16*, 3534. [CrossRef]

126. Shepherd, G.M. The dendritic spine: A multifunctional integrative unit. *J. Neurophysiol.* **1996**, *75*, 2197–2210. [CrossRef] [PubMed]

127. Bezchlibnyk, Y.B.; Stone, S.S.D.; Hamani, C.; Lozano, A.M. High frequency stimulation of the infralimbic cortex induces morphological changes in rat hippocampal neurons. *Brain Stimul.* **2017**, *10*, 315–323. [CrossRef] [PubMed]

128. Chakravarty, M.M.; Hamani, C.; Martinez-Canabal, A.; Ellegood, J.; Laliberté, C.; Nobrega, J.N.; Sankar, T.; Lozano, A.M.; Frankland, P.W.; Lerch, J.P. Deep brain stimulation of the ventromedial prefrontal cortex causes reorganization of neuronal processes and vasculature. *NeuroImage* **2016**, *125*, 422–427. [CrossRef] [PubMed]

129. Hering, H.; Sheng, M. Dendritic spines: Structure, dynamics and regulation. *Nat. Rev. Neurosci.* **2001**, *2*, 880. [CrossRef]

130. Kuem-Ju, L.; Sung-Jin, K.; Suk-Won, K.; Song-Hyen, C.; You-Chan, S.; Sang-Ha, P.; Bo-Hyun, M.; Eujin, C.; Min-Soo, L.; Sang-Hyun, C.; et al. Chronic mild stress decreases survival, but not proliferation, of new-born cells in adult rat hippocampus. *Exp. Amp; Mol. Med.* **2006**, *38*, 44.

131. Gulyaeva, N.V. Molecular Mechanisms of Neuroplasticity: An Expanding Universe. *Biochem. Mosc.* **2017**, *82*, 237–242. [CrossRef]

132. Chan, J.P.; Cordeira, J.; Calderon, G.A.; Iyer, L.K.; Rios, M. Depletion of central BDNF in mice impedes terminal differentiation of new granule neurons in the adult hippocampus. *Mol. Cell. Neurosci.* **2008**, *39*, 372–383. [CrossRef] [PubMed]

133. Reichardt, L.F. Neurotrophin-Regulated Signalling Pathways. *Philos. Trans. Biol. Sci.* **2006**, *361*, 1545–1564. [CrossRef]

134. Duman, R.S.; Voleti, B. Signaling pathways underlying the pathophysiology and treatment of depression: Novel mechanisms for rapid-acting agents. *Trends Neurosci.* **2012**, *35*, 47–56. [CrossRef] [PubMed]

135. Carlezon, W.A.; Duman, R.S.; Nestler, E.J. The many faces of CREB. *Trends Neurosci.* **2005**, *28*, 436–445. [CrossRef]

136. Öngür, D.; Drevets, W.C.; Price, J.L. Glial reduction in the subgenual prefrontal cortex in mood disorders. *Proc. Natl. Acad. Sci. USA* **1998**, *95*, 13290–13295. [CrossRef]

137. Bowley, M.P.; Drevets, W.C.; Öngür, D.; Price, J.L. Low glial numbers in the amygdala in major depressive disorder. *Biol. Psychiatry* **2002**, *52*, 404–412. [CrossRef]

138. Vostrikov, V.M.; Uranova, N.A.; Orlovskaya, D.D. Deficit of perineuronal oligodendrocytes in the prefrontal cortex in schizophrenia and mood disorders. *Schizophr. Res.* **2007**, *94*, 273–280. [CrossRef]

139. Stockmeier, C.A.; Mahajan, G.J.; Konick, L.C.; Overholser, J.C.; Jurjus, G.J.; Meltzer, H.Y.; Uylings, H.B.; Friedman, L.; Rajkowska, G. Cellular changes in the postmortem hippocampus in major depression. *Biol. Psychiatry* **2004**, *56*, 640–650. [CrossRef]

140. Rajkowska, G.; Miguel-Hidalgo, J.J.; Dubey, P.; Stockmeier, C.A.; Krishnan, K.R. Prominent reduction in pyramidal neurons density in the orbitofrontal cortex of elderly depressed patients. *Biol. Psychiatry* **2005**, *58*, 297–306. [CrossRef]

141. Airan, R.D.; Meltzer, L.A.; Roy, M.; Gong, Y.; Chen, H.; Deisseroth, K. High-Speed Imaging Reveals Neurophysiological Links to Behavior in an Animal Model of Depression. *Science* **2007**, *317*, 819. [CrossRef]

142. Srejic, L.R.; Hamani, C.; Hutchison, W.D. High-frequency stimulation of the medial prefrontal cortex decreases cellular firing in the dorsal raphe. *Eur. J. Neurosci.* **2015**, *41*, 1219–1226. [CrossRef] [PubMed]

143. Celada, P.; Puig, M.; Casanovas, J.; Guillazo, G.; Artigas, F. Control of Dorsal Raphe Serotonergic Neurons by the Medial Prefrontal Cortex: Involvement of Serotonin-1A, GABA sub(A), and Glutamate Receptors. *J. Neurosci.* **2001**, *21*, 9917–9929. [CrossRef]

144. Nambu, A.; Tokuno, H.; Takada, M. Functional significance of the cortico–subthalamo–pallidal 'hyperdirect' pathway. *Neurosci. Res.* **2002**, *43*, 111–117. [CrossRef]

145. Anderson, R.J.; Frye, M.A.; Abulseoud, O.A.; Lee, K.H.; McGillivray, J.A.; Berk, M.; Tye, S.J. Deep brain stimulation for treatment-resistant depression: Efficacy, safety and mechanisms of action. *Neurosci. Biobehav. Rev.* **2012**, *36*, 1920–1933. [CrossRef]

146. Deeb, W.; Giordano, J.J.; Rossi, P.J.; Mogilner, A.Y.; Gunduz, A.; Judy, J.W.; Klassen, B.T.; Butson, C.R.; Van Horne, C.; Deny, D.; et al. Proceedings of the Fourth Annual Deep Brain Stimulation Think Tank: A Review of Emerging Issues and Technologies. *Front. Integr. Neurosci.* **2016**, *10*, 38. [CrossRef]

147. Schermer, M. Ethical Issues in Deep Brain Stimulation. *Front. Integr. Neurosci.* **2011**, *5*. [CrossRef]

148. Bell, E.; Mathieu, G.; Racine, E. Preparing the ethical future of deep brain stimulation. *Surg. Neurol.* **2009**, *72*, 577. [CrossRef]

## 6

A Deep Brain Stimulation Trial Period for Treating Chronic Pain

Prasad Shirvalkar [1,2,3,*], **Kristin K. Sellers** [2], **Ashlyn Schmitgen** [2], **Jordan Prosky** [1], **Isabella Joseph** [2], **Philip A. Starr** [2] **and Edward F. Chang** [2]

[1]   Department of Anesthesiology (Pain Management), University of California San Francisco, San Francisco, CA 94143, USA; Jordan.Prosky@ucsf.edu

[2]   Department of Neurological Surgery, University of California San Francisco, San Francisco, CA 94143, USA; Kristin.Sellers@ucsf.edu (K.K.S.); Ashlyn.Schmitgen@ucsf.edu (A.S.); Isabella.Joseph@ucsf.edu (I.J.); Philip.Starr@ucsf.edu (P.A.S.); Edward.Chang@ucsf.edu (E.F.C.)

[3]   Department of Neurology, University of California San Francisco, San Francisco, CA 94143, USA

*   Correspondence: Prasad.Shirvalkar@ucsf.edu

Abstract: Early studies of deep brain stimulation (DBS) for various neurological disorders involved a temporary trial period where implanted electrodes were externalized, in which the electrical contacts exiting the patient's brain are connected to external stimulation equipment, so that stimulation efficacy could be determined before permanent implant. As the optimal brain target sites for various diseases (i.e., Parkinson's disease, essential tremor) became better established, such trial periods have fallen out of favor. However, deep brain stimulation trial periods are experiencing a modern resurgence for at least two reasons: (1) studies of newer indications such as depression or chronic pain aim to identify new targets and (2) a growing interest in adaptive DBS tools necessitates neurophysiological recordings, which are often done in the peri-surgical period. In this review, we consider the possible approaches, benefits, and risks of such inpatient trial periods with a specific focus on developing new DBS therapies for chronic pain.

Keywords: deep brain stimulation; chronic pain; lead externalization; trial period; stereoEEG

1. Introduction

Deep brain stimulation (DBS), which involves the insertion of electrical leads into important cortical or subcortical structures to treat various neurological diseases, is often performed in a single surgery where the leads are subsequently connected to an implanted stimulator. Alternatively, DBS can be performed in a two-staged surgery where the leads (or electrodes) are first implanted, externalized (i.e., the non-neural side of the electrode exits the body), and connected to an external stimulator for a trial period to assess therapeutic benefit over 3–10 days. DBS trials with lead externalization have been used extensively over the last 50 years specifically for treating chronic pain [1–3]. Lead externalization permits inpatient testing of stimulation effects prior to permanent implantation, which is especially important for novel or unapproved DBS indications to ensure successful therapeutic response. This is especially important for diseases that encompass broad domains of symptoms spanning from neuropsychiatric to somatic, such as chronic pain syndromes. Because optimal brain targets for chronic pain are still unknown, such trials offer a key opportunity for the exploration and validation of both targets and pulse parameters that may modulate activity in multiple, relevant brain networks underlying various symptoms. Further, such a trial period allows the recording of neurophysiological activity from critical brain regions to further research and understand the mechanisms of action of stimulation. Modern recordings have aimed to uncover key biomarkers of chronic pain states toward the development of adaptive (or "closed-loop") control algorithms where stimulation delivery is adjusted in response to biomarkers to increase efficacy or avert the development of long-term tolerance.

Such trial periods that allow patients to "test drive" the neuromodulation therapy are used even when the general target regions are known, such as in spinal cord stimulation (SCS) [4]. A trial period is often necessary because of the large heterogeneity in patient response, to assess safety, and for the fine tuning of electrode position relative to the neural target so that patient benefit can be maximized before committing to an expensive therapy. It is worth pointing out that a short trial period to determine chronic brain stimulation targets assumes that an acute response to stimulation can be found (within minutes or hours of stimulation) and that these effects will translate to long-term efficacy. It remains to be determined whether this is the case for chronic pain.

The global burden of chronic pain is significant and growing alongside that of non-communicable diseases, which account for 78.6% of years lived with disability worldwide [5]. The economic impact of chronic neurological conditions such as chronic pain and epilepsy is greater than that of many other health conditions due to absenteeism, reduced levels of productivity, and increased risk of leaving labor markets, indicating that there is a significant indirect economic cost associated with these conditions [6]. Chronic pain also poses a significant cost to the healthcare system; analysis of a Canadian database indicates that the costs attributed to the healthcare of patients with painful neuropathic disorders were considerably higher than those in patients without chronic pain in the same age and sex demographics [6]. Perhaps most importantly, chronic neurological conditions have a significant debilitating effect on the overall quality of life of patients and are associated with some of the poorest quality-of-life indices, with the potential to impact social relationships, economic participation, and mental health. DBS for pain is still performed with a very limited trial period (off-label in the U.S.) resulting in highly variable success rates across patients.

In this review, we outline important considerations for DBS trial periods for chronic pain including possible brain targets for stimulating and recording. We then propose an argument for the use of stereoelectroencephalography (sEEG) in the trial and discuss possible trial related risks. An sEEG based approach is elaborated in the context of characterizing pain biomarkers and neurophysiological effects of stimulation. Finally, we offer practical advice for conducting a trial, including mitigating the placebo effect and rigorously ensuring therapeutic efficacy before permanent implantation.

2. Anatomical Targets/Considerations

Determining the optimal neural targets for stimulation-induced pain relief is a key goal of the DBS trial period. The trial period affords the opportunity to explore multiple pain-relevant brain regions based on pre-clinical and human experience to select the sites most appropriate for the pain syndrome and patient. In a survey of the current state of DBS for chronic pain, Farrell et al. focus on three prominent brain targets that have been tested most frequently: the ventral posterolateral/medial thalamus (VPL/VPM), the periventricular/periaqueductal grey (PVG/PAG), and the anterior cingulate cortex (ACC) across a wide variety of chronic pain syndromes [7]. Most studies highlighted in that review used a simple readout of somatic pain intensity (numeric or visual analog rating scale (NRS, VAS)); however, this approach fails to measure changes in the affective or cognitive domains of pain. Numerous other targets have been proposed such as motor cortex, ventral striatum, and insula. We will briefly discuss the most promising candidates below in the context of how these targets may offer pain relief across multiple dimensions of the pain experience. Importantly, the target efficacy for pain relief depends on the class of pain syndrome being treated and the unique qualities of the patient.

The motivation for treating intractable pain with brain surgery began with early results [8] demonstrating analgesia after thalamotomy and selective ablation. Following development by Mazars [9], Hosobuchi et al. used thalamic stimulation to produce successful masking of facial pain with electrically induced paresthesia in four of five patients, with pain relieving effects observed after a few minutes of stimulation [10]. Similar paresthesia-based analgesia for phantom limb pain has been reported previously [11]. Whereas VPL/VPM stimulation induces a phenomenon of purportedly "pleasant" paresthesia, PVG/PAG has been shown to induce a sense of warmth in painful areas. The pain relief following PAG/PVG stimulation has been attributed to the release of endogenous opioids as evidenced by abolished effect after naloxone [12]. In contrast, a study of 45 patients receiving chronic PAG or PVG stimulation for a wide variety of pain syndromes for one year demonstrated that despite the development of long-term tolerance to stimulation in twelve patients, there was no cross-tolerance with morphine [13]. This suggests that pain relief with PAG/PVG stimulation may not exclusively depend on an endogenous opioid mechanisms. Regardless, two large clinical trials evaluating combined VPL/PAG stimulation for chronic pain of various syndromes failed to meet therapeutic endpoints, though these studies were fraught with design and follow-up problems (see [14] for a discussion). Specifically, these trials targeted the same two brain regions across hundreds of patients with vastly different pain syndromes without placebo or randomized design. Notably, a significant portion of patients were lost to follow-up; the resulting patient attrition severely reduced power to detect a clinically meaningful effect and resulted in no significant benefit using an intention-to-treat analysis. These flaws highlight the need for individualized brain targeting based on etiology and the use of endpoints that measure multiple dimensions of pain.

Studies from Aziz and colleagues have ignited interest in targeting the affective dimension of pain by targeting the dorsal ACC. Patients suffering from a variety of chronic neuropathic pain syndromes were followed for up to 3 years, and significant benefit was found at the 6-month time point [2], though no significant effect was found on further follow-up. Further ACC stimulation at the wide pulse widths and high amplitudes required for analgesia was associated with de novo epilepsy in a handful of patients [15]. However, pain relief with ACC stimulation has been reported to have a long wash-in period (hours to 3 days), which may limit the ability to detect a beneficial effect in shorter timescales (however, see [16]). Nonetheless, the novelty of the ACC as a target has inspired a renewed interest in modulating the affective dimension of pain and basic research into pain-relevant mechanisms in the ACC. It is still unknown whether targeting other regions of the ACC may be beneficial for chronic pain despite functional imaging evidence that more anterior or posterior regions may be involved [16,17]; such alternative regions of the cingulate merit exploration for therapeutic DBS in a potential trial period.

Motor cortex stimulation (MCS) has also been studied for pain relief using both non-invasive [18] and direct cortical stimulation [19]. In a meta-analysis, 54% of 117 patients with central pain and 68% of 44 patients with trigeminal neuropathic pain experienced a greater than 40% reduction in pain scores, suggesting efficacy for neuropathic pain syndromes [20]. In contrast, double-blinded studies of MCS failed to show significant analgesia for the treatment of hemi-body post-stroke pain or post-herpetic neuralgia pain, while noting that patients suffering from facial pain and upper limb pain may obtain relief (e.g., see [21]). Potential mechanisms of analgesia resulting from MCS are still debated. Other targets such as the posterior insula have demonstrated increased thermal pain thresholds in epilepsy patients without chronic pain, though generalization to clinical pain states is unknown [22].

When selecting neural targets for deep brain stimulation trial periods, it is important to consider the specific type of chronic pain that the patient is suffering from. Certain types of pain such as facial and upper limb neuropathic pain may warrant targeting the contralateral motor cortex, while inflammatory pain syndromes may benefit relatively more from targeting the PAG. Stimulation of the ACC or insula are other potentially promising targets, though no systematic study has been able to demonstrate long-term pain relief through DBS, suggesting neural adaptation as a key obstacle. The only double-blind sham-controlled clinical trial for post-stroke pain targeted the ventral striatum/capsular region and aimed to mitigate the affective component of pain to improve pain-related disability [23]. At present, while there are numerous individual anecdotes of patients obtaining pain relief from the stimulation of various targets, there is a lack of clear evidence pointing to reliable targets for long-term pain relief. Advances in longitudinally stable pain biomarker detection will ideally inform next-generation closed-loop DBS therapy for chronic pain that may avert long-term tolerance [19,20,24].

The hope is that through individual "N-of-1" DBS trial periods, we may find brain targets that produce acute pain relief that further extends to longer time periods.

3. DBS Trial Period Safety and Risks

Trialing deep brain stimulation therapy in advance of a permanent implant can pose additional patient-specific and systemic risks both in relation to the surgery and potential success of this therapy as an option of last resort. Specifically, a DBS trial period may introduce the added risk of possible infection and additional costs of extended inpatient evaluation.

Beyond the risks from intracranial implantation, which can be mitigated with strict planning and surgical protocols, it is important to consider the costs of a temporary implant and inpatient trial period from a holistic perspective. For example, while we are studying the effects of DBS on pain, it is important to control for external factors, such as the effects of financial stress, social isolation, and physical restrictions that are associated with prolonged inpatient stay. However, by accounting for these effects, testing DBS in a temporary, resource-rich environment, and applying the predictive power of an inpatient trial, we may avoid the unnecessary financial and psychosocial burden of a long-term implant for unsuccessful trial patients. Thus, when assessing potential patients for DBS therapy for chronic pain, it is useful to consider the safety, appropriateness, fiscal neutrality, and effectiveness (SAFE) principles for neuromodulation therapies [25].

The SAFE (safety, appropriateness, fiscal neutrality, and effectiveness) principles can be used as an evidence-based algorithm to guide the selection of appropriate pain syndromes and DBS targets for individual patients. These principles further support using a minimally biased trial period to evaluate for benefit, similar to techniques used in SCS for chronic pain treatment. For example, studies using effective psychosocial screening for SCS trials produced a higher rate and longer duration of pain relief than studies in which no psychosocial screening was performed. Further, disregarding these psychosocial factors may increase the risk of injury to patients while creating unnecessary costs from ineffective therapeutic interventions. Thus, performing a well-designed, comprehensive inpatient trial in line with the SAFE principles, as described, can increase the chances of long-term success of DBS for chronic pain. By closely examining each of these guiding principles, as demonstrated below, both patients and researchers can perform a more thorough and personalized approach to trial DBS candidacy.

Safety: Reports of infection rates involved in temporary lead externalization have been mixed. An early single center, prospective analysis over a four-year period found an increased rate of infection when DBS for Parkinson's disease was performed using a staged procedure with externalization (15.3% vs. 4.2% for one-stage) [26]. However, in a two-stage surgical procedure, Rosa et al. found that lead externalization for 2–7 days did not increase post-operative infection risk following Stage I bilateral DBS lead implant when oral antibiotics were used for 5 days after Stage II lead extender and internal pulse generator (IPG) placement [27]. In this study of 105 patients, the rate of infection from this two-stage surgery (2.8%) was consistent with post-operative risk of infection in the literature. Bojanic et al. similarly observed no increased risk of infection when directly comparing externalized trial vs. one-stage DBS surgery [28]. Of 60 patients undergoing single-stage surgery, they observed 7 infections, while 86 patients undergoing an externalized trial resulted in 3 infections.

Appropriateness and efficacy: A temporary trial stage presents a measurable predictor of long-term clinical benefit. In order to ensure that the trial has realistic predictive value, however, it is critical to ensure a clinically meaningful benefit. Observation of a clinically significant benefit (a 12-point improvement on the 100-point visual analog scale [29]) relies on the consideration of intrinsic factors such as patient attentional biases, motivations, and study expectations. The expectation effects of pain or benefit from DBS can be understood through a motivation–decision model of pain, in which the threat of pain or promise of relief is a consequence of a computed decision to respond to or ignore this pain signal [30]. This is an especially important consideration when working with patients with chronic pain, who have been shown to bias expectations toward pain escape/avoidance and, thus, increase perceived pain intensity through top–down modulatory circuits. In fact, the patient's expectation of improvement at trial entry may be the single most robust predictor of reported pain reduction. Since anticipation of pain often becomes a self-fulfilling prophecy, addressing patient expectations should be incorporated into the trial plan. The trial stage presents an extended opportunity to use comprehensive psychosocial assessments, including the Structured Clinical Interview for DSM-5 (Diagnostic and Statistical Manual of Mental Disorders—Fifth Edition, SCID-5), Hamilton Depression Rating Scale, West Haven Yale Multidimensional Pain Inventory (WHYPI), Pain Catastrophizing Scale, Beck Depression Inventory, and Beck Anxiety Inventory, in addition to cognitive and behavioral testing to provide a more complete picture of patient outcomes.

Psychosocial components of pain, such as attention, culture, anxiety, and depression, similarly influence the perception of pain and the outcomes of therapies. Despite meeting all clinical criteria, sound surgical approaches, and even early signs of clinical benefit, a significant number of patients continue to fail neuromodulation therapy in the long term. This suggests that the inherent characteristics of patients are a strong factor in determining neuromodulation efficacy. Strict inclusion and exclusion criteria and extensive psychological evaluation are critical prior to trial enrollment [31]. Studies suggest that a comprehensive program consisting of pre-operative psychosocial assessment and consistent psychological and rehabilitative support throughout the trial phase and subsequent therapy are key elements for the success of neurostimulation.

Fiscal neutrality: Bojanic et al. found that despite the extra costs of seven additional inpatient days (up to £11,200), there were significant cost savings when compared to committing patients to a potentially ineffective implant (up to £147,000), particularly when the indication was chronic pain. At our institution, a similar DBS trial period of 7 days presents an actual cost of $34,000 including imaging, surgery, device, and inpatient costs ($150,000 billed to private insurance) versus a cost for a one-stage DBS implant of $90,000 ($203,000 billed to private insurance). With a trial to permanent implant conversion ratio of 50% (higher end), this represents a cost savings of up to $56,000 per every 2 patients ($53,000 when billed to private insurance). The concept of fiscal neutrality (maximizing the neuromodulation approach to be cost neutral in the long term), supports performing adequate trials for DBS for treating pain.

4. Motivation for a StereoEEG Trial in Patients with Chronic Pain

sEEG is most commonly used as a diagnostic tool for patients with refractory epilepsy. Localization of seizure onset zones is achieved using multi-contact depth electrodes, which are placed through burr holes targeting both cortical and deep structures of the brain. Continuous recording can provide a three-dimensional view of the origin and spread of epileptic seizures [32]. sEEG has been used to guide treatment of refractory epilepsy when non-invasive treatments such as pharmacology, diet, or other alternative therapeutic options are ineffectual. Similarly, we propose using sEEG in patients with chronic pain who have failed to achieve relief of symptoms with pharmacological interventions or spinal cord stimulators.

sEEG has been widely adopted internationally, with global studies generating extensive data in support of sEEG with potential synergistic applications in cognitive neurophysiology research. sEEG is an invasive monitoring technique, and a major concern is the potential for hemorrhagic complications, which can lead to neurological deficits or death. However, rates of clinically significant hemorrhage and other infections occur at much lower rates in sEEG compared to those in other neurophysiological surgical approaches (e.g., subdural strip and grid electrode implants). sEEG is often a highly efficacious and cost-efficient procedure with a low associated morbidity that has demonstrated success in network characterization for thousands of epilepsy patients worldwide.

sEEG is an appealing approach for neural circuit mapping and testing acute stimulation efficacy, which we propose can be used to identify optimal brain regions in candidate patients who are most likely to respond when a chronic DBS device is implanted. Specifically, for chronic pain, which engages multiple well-established nodes across a widespread pain network, an sEEG trial can be used to target multiple brain regions based on converging evidence from pre-clinical and human brain mapping studies (Figure 1, see Section 2, Anatomical Targets/Considerations). Similar prior efforts have been successful for epilepsy and even facilitated the development of new responsive brain stimulation therapy [33]. As sEEG is beneficial for intracranial investigations that require sampling from superficial and deep structures simultaneously across both hemispheres, we propose using sEEG as both a clinical tool and to advance research on the fundamental mechanisms of chronic pain processing in patients.

Figure 1. Stereoelectroencephalography (sEEG) targeting for deep brain stimulation (DBS) for chronic pain during the inpatient trial period. Top row depicts left lateral, posterior, and right lateral views in an example patient with post-stroke pain. Eight images across rows 2 and 3 depict individual electrode trajectories targeting labeled regions of interest. R/LSGC: right /left subgenual cingulate cortex, R/LACC: right/left anterior cingulate cortex, RVPN: right ventral posterior thalamic nucleus, LAINS: left anterior insula, LPINS: left posterior insula, LVCVS: left ventral capsule and ventral striatum.

The main benefit of sEEG over other approaches lies in the potential for focal stimulation combined with pain-related network discovery. Methods such as functional magnetic resonance imaging (fMRI) and magnetoencephalography (MEG) can be informative and useful in network discovery, potentially prior to a trial period, to discover optimal targets in each individual patient prior to electrode implantation. Regarding network discovery with other modalities, blood oxygen level dependent (BOLD) signals in fMRI can provide whole-brain localization and temporal tracking of neural activity correlated with pain states [34,35]. However, fMRI-based signals cannot be detected in the ambulatory setting, limiting their use in clinically relevant timescales for chronic pain therapy (however, see [36] for longitudinal fMRI). For example, due to the limitations of patient tolerance and equipment availability, fMRI cannot feasibly be used continuously over a period of hours, making it unrealistic for evaluating clinically relevant spontaneous pain fluctuations. Likewise, prior work has used simultaneous stimulation (with DBS or transcranial magnetic stimulation (TMS)) and recording with magnetoencephalography (MEG) [37] or scalp EEG [38] to identify predictive biomarkers of subjective pain experience without the associated risks of trial surgery. Studies evaluating network effects of DBS with EEG/MEG nonetheless require permanent DBS surgery, which poses greater risks than sEEG. Prior efforts to identify biomarkers of stimulation using TMS/EEG require averaging over larger volumes of tissue and can suffer more from stimulation artifact during simultaneous neural recording. Furthermore, TMS itself can be painful, confounding interpretation of any putative pain-relevant biomarkers. Non-invasive approaches remain an important complement to sEEG and, in theory, could even be used to identify key anatomical pain nodes in the future. For example, studies aiming to decode subjective pain intensity have been able to use MEG successfully to identify local field potential (LFP)-based biomarkers of pain, which are often reproducible within subjects [39];

such individualized MEG mapping may serve a useful pre-surgical step for target planning. While sEEG is limited by the number of electrodes and sampled regions per patient when compared to more global brain network approaches such as fMRI or MEG [40], it can better facilitate the characterization of biomarkers of clinical pain and stimulation with high spatiotemporal resolution.

5. Detecting Biomarkers of Chronic Pain and Stimulation-Related Pain Relief

While considerable effort has been devoted to identifying intracranial biomarkers of pain, the vast majority of studies to date have focused on experimental pain states in healthy individuals, which do not necessarily translate to altered brain dynamics seen in patients with chronic pain [34,41]. Rather than focusing exclusively on signatures of evoked pain, we suggest that studying the dynamics of spontaneous pain can be more informative. By further combining simultaneous recording and stimulation, it may be possible to dissociate neural correlates of the pain state from those of stimulation-related pain relief. Such converging evidence would help to develop practical approaches to personalized, adaptive neurostimulation.

5.1. Biomarkers of Chronic Pain and Network Discovery

Chronic pain is associated with both spontaneous and evoked pain, which are associated with distinct underlying brain activity. The chronic pain experience is almost certainly a network-wide phenomenon, but focusing on critical nodes of this network has pointed to brain regions that may harbor useful biomarkers [42]. fMRI studies provide evidence that brain activation patterns of sustained chronic pain states do not overlap with those of stimulus-evoked acute pain states in both patients and healthy subjects [43]. Baliki et al. found a double dissociation where sustained chronic low back pain in patients was associated with increased BOLD activity in the medial prefrontal cortex (mPFC) and rostral cingulate, while thermal experimental pain preferentially activated the insula both in patients and healthy controls. Further, the posterior thalamus and bilateral dorsolateral prefrontal cortex (DLPFC) exhibit atrophy over time in chronic pain [44]; pain-related activation of the DLPFC is also related to activity in the mPFC, but not in the insula [43]. The duration of experienced pain also influences brain representation of pain. Compared to patients experiencing subacute low back pain for only 2 months, patients with chronic back pain lasting >10 years show increased brain activity in the mPFC, orbitofrontal cortex, precuneus, and amygdala [45]. These authors and others have argued that the chronification of pain shifts brain representations from nociceptive to emotional circuits. Therefore, long-term chronic pain is associated with network-level changes in pain processing that cannot necessarily be inferred from solely studying evoked pain in healthy patients using experimental stimuli such as laser-evoked potentials or the thermal grill illusion. These data suggest that the sensory, cognitive, and emotional phenomenology of real-world chronic pain is distinct from that of experimentally induced pain. As such, the mPFC, rostral ACC, and DLPFC may be sensible targets to detect biomarkers of the chronic pain state.

Recordings of LFP from brain regions that are likely to harbor chronic-pain-relevant signals (e.g., mPFC, ACC, DLPFC) can be used to further understand mechanisms of pain and devise control strategies for closed-loop algorithms. Two brain stimulation devices with closed-loop functionality are current available: Neuropace® RNS (Neuropace, Mountain View, CA, USA) [46] and Medtronic® Percept (Medtronic, Minneapolis, MN, USA) (recently approved for sensing and stimulation [47] and full closed-loop functionality is anticipated soon). Theses device are capable of using neural power band-limited time series signals (e.g., alpha band power) as inputs to an embedded closed-loop controller that can modify stimulation parameters to optimize therapy. For this reason, we focus on band powers of interest that have previously been associated with predicting pain states.

Despite the limitations of interpreting biomarkers of acute/evoked pain state, there is an abundance of such data using sEEG, MEG, and EEG, which can provide a starting point. The most commonly reported neural features predictive of a high pain state have been a decrease in the central alpha band (8–12 Hz) power [48–50] and an increase in the parietal or prefrontal gamma band (>30 Hz) power [51,52]. Importantly, recent studies have distinguished neural correlates of painful stimuli from nonpainful stimuli, providing greater selectivity for pain states. Using sEEG, Liu et al. found significant evoked-pain-related cross-frequency coupling between theta (4–8 Hz) and gamma band activity in the amygdala and hippocampus, which can be tested for validity as a chronic pain biomarker [53]. While most studies of neural pain biomarkers seek to predict the pain VAS, it will be important for future research to identify what power bands may support different dimensions of pain (i.e., somatosensory, affective, cognitive) by analyzing alternative metrics (e.g., McGill Pain Questionnaire (MPQ) or pain unpleasantness). There remains a large gap in characterizing such power-band based biomarkers of naturalistic, spontaneous chronic pain; an sEEG trial can fill this gap. Ultimately, by combining recording with simultaneous stimulation in these areas, an sEEG trial period could inform adaptive DBS algorithms (for a thorough discussion of brain-based pain biomarkers see [42,54]).

5.2. Biomarkers of Stimulation-Induced Pain Relief

Beyond biomarkers that predict the chronic pain state, it is critical to characterize neural signals resulting from the electrical stimulation of various sites across many parameters. There are at least three strategies for detecting biomarkers of stimulation-induced pain relief. First, by recording LFPs from multiple brain regions either during or immediately after pain-relieving stimulation (see Section 6, Practical Considerations), spectral power within the frequency bands of interest can be compared to validate putative pain biomarkers that were detected in the absence of stimulation. For example, if ACC theta power was positively correlated with a high reported pain state, therapeutic stimulation would be expected to decrease ACC theta power if this biomarker was causal. Such a biomarker could be incorporated into a closed-loop algorithm using a simple threshold; for example, one algorithm could initiate stimulation when ACC theta power increased beyond some prespecified threshold power value. Second, neural activity in certain frequencies recorded at the site of stimulation may help predict whether and when stimulation may be beneficial. In a notable study, mechanistic evidence supporting the VPL/M as a target for both recording and stimulation was provided by Huang et al. in thirteen patients with chronic pain [55]. Distinct thalamic theta, alpha, high beta, and high gamma oscillations were correlated with pain relief and, thereby, suggested possible biomarkers by which one may identify individual patients who may benefit from VPL/M stimulation. Third, simultaneous recordings across multiple electrodes could provide a readout of functional connectivity in the pain network, which could be "pinged" by delivering intermittent single-pulse electrical stimulation (SPES) at various sites. SPES has previously been used to probe cortico-cortical connections and intra-areal plasticity by averaging LFP time-locked to the stimuli using sEEG in epilepsy patients [56]. The averaged LFP reflects cortico-cortical evoked potentials that can be recorded in adjacent and remote sites during periods of high and low pain states to provide a connectome representation of network changes related to chronic pain. Similar biomarkers of stimulation-induced pain relief can help to narrow down final candidate brain targets for permanent DBS implantation.

6. Practical Considerations for Chronic Pain DBS Trial Period

There are numerous factors to consider in the experimental design of a trial period: the duration of a trial period, how many patients to enroll, and outcome metrics of interest. Indeed, prior studies of DBS and chronic pain may have failed to reach primary endpoints because of nonrandomized design, heterogeneous patient populations, subjective assessment of patient outcomes, lack of measuring "meaningful" changes in symptoms, inconsistencies in sites stimulated, and other factors (see review [7]). Practical considerations should not be left to last minute planning. Common understanding of goals and procedures is needed across clinical specialties including neurological surgery, neurology, and pain management. The research team must work closely with neurosurgeons to map the targeting of electrodes for implantation; the administration of pain medications must be coordinated across pain providers, nursing staff, and research team so testing can be timed appropriately; patient care assistants and monitoring staff must be appraised of patient needs that differ from standard inpatient care on their unit; and research staff not accustomed to inpatient care must be oriented to the environment. We have found that participating in nursing staff meetings prior to patient implant is an effective way to coordinate activities and communicate DBS trial period goals between research staff, clinical personnel, and candidate patients.

The overall duration of implant for each patient should carefully weigh experimental need, insertional effect, patient tolerance, and infection risk (discussed further above). Experimental need can be broken down into multiple categories: resting-state biomarker discovery, stimulation efficacy, and modulation of task performance (task-based biomarker discovery/stimulation effects on task performance). Further, the insertional effect, or stun effect, which has been well-studied in Parkinson's disease patients undergoing trial periods for DBS, can often be described as a temporary improvement in disease symptoms in response to DBS lead placement [57]. The positive effect can often persist 6 months following surgical implantation and before the onset of stimulation. The insertional effect has been similarly described in chronic pain patients, in which some patients (43% of 21 patients) experience a substantial reduction in their pain immediately following lead implant [58]. While the cause and predisposing conditions of this insertional effect are not well understood, Hamani et al. found that a positive insertional effect was correlated with a successful stimulation period.

An emerging trend has been to use the inpatient DBS trial period to both test stimulation and record neural activity that may guide biomarker discovery toward developing closed-loop DBS algorithms. Resting-state biomarker discovery is best served by recording periods of brain activity during wakefulness in the absence of stimulation or tasks and across varying levels of reported pain metrics. Level of pain may be assessed using a collection of surveys or verbal reports that are repeatedly administered throughout the trial period. The dynamics of subjective pain experience varies widely across patients and pain subtypes [59]. As the timescale of pain predictability based on neural activity is relatively unknown, we opt to study brain activity for relatively long periods (e.g., 30 min) around each survey point to provide a starting point on studying individual dynamics/timescales. Each time a survey is administered translates to one data point; this should be repeated multiple times throughout the entire trial period. At least 10 data points, but preferably many more, are needed for a statistically valid association of neural activity with the symptom reports, necessitating a total trial duration of at least 3 days.

Evaluating for stimulation efficacy should involve testing at least two different stimulation locations and various parameters in order to identify putative therapeutic targets for permanent implant. Two critical factors should be considered during the design of stimulation efficacy testing: placebo effect and expected wash-in and wash-out durations. The placebo effect is an important confounder during DBS [60], and while it may be advantageous in the long-term treatment of chronic pain, care should be taken to control for short-term placebo effect during trial DBS. In order to account for this, double-blind, sham-controlled stimulation testing is needed. By design, when using clinically approved devices, the operator of the stimulator cannot be blinded to the stimulation condition. Thus, during double-blind stimulation testing, the individual operating the DBS stimulator should not interact with the patient in any way, and ideally should not be visible to the patient. All other people in the room (including the patient) should be blinded to the stimulation condition. Furthermore, it can be useful for all other people in the room and the patient to be naïve of stimulation (sham) onset and offset times. This may further mitigate expectation or anxiety associated with anticipated effects of stimulation, which may offer better predictive value of long-term success. Having a sham block paired with each verum stimulation block doubles testing time but provides more robust and interpretable results. If possible, having the patient self-administer surveys at cued times, with no researchers in the room, may also decrease Hawthorne effects [61]. This may not always be feasible due to safety considerations and the need for active monitoring of intracranial recordings during stimulation. The duration of stimulation and the wash-out period between testing sham/verum blocks or between stimulation locations should be determined as a function of expected wash-in and wash-out effects. While stimulation of some targets such as the VPL or PAG can produce rapid pain relief over seconds to minutes, the ACC or other sites may have much longer wash-in times over days. This remains an area of active investigation and varies as a function of disease duration and specific behavior/symptom assessed [16,62–64]. Longer wash-out periods provide more confidence that effects observed for subsequent stimulation parameters cannot be attributed to carryover effects from prior stimulation conditions. All candidate stimulation targets should be tested multiple times, so counterbalancing test order can also help mitigate carryover effects. Early in target discovery, it may be beneficial to stimulate different parameters within the same region (e.g., low vs. high pulse width or frequency) with shorter wash out; if a candidate brain region or parameter set for therapeutic efficacy is found, it is useful to retest it with longer wash out.

Recording neural activity during behavioral tasks, in the presence and absence of stimulation, can serve multiple purposes. Specifically, we propose using behavioral tasks that systematically assess various domains of the pain experience including somatic, affective, and cognitive ones. Tasks that are particularly relevant include quantitative sensory testing with thermal stimuli including pain thresholds [65] and mechanical pain thresholds with Von Frey filaments [66] (somatic); the emotional Stroop [67] and emotional facial recognition tasks (affective judgment and interference); and the oddball [68]; and Iowa gambling tasks [69] (cognitive attention and decision making). Task-based biomarkers can be used to track symptom status and treatment efficacy or identify brain regions that may be best targeted by stimulation for therapeutic benefit [70]. Machine learning methods can be applied to identify spectral properties that could serve as biomarkers for specific symptoms or induced states [71]. Variation in task performance may also more directly indicate the efficacy of stimulation. In order to make such conclusions, patients must be familiarized with tasks in order to prevent test–retest effects from skewing the results. Initial familiarization with tasks can be conducted prior to implant. Following implantation, tasks must be conducted multiple times (e.g., with and without stimulation) in order to determine baseline activity vs. potential changes induced by stimulation.

Not to be underestimated, patient tolerance and ability to actively participate during the trial period is critical for success. Detailed informed consent, ideally implementing teach-to-goal methods [72], should include clearly detailed information about what to expect during the trial period. In addition, we have found that having the patient complete questionnaire surveys (similar to those subsequently administered during the trial period) in his/her home environment prior to implant can decrease frustration with completing the same metric repeatedly. Continued clear communication with the patient and family members is vital. Having well-defined times when family members can visit or share a meal provides needed breaks in long days of testing. The depth of scientific discussion will need to be tailored to each patient's interest and level of understanding, but overall, we have found that patients are much more engaged when they clearly understand the need for each study and the role each test plays in the larger picture.

The selection of which metrics should be administered to assess pain and how often is again tied to both scientific need and patient tolerability. Patients experience survey fatigue in answering the same surveys repeatedly (e.g., upward of 50 times a day), which can hinder accurate communication of symptoms. Individual patents also differ in their adeptness of communicating pain through numeric ratings, free speech dialog, pain maps [73], or standardized surveys. Different methods of collecting information about pain symptoms also tap into different aspects of the pain experience [74], such as quantitative pain measures (e.g., numerical rating), pain experience (e.g., unpleasant sensory or emotional experience), and pain expression (e.g., qualitative words, pain narrative, and behavior to communicate pain, pain behavior). We found that a combination of metrics was the most useful, with short versions administered more frequently and long versions administered about three times per day.

When deciding how many people to enroll in a trial period, overall expense, and expected trial to permanent conversion ratio must be taken into consideration. Expense (both in time and money) impose a cap on the total number of patients who can be enrolled. A meta-analysis review of spinal cord stimulation showed a 41% conversion ratio from a trial period to a permanent implant [4]. While a higher conversion ratio may seem preferable, imposing increasingly strict inclusion criteria on a trial period may prevent testing in a broader population who could ultimately benefit from the therapy. Regardless, given the intensiveness of the trial period and subsequent management of patients with implanted devices, the size of DBS trials for chronic pain will likely remain small (<30 individuals) for the foreseeable future, until the therapy is sufficiently developed to obtain regulatory approval.

Lastly, we must balance the goal of full mechanistic understanding of neural circuitry underlying chronic pain vs. the identification of effective therapy. It is not practical to require the former as a prerequisite for providing treatment options for patients currently suffering from chronic pain. Rather, we recommend incorporating our current knowledge of pain circuits and using this as a starting point for where to implant electrodes for biomarker discovery. This approach has the benefit of not only being ready for implementation now but also being mechanistically informed according to current state of knowledge. Existing therapies, including spinal cord stimulation, have been shown to be effective at alleviating chronic pain in many individuals, but the mechanisms remain debated. Most important for clinical treatment is the efficacy of the therapy. While the number of patients implanted remains modest, it is likely more feasible to focus on a more individualized approach. Recording from implicated regions affords the relatively rare opportunity to identify correlative or causal factors that predict pain or pain relief in individual subjects. However, as the cohort of patients grow, looking for trends across patients will be incredibly valuable to determine whether patients share common biomarker features. This may be particularly fruitful to separate cohorts with different pain etiologies, pain dynamics, or even based on syndrome subtypes.

Author Contributions: Conceptualization P.S., E.F.C., and P.A.S.; writing—review and editing, P.S., K.K.S., A.S., J.P., I.J., E.F.C., and P.A.S.; funding acquisition, P.A.S., E.C., and P.S. All authors have read and agreed to the published version of the manuscript.

References

1. Ben-Haim, S.; Mirzadeh, Z.; Rosenberg, W.S. Deep brain stimulation for intractable neuropathic facial pain. *Neurosurg. Focus* **2018**, *45*, E15. [CrossRef]
2. Boccard, S.G.J.; Pereira, E.A.C.; Moir, L.; Aziz, T.Z.; Green, A.L. Long-term Outcomes of Deep Brain Stimulation for Neuropathic Pain. *Neurosurgery* **2013**, *72*, 221–231. [CrossRef]
3. Levy, R.M.; Lamb, S.; Adams, J.E. Treatment of chronic pain by deep brain stimulation: Long term follow-up and review of the literature. *Neurosurgery* **1987**, *21*, 885–893. [CrossRef]
4. Huang, K.T.; Martin, J.; Marky, A.; Chagoya, G.; Hatef, J.; Hazzard, M.A.; Thomas, S.M.; Lokhnygina, Y.; Lad, S.P. A National Survey of Spinal Cord Stimulation Trial-to-Permanent Conversion Rates. *Neuromodul. Technol. Neural Interface* **2015**, *18*, 133–140. [CrossRef]
5. Jackson, T.; Thomas, S.; Stabile, V.; Shotwell, M.; Han, X.; McQueen, K. A Systematic Review and Meta-Analysis of the Global Burden of Chronic Pain without Clear Etiology in Low- and Middle-Income Countries: Trends in Heterogeneous Data and a Proposal for New Assessment Methods. *Anesth. Analg.* **2016**, *123*, 739–748. [CrossRef]
6. Phillips, C.J. The Cost and Burden of Chronic Pain. *Rev. Pain* **2009**, *3*, 2–5. [CrossRef]
7. Farrell, S.; Green, A.; Aziz, T. The Current State of Deep Brain Stimulation for Chronic Pain and Its Context in Other Forms of Neuromodulation. *Brain Sci.* **2018**, *8*, 158. [CrossRef]
8. Pool, J.L. Psychosurgery in Older People. *J. Am. Geriatr. Soc.* **1954**, *2*, 456–466. [CrossRef]
9. Mazars, G.; Roge, R.; Mazars, Y. Results of the stimulation of the spinothalamic fasciculus and their bearing on the physiopathology of pain. *Rev. Neurol.* **1960**, *103*, 136–138.
10. Hosobuchi, Y.; Adams, J.E.; Rutkin, B. Chronic Thalamic Stimulation for the Control of Facial Anesthesia Dolorosa. *Arch. Neurol.* **1973**, *29*, 158–161. [CrossRef]
11. Nandi, D.; Yianni, J.; Humphreys, J.; Wang, S.; O'sullivan, V.; Shepstone, B.; Stein, J.F.; Aziz, T.Z. Phantom limb pain relieved with different modalities of central nervous system stimulation: A clinical and functional imaging case report of two patients. *Neuromodul. J. Int. Neuromodul. Soc.* **2004**, *7*, 176–183. [CrossRef]

12. Adams, J.E. Naloxone reversal of analgesia produced by brain stimulation in the human. *Pain* **1976**, *2*, 161–166. [CrossRef]
13. Young, R.F.; Chambi, V.I. Pain relief by electrical stimulation of the periaqueductal and periventricular gray matter: Evidence for a non-opioid mechanism. *J. Neurosurg.* **1987**, *66*, 364–371. [CrossRef]
14. Coffey, R.J. Deep brain stimulation for chronic pain: Results of two multicenter trials and a structured review. *Pain Med. Malden Mass* **2001**, *2*, 183–192. [CrossRef]
15. Maslen, H.; Cheeran, B.; Pugh, J.; Pycroft, L.; Boccard, S.; Prangnell, S.; Green, A.L.; FitzGerald, J.; Savulescu, J.; Aziz, T. Unexpected Complications of Novel Deep Brain Stimulation Treatments: Ethical Issues and Clinical Recommendations. *Neuromodul. Technol. Neural Interface* **2018**, *21*, 135–143. [CrossRef] [PubMed]
16. Bijanki, K.R.; Manns, J.R.; Inman, C.S.; Choi, K.S.; Harati, S.; Pedersen, N.P.; Drane, D.L.; Waters, A.C.; Fasano, R.E.; Mayberg, H.S.; et al. Cingulum stimulation enhances positive affect and anxiolysis to facilitate awake craniotomy. *J. Clin. Investig.* **2019**, *129*. [CrossRef] [PubMed]
17. Spisak, T.; Kincses, B.; Schlitt, F.; Zunhammer, M.; Schmidt-Wilcke, T.; Kincses, Z.T.; Bingel, U. Pain-free resting-state functional brain connectivity predicts individual pain sensitivity. *Nat. Commun.* **2020**, *11*, 187. [CrossRef]
18. Lefaucheur, J.-P.; Drouot, X.; Cunin, P.; Bruckert, R.; Lepetit, H.; Créange, A.; Wolkenstein, P.; Maison, P.; Keravel, Y.; Nguyen, J.-P. Motor cortex stimulation for the treatment of refractory peripheral neuropathic pain. *Brain* **2009**, *132*, 1463–1471. [CrossRef] [PubMed]
19. Nandi, D.; Smith, H.; Owen, S.; Joint, C.; Stein, J.; Aziz, T. Peri-ventricular grey stimulation versus motor cortex stimulation for post stroke neuropathic pain. *J. Clin. Neurosci.* **2002**, *9*, 557–561. [CrossRef]
20. Fontaine, D.; Hamani, C.; Lozano, A. Efficacy and safety of motor cortex stimulation for chronic neuropathic pain: Critical review of the literature: Clinical article. *J. Neurosurg.* **2009**, *110*, 251–256. [CrossRef]
21. Nguyen, J.-P.; Velasco, F.; Brugières, P.; Velasco, M.; Keravel, Y.; Boleaga, B.; Brito, F.; Lefaucheur, J.-P. Treatment of chronic neuropathic pain by motor cortex stimulation: Results of a bicentric controlled crossover trial. *Brain Stimulat.* **2008**, *1*, 89–96. [CrossRef] [PubMed]
22. Denis, D.J.; Marouf, R.; Rainville, P.; Bouthillier, A.; Nguyen, D.K. Effects of insular stimulation on thermal nociception. *Eur. J. Pain* **2016**, *20*, 800–810. [CrossRef] [PubMed]
23. Lempka, S.F.; Malone, D.A.; Hu, B.; Baker, K.B.; Wyant, A.; Ozinga, J.G.; Plow, E.B.; Pandya, M.; Kubu, C.S.; Ford, P.J.; et al. Randomized clinical trial of deep brain stimulation for poststroke pain. *Ann. Neurol.* **2017**, *81*, 653–663. [CrossRef] [PubMed]
24. Shirvalkar, P.; Veuthey, T.L.; Dawes, H.E.; Chang, E.F. Closed-Loop Deep Brain Stimulation for Refractory Chronic Pain. *Front. Comput. Neurosci.* **2018**, *12*. [CrossRef]
25. Krames, E.S.; Monis, S.; Poree, L.; Deer, T.; Levy, R. Using the SAFE principles when evaluating electrical stimulation therapies for the pain of failed back surgery syndrome. *Neuromodul. J. Int. Neuromodul. Soc.* **2011**, *14*, 299–311, discussion 311. [CrossRef]
26. Constantoyannis, C.; Berk, C.; Honey, C.R.; Mendez, I.; Brownstone, R.M. Reducing hardware-related complications of deep brain stimulation. *Can. J. Neurol. Sci. J. Can. Sci. Neurol.* **2005**, *32*, 194–200. [CrossRef]
27. Rosa, M.; Scelzo, E.; Locatelli, M.; Carrabba, G.; Levi, V.; Arlotti, M.; Barbieri, S.; Rampini, P.; Priori, A. Risk of Infection After Local Field Potential Recording from Externalized Deep Brain Stimulation Leads in Parkinson's Disease. *World Neurosurg.* **2017**, *97*, 64–69. [CrossRef]
28. Bojanic, S.; Sethi, H.; Hyam, J.; Yianni, J.; Nandi, D.; Joint, C.; Carter, H.; Gregory, R.; Bain, P.; Aziz, T.Z. Externalising deep brain electrodes: An increased risk of infection? *J. Clin. Neurosci.* **2004**, *11*, 732–734. [CrossRef]
29. Hawker, G.A.; Mian, S.; Kendzerska, T.; French, M. Measures of adult pain: Visual Analog Scale for Pain (VAS Pain), Numeric Rating Scale for Pain (NRS Pain), McGill Pain Questionnaire (MPQ), Short-Form McGill Pain Questionnaire (SF-MPQ), Chronic Pain Grade Scale (CPGS), Short Form-36 Bodily Pain Scale (SF-36 BPS), and Measure of Intermittent and Constant Osteoarthritis Pain (ICOAP). *Arthritis Care Res.* **2011**, *63*, S240–S252. [CrossRef]
30. Fields, H.L. How expectations influence pain. *Pain* **2018**, *159* (Suppl. 1), S3–S10. [CrossRef]
31. Beltrutti, D.; Lamberto, A.; Barolat, G.; Bruehl, S.P.; Doleys, D.; Krames, E.; Meglio, M.; North, R.; Olson, K.; Reig, E.; et al. The Psychological Assessment of Candidates for Spinal Cord Stimulation for Chronic Pain Management. *Pain Pract.* **2004**, *4*, 204–221. [CrossRef] [PubMed]

32.   Almeida, A.N.; de Olivier, A.; Quesney, F.; Dubeau, F.; Savard, G.; Andermann, F. Efficacy of and morbidity associated with stereoelectroencephalography using computerized tomography—Or magnetic resonance imaging—Guided electrode implantation. *J. Neurosurg.* **2006**, *104*, 483–487. [CrossRef] [PubMed]

33.   Kossoff, E.H.; Ritzl, E.K.; Politsky, J.M.; Murro, A.M.; Smith, J.R.; Duckrow, R.B.; Spencer, D.D.; Bergey, G.K. Effect of an external responsive neurostimulator on seizures and electrographic discharges during subdural electrode monitoring. *Epilepsia* **2004**, *45*, 1560–1567. [CrossRef] [PubMed]

34.   Wager, T.D.; Atlas, L.Y.; Lindquist, M.A.; Roy, M.; Woo, C.-W.; Kross, E. An fMRI-Based Neurologic Signature of Physical Pain. *N. Engl. J. Med.* **2013**, *368*, 1388–1397. [CrossRef] [PubMed]

35.   Rosa, M.J.; Seymour, B. Decoding the matrix: Benefits and limitations of applying machine learning algorithms to pain neuroimaging. *Pain* **2014**, *155*, 864–867. [CrossRef]

36.   Apkarian, A.V.; Baliki, M.N.; Farmer, M.A. Predicting transition to chronic pain. *Curr. Opin. Neurol.* **2013**, *26*, 360–367. [CrossRef]

37.   Gopalakrishnan, R.; Burgess, R.C.; Malone, D.A.; Lempka, S.F.; Gale, J.T.; Floden, D.P.; Baker, K.B.; Machado, A.G. Deep brain stimulation of the ventral striatal area for poststroke pain syndrome: A magnetoencephalography study. *J. Neurophysiol.* **2018**, *119*, 2118–2128. [CrossRef]

38.   Lefaucheur, J.-P.; Jarry, G.; Drouot, X.; Ménard-Lefaucheur, I.; Keravel, Y.; Nguyen, J.-P. Motor cortex rTMS reduces acute pain provoked by laser stimulation in patients with chronic neuropathic pain. *Clin. Neurophysiol.* **2010**, *121*, 895–901. [CrossRef]

39.   Gross, J.; Schnitzler, A.; Timmerman, L.; Ploner, M. Gamma oscillations in human primary somatosensory cortex reflect pain perception. *PLoS Biol.* **2007**, *5*. [CrossRef]

40.   Bartolomei, F.; Lagarde, S.; Wendling, F.; McGonigal, A.; Jirsa, V.; Guye, M.; Benar, C. Defining epileptogenic networks: Contribution of SEEG and signal analysis. *Epilepsia* **2017**, *58*, 1131–1147. [CrossRef]

41.   Coghill, R.C.; McHaffie, J.G.; Yen, Y.-F. Neural correlates of interindividual differences in the subjective experience of pain. *Proc. Natl. Acad. Sci. USA* **2003**, *100*, 8538–8542. [CrossRef] [PubMed]

42.   Tracey, I.; Woolf, C.J.; Andrews, N.A. Composite Pain Biomarker Signatures for Objective Assessment and Effective Treatment. *Neuron* **2019**, *101*, 783–800. [CrossRef] [PubMed]

43.   Baliki, M.N.; Chialvo, D.R.; Geha, P.Y.; Levy, R.M.; Harden, N.; Parrish, T.B.; Apkarian, A.V. Chronic Pain and the Emotional Brain: Specific Brain Activity Associated with Spontaneous Fluctuations of Intensity of Chronic Back Pain. *J. Neurosci.* **2006**, *26*, 12165–12173. [CrossRef] [PubMed]

44.   Apkarian, A.V.; Sosa, Y.; Sonty, S.; Levy, R.M.; Harden, R.N.; Parrish, T.B.; Gitelman, D.R. Chronic Back Pain Is Associated with Decreased Prefrontal and Thalamic Gray Matter Density. *J. Neurosci.* **2004**, *24*, 10410–10415. [CrossRef] [PubMed]

45.   Hashmi, J.A.; Baliki, M.A.; Huang, L.; Baria, A.T.; Torbey, S.; Hermann, K.M.; Schnitzer, T.J.; Apkarian, A.V. Shape shifting pain: Chronification of back pain shifts brain representation from nociceptive to emotional circuits. *Brain* **2013**, *136*, 2751–2768. [CrossRef]

46.   Sun, F.T.; Morrell, M.J. The RNS System: Responsive cortical stimulation for the treatment of refractory partial epilepsy. *Expert Rev. Med. Devices* **2014**, *11*, 563–572. [CrossRef]

47.   Medtronic FDA Approves Percept DBS Device. Available online: https://www.medtronic.com/us-en/about/news/fda-approval-percept.html (accessed on 20 September 2020).

48.   Ploner, M.; Gross, J.; Timmermann, L.; Pollok, B.; Schnitzler, A. Oscillatory activity reflects the excitability of the human somatosensory system. *NeuroImage* **2006**, *32*, 1231–1236. [CrossRef]

49.   Mouraux, A.; Guérit, J.M.; Plaghki, L. Non-phase locked electroencephalogram (EEG) responses to CO_2 laser skin stimulations may reflect central interactions between A partial partial differential- and C-fibre afferent volleys. *Clin. Neurophysiol. Off. J. Int. Fed. Clin. Neurophysiol.* **2003**, *114*, 710–722. [CrossRef]

50.   Babiloni, C.; Brancucci, A.; Del Percio, C.; Capotosto, P.; Arendt-Nielsen, L.; Chen, A.C.N.; Rossini, P.M. Anticipatory electroencephalography alpha rhythm predicts subjective perception of pain intensity. *J. Pain Off. J. Am. Pain Soc.* **2006**, *7*, 709–717. [CrossRef]

51.   Zhang, Z.G.; Hu, L.; Hung, Y.S.; Mouraux, A.; Iannetti, G.D. Gamma-Band Oscillations in the Primary Somatosensory Cortex—A Direct and Obligatory Correlate of Subjective Pain Intensity. *J. Neurosci.* **2012**, *32*, 7429–7438. [CrossRef]

52.   Chien, J.H.; Liu, C.C.; Kim, J.H.; Markman, T.M.; Lenz, F.A. Painful cutaneous laser stimuli induce event-related oscillatory EEG activities that are different from those induced by nonpainful electrical stimuli. *J. Neurophysiol.* **2014**, *112*, 824–833. [CrossRef] [PubMed]

53. Liu, C.C.; Chien, J.H.; Kim, J.H.; Chuang, Y.F.; Cheng, D.T.; Anderson, W.; Lenz, F.A. Cross-frequency coupling in deep brain structures upon processing the painful sensory inputs. *Neuroscience* **2015**, *303*, 412–421. [CrossRef] [PubMed]

54. Davis, K.D.; Aghaeepour, N.; Ahn, A.H.; Angst, M.S.; Borsook, D.; Brenton, A.; Burczynski, M.E.; Crean, C.; Edwards, R.; Gaudilliere, B.; et al. Discovery and validation of biomarkers to aid the development of safe and effective pain therapeutics: Challenges and opportunities. *Nat. Rev. Neurol.* **2020**, *16*, 381. [CrossRef] [PubMed]

55. Huang, Y.; Green, A.L.; Hyam, J.; Fitzgerald, J.; Aziz, T.Z.; Wang, S. Oscillatory neural representations in the sensory thalamus predict neuropathic pain relief by deep brain stimulation. *Neurobiol. Dis.* **2018**, *109*, 117–126. [CrossRef]

56. Matsumoto, R.; Kunieda, T.; Nair, D. Single pulse electrical stimulation to probe functional and pathological connectivity in epilepsy. *Seizure Eur. J. Epilepsy* **2017**, *44*, 27–36. [CrossRef]

57. Mestre, T.A.; Lang, A.E.; Okun, M.S. Factors influencing the outcome of deep brain stimulation: Placebo, nocebo, lessebo, and lesion effects. *Mov. Disord.* **2016**, *31*, 290–298. [CrossRef]

58. Hamani, C.; Schwalb, J.M.; Rezai, A.R.; Dostrovsky, J.O.; Davis, K.D.; Lozano, A.M. Deep brain stimulation for chronic neuropathic pain: Long-term outcome and the incidence of insertional effect. *Pain* **2006**, *125*, 188–196. [CrossRef]

59. Foss, J.M.; Apkarian, A.V.; Chialvo, D.R. Dynamics of Pain: Fractal Dimension of Temporal Variability of Spontaneous Pain Differentiates Between Pain States. *J. Neurophysiol.* **2006**, *95*, 730–736. [CrossRef]

60. Mercado, R.; Constantoyannis, C.; Mandat, T.; Kumar, A.; Schulzer, M.; Stoessl, A.J.; Honey, C.R. Expectation and the placebo effect in Parkinson's disease patients with subthalamic nucleus deep brain stimulation. *Mov. Disord. Off. J. Mov. Disord. Soc.* **2006**, *21*, 1457–1461. [CrossRef]

61. McCambridge, J.; Witton, J.; Elbourne, D.R. Systematic review of the Hawthorne effect: New concepts are needed to study research participation effects. *J. Clin. Epidemiol.* **2014**, *67*, 267–277. [CrossRef]

62. Cooper, S.E.; McIntyre, C.C.; Fernandez, H.H.; Vitek, J.L. Association of Deep Brain Stimulation Washout Effects with Parkinson Disease Duration. *JAMA Neurol.* **2013**, *70*, 95–99. [CrossRef] [PubMed]

63. Cooper, S.E.; Driesslein, K.G.; Noecker, A.M.; McIntyre, C.C.; Machado, A.M.; Butson, C.R. Anatomical targets associated with abrupt versus gradual washout of subthalamic deep brain stimulation effects on bradykinesia. *PLoS ONE* **2014**, *9*, e99663. [CrossRef] [PubMed]

64. Perera, T.; Yohanandan, S.A.C.; Vogel, A.P.; McKay, C.M.; Jones, M.; Peppard, R.; McDermott, H.J. Deep brain stimulation wash-in and wash-out times for tremor and speech. *Brain Stimul. Basic Transl. Clin. Res. Neuromodul.* **2015**, *8*, 359. [CrossRef]

65. Rolke, R.; Magerl, W.; Campbell, K.A.; Schalber, C.; Caspari, S.; Birklein, F.; Treede, R.D. Quantitative sensory testing: A comprehensive protocol for clinical trials. *Eur. J. Pain* **2006**, *10*, 77–88. [CrossRef]

66. Dualé, C.; Daveau, J.; Cardot, J.-M.; Boyer-Grand, A.; Schoeffler, P.; Dubray, C. Cutaneous Amitriptyline in Human VolunteersDifferential Effects on the Components of Sensory Information. *Anesthesiol. J. Am. Soc. Anesthesiol.* **2008**, *108*, 714–721. [CrossRef]

67. Andersson, G.; Haldrup, D. Personalized pain words and Stroop interference in chronic pain patients. *Eur. J. Pain* **2003**, *7*, 431–438. [CrossRef]

68. Fichtenholtz, H.M.; Dean, H.L.; Dillon, D.G.; Yamasaki, H.; McCarthy, G.; LaBar, K.S. Emotion–attention network interactions during a visual oddball task. *Cogn. Brain Res.* **2004**, *20*, 67–80. [CrossRef]

69. Bechara, A.; Damasio, A.R.; Damasio, H.; Anderson, S.W. Insensitivity to future consequences following damage to human prefrontal cortex. *Cognition* **1994**, *50*, 7–15. [CrossRef]

70. Reckziegel, D.; Vachon-Presseau, E.; Petre, B.; Schnitzer, T.J.; Baliki, M.; Apkarian, A.V. Deconstructing biomarkers for chronic pain: Context and hypothesis dependent biomarker types in relation to chronic pain. *Pain* **2019**, *160*, S37–S48. [CrossRef]

71. Vijayakumar, V.; Case, M.; Shirinpour, S.; He, B. Quantifying and Characterizing Tonic Thermal Pain Across Subjects From EEG Data Using Random Forest Models. *IEEE Trans. Biomed. Eng.* **2017**, *64*, 2988–2996. [CrossRef]

72. Chiong, W.; Leonard, M.K.; Chang, E.F. Neurosurgical Patients as Human Research Subjects: Ethical Considerations

in Intracranial Electrophysiology Research. *Neurosurgery* **2018**, *83*, 29–37. [CrossRef] [PubMed]

73. Andreassen Jaatun, E.A.; Hjermstad, M.J.; Gundersen, O.E.; Oldervoll, L.; Kaasa, S.; Haugen, D.F. Development and Testing of a Computerized Pain Body Map in Patients With Advanced Cancer. *J. Pain Symptom Manag.* **2014**, *47*, 45–56. [CrossRef] [PubMed]

74. Wideman, T.H.; Edwards, R.R.; Walton, D.M.; Martel, M.O.; Hudon, A.; Seminowicz, D.A. The Multimodal Assessment Model of Pain. *Clin. J. Pain* **2019**, *35*, 212–221. [CrossRef] [PubMed]

## 7

Bilateral Subthalamic Nucleus Deep Brain Stimulation under General Anesthesia

Hye Ran Park [1], Yong Hoon Lim [2], Eun Jin Song [2], Jae Meen Lee [3], Kawngwoo Park [4], Kwang Hyon Park [5], Woong-Woo Lee [6], Han-Joon Kim [7], Beomseok Jeon [7] and Sun Ha Paek [2,*]

[1] Department of Neurosurgery, Soonchunhyang University Seoul Hospital, Seoul 04401, Korea; c99867@schmc.ac.kr
[2] Department of Neurosurgery, Seoul National University Hospital, Seoul 03080, Korea; lim.yh@daum.net (Y.H.L.); moineun@daum.net (E.J.S.)
[3] Department of Neurosurgery, Pusan National University Hospital, Busan 49241, Korea; geosung1@naver.com
[4] Department of Neurosurgery, Gachon University Gil Medical Center, Incheon 21565, Korea; medicwoo@gmail.com
[5] Department of Neurosurgery, Chuungnam National University Sejong Hospital, Sejong 30099, Korea; tooez4me@naver.com
[6] Department of Neurology, Nowon Eulji Medical Center, Eulji University, Seoul 01830, Korea; w2pooh@hanmail.net
[7] Department of Neurology, Seoul National University Hospital, Seoul 03080, Korea; movement@snu.ac.kr (H.-J.K.); brain@snu.ac.kr (B.J.)
*   Correspondence: paeksh@snu.ac.kr

Abstract: Bilateral subthalamic nucleus (STN) Deep brain stimulation (DBS) is a well-established treatment in patients with Parkinson's disease (PD). Traditionally, STN DBS for PD is performed by using microelectrode recording (MER) and/or intraoperative macrostimulation under local anesthesia (LA). However, many patients cannot tolerate the long operation time under LA without medication. In addition, it cannot be even be performed on PD patients with poor physical and neurological condition. Recently, it has been reported that STN DBS under general anesthesia (GA) can be successfully performed due to the feasible MER under GA, as well as the technical advancement in direct targeting and intraoperative imaging. The authors reviewed the previously published literature on STN DBS under GA using intraoperative imaging and MER, focused on discussing the technique, clinical outcome, and the complication, as well as introducing our single-center experience. Based on the reports of previously published studies and ours, GA did not interfere with the MER signal from STN. STN DBS under GA without intraoperative stimulation shows similar or better clinical outcome without any additional complication compared to STN DBS under LA. Long-term follow-up with a large number of the patients would be necessary to validate the safety and efficacy of STN DBS under GA.

Keywords: general anesthesia; intraoperative computed tomography; intraoperative magnetic resonance imaging; local anesthesia; microelectrode recording; Parkinson's disease; subthalamic nucleus; deep brain stimulation

1. Introduction

Parkinson's disease (PD) is the second most common neurodegenerative disease following Alzheimer's disease, characterized by bradykinesia, rigidity, resting tremor and postural instability [1]. The long-term use of anti-Parkinsonian drugs has been found to be associated with dyskinesia and symptom fluctuation. Since the introduction of deep brain stimulation (DBS) in 1980s, DBS has been accepted as a preferred surgical treatment for PD [2]. Internal globus pallidus (GPi) and subthalamic nucleus (STN) are the main stimulation targets [3]. In particular, bilateral STN DBS is known to significantly improve not only primary motor symptoms, but also non-motor symptoms, such as sensory symptoms and sleep disturbances [4,5].

Traditionally, DBS surgery is performed under local anesthesia (LA) and conscious sedation to evaluate clinical benefit and side effects by localizing electrophysiological target using microelectrode recording (MER) and/or intraoperative test stimulation while the patient is awake [6–15]. STN DBS has several advantages when implemented under LA. The spike features of MER can be analyzed, and symptom relief or side effects by stimulation can be evaluated with intraoperative macrostimulation. In addition, by using electrophysiological targeting using MER, it is possible to compensate for errors from planning based on preoperative imaging, which is caused by brain shift due to cerebrospinal fluid (CSF) leakage after dura opening. However, MER under LA requires PD patients to withstand surgical procedure with approximately 18 h of antiparkinsonian medication discontinued. Most PD patients are old age and have severe multiple neuro-skeleto-muscular symptoms due to comorbidity, such as spinal stenosis and herniated intervertebral disc. Moreover, patients have to wear a frame on their head during the entire procedure and undergo surgery with the frame fixed to the operation table; thus, the patients may suffer from intolerable pain and psychological sequelae. The risk of hemorrhage risk also increases if an unintended large motion occurs due to cough or tremor during surgery. Patient cooperation is one of the factors that may influence the outcome after surgery.

Because of these concerns, many authors have consistently tried STN DBS under GA and reported that the clinical outcome is not inferior compared to under LA. However, there have been no randomized trials comparing DBS surgery under LA and GA due to logistical concerns. Only class II evidence has been compared through retrospective data analysis [16]. Here, we aimed to review previously published literature on STN DBS under GA as an alternative to STN DBS under LA. The technique and clinical outcome using intraoperative imaging and MER in DBS under GA are thoroughly reviewed along with the introduction of single-center experience of our institution.

2. STN DBS Using Intraoperative Imaging or Microelectrode Recording Under GA

The DBS surgical procedure can be divided into two stages: the intracranial implantation of DBS electrodes and the implantation of implantable pulse generator (IPG). In the case of IPG implantation, GA is generally preferred because tunneling is required subcutaneously. For intracranial electrode implantation, the STN DBS procedure under LA and GA are similar, but the specific details are different. The main difference between the STN DBS surgical procedure under LA and GA is the intraoperative verification method for the intended target acquisition, i.e., test stimulation or intraoperative imaging with or without MER. An accurate electrode location is a key factor to determine the postoperative prognosis after STN DBS surgery [17–20]. Image verification of the lead position is an important step, whether intra- or postoperatively [21]. For STN DBS under GA, some centers perform intraoperative verification using MER even under GA, and other centers use intraoperative imaging without MER. We reviewed each method of STN DBS under GA using intraoperative imaging or MER, respectively (Table 1).

Table 1. Summary data of published literature presenting clinical outcome effect of after subthalamic nucleus deep brain stimulation under general anesthesia in patients with Parkinson's disease.

Author	Year	No. of Patients	Age (yrs)	Disease Duration (yrs)	Follow-Up Months	UPDRS III Medication Off				LEDD			
						Baseline	Follow-Up *	% Change	p-Value	Baseline	Follow-Up *	% Change	p-Value
Intraoperative imaging													
Interventional MRI													
Starr et al. [22]	2010	29	58 ± 8.1	NR	9	49 ± 13	19 ±14	60%	0.0001	NR	NR	NR	NR
Foltynie et al. [23]	2011	79	58.9±7.7	11.5 ± 7	14	51.5 ± 14.9	23.8 ± 11.2	52%	0.0001	NR	NR	NR	NR
Nakajima et al. [24]	2011	14	56.1 ± 6.5	13.8 ± 8.1	12 ± 6.1	57.9 ± 16.6	27.3 ± 11.8	53%	0.0001	1505 ± 764	764 ± 435	49.20%	<0.01
Ostrem et al. [25]	2013	17	59.8	11.1	6	44.5 ± NA	22.5	49.44%	0.001	1337 ± 482	NR	24.70%	0.003
Saleh et al. [26]	2015	14	64 ± 11.9	10.9 ± 3.8	5.86 ± 1.15	NR	NR	NR	NR	NR	NR	49.27%	0.0031
Ostrem et al. [27]	2016	20	63.2 ± 6.8	10.8 ± 2.9	12	40.75 ± 10.9	24.35 ± 8.8	40.20%	0.001	1072.5 ± 382	828.25 ± 492	21.13%	0.046
Sidiropoulous et al. [28]	2016	12	64.7 ± 5.9	11.9 ± 3.7	13.5 ± 3.7	37.2	20.2	46.2%	0.03	1458 ± 653	1337 ± 733	8.3%	0.7
Chircop et al. [29]	2018	26	60.2 ± 9.3	8.8 ± 2.7	12	45.9 ± 14.3	26.7 ± 11.5	41.70%	<0.001	863 ± 211	599 ± 273	30.60%	<0.001
Matias et al. [30]	2018	33	67.2 ± 6.4	12.7 ± 6.9	9.1	52.8 ± 14.9	28.6 ± 11.9	45.8%	<0.001	NR	NR	NR	NR
Intraoperative CT													
Mirzadeh et al. [31]	2016	35	61.1	10.7	6	48.4 ± 13.8	28.9 ± 12.5	40.30%	<0.0001	1207 ± 733	1035 ± 478	14%	0.004
Microelectrode recording													
Hertel et al. [32]	2006	9	70.7 ± 3.6	13.6 ± 6.0	3	43.0 ± NR	19 ± NR	55.80%	NR	NR	NR	NR	NR
Lefaucheur et al. [33]	2008	30	57.7 ± 11.1	14.0 ± 4.0	12	47.9 ± 13.6	48.6 ± 19.0	69.10%	0.87	1470.8 ± 729.5	NR	66.4 ± 17.2	NR
Lin et al. [34]	2008	10	58.9 ± 9.9	8.8 ± 3.7	6	50.2 ± 12.9	25.6 ± 11.68	48.85%	<0.05	NR	NR	NR	NR
Fluchere et al. [35]	2014	188	61 ± 7	12 ± 4	12	33.6 ± 13.3	13.2 ± 9.1	61.00%	<0.001	1173 ± 495	636 ± 376	46.00%	<0.001
This study	2020	90	57.43 ± 7.85	11.67 ± 4.75	6	38.11 ± 13.96	21.48 ± 12.33	43.60%	<0.001	1448.0 ± 546.93	483.99 ± 330.42	66.60%	<0.001

Data are presented as: mean ± standard deviation UPDRS, Unified Parkinson's Disease Rating Scale; LEDD, Levodopa equivalent daily dose; NR, Not reported. * On stimulation.

2.1. Using Intraoperative Imaging

With the development of the quality of magnetic resonance imaging (MRI) over the past decades, it has become feasible to identify the STN boundary can to easily implement DBS under GA using direct targeting using advanced imaging [36]. The combination of direct targeting based on MRI visualization of anatomical structures and intraoperative imaging used to confirm accurate lead placement enables surgeons to accurately identify STN targets. It may allow STN DBS procedure to be performed in an asleep state under general anesthesia (GA) without neurophysiological test [37–39].

Successful clinical results on the intraoperative imaging to verify the accuracy of STN lead position instead of electrophysiological structure mapping or stimulation tests during DBS surgery have been reported [23,29,31,37,40–44]. In recent studies on the advancement of intraoperative imaging, no significant clinical results were found when compared to awake DBS [16,30,37,45,46]. However, most of these studies are retrospective analyses with a small number of patients and significant heterogeneity in anesthesia and surgical techniques. In addition, most of the studies were conducted in highly specialized centers with considerable experience in intraoperative imaging. Although these results may not be generalized to all DBS centers for these reasons, current results of STN DBS under GA are promising.

2.1.1. Intraoperative CT

In some centers, intraoperative computed tomography (iCT) during surgery is used to verify the accuracy of lead placement (Table 1). This is achieved through fusion of iCT scans and preoperative MRI scans after intracranial electrode implantation [31,37,41,44,47]. In awake DBS surgery with MER guidance, iCT provides useful information, such as hemorrhage and a general idea of electrode location when fused with preoperative MRI [21]. According to a study about the accuracy of microelectrode trajectory in patients receiving MER-guided awake DBS using iCT, median (IQR) radial error 0.59 (0.64) mm, and median (IQR) absolute x and y coordinate errors were 0.29 (0.52) and 0.38 (0.44) mm, respectively [21]. Burchiel et al. fused and compared iCT and trajectory planning images after electrode implantation for various targets [37]. The mean vector error and mean deviation of trajectory was 1.59 ± 1.11 mm and 1.24 ± 0.87 mm, respectively, and the intraoperative replacement was performed on one electrode with a vector error of more than 3 mm. There was a significant correlation between the distance from the ventricle and the error. Kremer et al. stated that the mean difference between lead tips was 0.98 ± 0.49 mm, and the upper confidence interval did not exceed the non-inferiority margin described when comparing postoperative MRI with iCT [48].

Some centers use MER without test stimulation but with intraoperative imaging to verify the intended target acquisition in STN DBS surgery under GA [32,49–58]. A recent study compared the mean errors of MER-guided electrode implantation in DBS surgery under LA and those of iCT scan-guided intracranial electrode implantation in STN DBS surgery under GA [42]. When targeting STN, mean radial errors of the LA and GA group was about 0.9 ± 0.3 mm without significant difference (P = 0.70). The average number of brain penetration for electrode implantation in DBS surgery under LA and GA was similar (1.1 ± 0.2 and 1.1 ± 0.3 penetrations, $p = 0.97$). Brodsky et al. compared 6-months of the clinical outcomes between the group of LA and GA with iCT [59]. There was no significant difference in the improvement in UPDRS III and II, but the improvement in summary index ($p = 0.004$), subscores for cognition ($p = 0.011$), communication ($p < 0.001$), and speech outcome (category, $p = 0.0012$; phonemic fluency, $p = 0.038$) was found better in the GA group.

A few authors have published the results of a study using the intraoperative O-arm. Sharma et al. performed STN DBS surgery under GA using intraoperative O-arm without MER for various targets, and no significant targeting error due to incorporation of iCT images into preoperative CT or MRI was observed [60]. Carlson et al. also reported that intraoperative O-arm images provided a higher accuracy in determining the location of STN DBS electrodes than postoperative CT and MRI images [61].

2.1.2. Intraoperative MRI

Other centers use intraoperative (interventional) MRI (iMRI) to guide DBS electrode placement to the STN (Table 1) [23–29,44,62–64]. For example, the UCSF group reported their experience about bilateral STN DBS in PD patients using a first-generation MRI system (Nexframe, high-field interventional MR-imaging) [25] and ClearPoint system (ClearPoint interventional MRI) [27]. There have been few published studies on the use of intraoperative MRI [23,24,26–28,44,62–67]. One of the reported advantages of iMRI is that it provides a real-time image acquisition to prospectively guided both trajectory planning and intended target verification prior to electrode placement [66]. Therefore, iMRI is one of the most useful methods for DBS targeting that allows precise validation of the real location of electrodes relative to the intended targets [66].

Researches using iMRI with or without stereotactic frame have shown that an accuracy of less than 1 mm can be achieved with mean error close to 0.7 ± 0.3 mm [22,23,25,27,64,66]. The main advantage of electrode implantation using iMRI is that electrode trajectory can be accurately implanted and adjusted before final placement by visualizing the intended target [66]. The error after correcting the electrode location using iMRI under GA without MER was similar to the error of using MER [30]. When comparing the electrode location on both sides, the error was smaller in the second insertion side than in the first insertion side, which is presumed to be due to the correction based on the iMRI result after the first insertion. Sidiropoulos et al. performed STN and GPi DBS surgery in advanced PD patients using the ClearPoint system and found that the mean radial error was 1.2 ± 0.7 mm in the STN group and 0.8 ± 0.3 mm in the GPi group [28]. Starr et al. et al. demonstrated a significantly lower rate of radial error compared to when inserted using the traditional frame-based stereotaxy (3.1 ± 1.41 mm) in the iMRI-guided placement group (1.2 ± 0.65 mm) through burr hole-mounted trajectory guide [22]. They explained that the possibility of brain shift-related errors was reduced because iMRI was performed after burr hole creation and intracranial air flow. Clinically, the UPDRS III "off" medication score and LEDD improved one year after surgery with iMRI [27].

2.1.3. Targeting Accuracy

The theoretical assumption of STN DBS under GA surgery is that the accuracy in targeting STN is not less and the results are better than STN DBS surgery under LA using MER. Kochanski et al. analyzed MER trajectories after STN DBS using 227 iCTs and found that 1.2 ± 0.2mm of radial error occurred in comparison with the location of the intended targets [68]. These errors may be related to the mechanical errors related with the frame, arc, guide tube, and frame, which can lead to lead deviation [69]. In a large-scale study of DBS patients who underwent surgery using iCT, there were greater Euclidean error and greater medial deviation in the trajectory targeting Vim. The authors found that there are systematic tendencies in stereotactic error that differ with respect to the structure targeted [70]. In the study analyzing stereotactic accuracy of iMRI, the DBS lead placement using iMRI guidance showed a radial targeting error of 0.6–1.2 mm, while the error using iCT was 0.8–1.24 mm [22,25,27,28,31,37,71]. STN DBS surgery under GA using confirmatory iCT is based on the assumption that CT-MRI merge was performed correctly, but there may be some errors in the fusion of imaging modality, which may lead to suboptimal targeting [38,72,73]. The advantage of STN DBS surgery with iMRI guidance is that it has less dependence on image fusion and can reflect brain shift after dura opening. Analysis of the iMRI study revealed that the deep brain structure moves about 2 mm after opening the dura [74].

2.2. Using Microelectrode Recording

2.2.1. Is MER Mandatory for STN DBS Surgery?

In the standard STN DBS procedure under LA, MER is used during surgery to obtain a signal to identify the deep structure [75]. The final site of electrode implantation is determined by considering both MER and intraoperative test stimulation [7–9,11,13–15]. Sedative drugs, such as propofol, dexmedetomidine, and remifentanil, are given to patients when it is not necessary for them to be awake [76,77]. The goal of using MER in STN DBS surgery is to obtain high accuracy in radiographic and neurophysiological targeting. Theoretically, the ideal target should be one and the same, but several important factors can lead to errors in targeting, resulting in inconsistency between optimal radiographic and neurophysiological targets. In the report on awake STN DBS, about 25% (38/150) of the electrodes were found very accurately located on the intended target very accurately with an error of less than 1mm, but electrophysiological recording did not match with the target in MER and/or intraoperative stimulation, or showed an unacceptably low side-effect threshold by stimulation [68]. Although these findings may be explained by brain shifts, these cases indicate that MER is essential for target confirmation during DBS surgery. Even small merge error combined with brain shift can lead to discrepancies between optimal radiographic and neurophysiological targets [38,72,74,78–80]. The advantage of this method is that it is possible to observe the changes in MER related to passive motion during surgery, and immediately evaluate the effects and side effects through test stimulation [9,81]. By reflecting this result and modifying the electrode position, the effect can be maximized while the complications of stimulation can be minimized.

MER signals may be mixed with many noises which may be caused by snoring or movements of the patient. The reliability and usefulness of MER during STN DBS surgery under LA are still being investigated. However, awake surgery may not be possible for some patients with severe anxiety, fear, reduced cooperation, severe pain, respiration difficulties and so on.

MER may increase the risk of intracranial hemorrhage and cognitive decline [82]. Binder et al. reported a bleeding rate of 3.3% and a risk of permanent defects 0.6% [83]. The number of MER trajectory was found slightly higher in patients with hemorrhage without statistical significance than the patients without hemorrhage [84]. Some researchers have also questioned whether MER has a real significant impact on target refinement [8]. They argued that a short MER-determined STN length alone cannot predict the occurrence of stimulation-related side effect [18]. Moreover, the MER procedure increases both surgical time and the cost [8,85].

Macrostimulation test cannot be performed if the patients are asleep during the operation. There is also controversy about whether intraoperative stimulation is needed during DBS surgery. Some researchers believe that it is necessary to confirm the effectiveness of the stimulus. On the other hand, some argued that discontinuation of the drug in LA makes the results less reliable, especially if it is not located in the correct position within the STN, the effect can be easily observed and difficult to distinguish from the lesion effect [86].

Due to the improved image quality of preoperative imaging, determining the final electrode location by imaging alone without MER does not negatively affect motor improvement and LEDD, and does not aggravate surgical complications [24,26,29,42,87]. The UPDRS III reduction rate at postoperative 3 months was higher in the group of STN DBS under LA with MER cohort ($p = 0.006$), but there was no significant difference at 1 year ($p = 0.18$), as well as in dysarthria, capsular, oculomotor, and sensory side effects [87]. Chen et al. also reported that there was no difference in the UPDRS III reduction rate and score 6 months after STN DBS surgery between the MER group and the non-MER group [42]. In addition to frequently used imaging sequences, direct targeting can be used with quantitative susceptibility mapping (QSM) and diffusion tensor imaging (DTI) [68].

2.2.2. Is MER Possible Under GA?

STN DBS under GA has traditionally been used in patients who are unable to tolerate awake surgery including pediatric patients, or in patients who do not require clinical testing, such as obsessive-compulsive disorder or epilepsy. The biggest concern with STN DBS surgery under GA for movement disorder is the possibility of diminution of MER signals. A few small-sized retrospective studies have reported that MER obtained from STN, GPi, substantia nigra in STN DBS surgery under GA with both volatile and intravenous anesthetics in PD and dystonia patients showed no significant difference compared with patients awake during the procedure [54,88–91]. Notably, the neural activity of typical burst pattern disappeared when higher anesthetic doses were used. However, the results of these studies are controversial given the small sample size and heterogeneity of the anesthetic used. A prospective, double-blinded study is needed to compare the effects of anesthetic agents on MER quality in patients undergoing STN DBS surgery under GA.

The next concern is that since intraoperative stimulation cannot be performed under GA, immediate response of clinical effects and adverse effects associated with stimulation cannot be assessed during the STN DBS surgery. Several trials of MER in deep sedation have been performed without intraoperative stimulation [32,33,89]. In these studies, propofol or remifentanil tended to interfere with the electrophysiological signal, but there were no significant differences in terms of exact targeting, clinical effectiveness, and adverse event profiles. Other authors also reported that although there was significant MER signal attenuation in deep sedation with propofol, it did not interfere with the optimal approach to the target [32,33,92,93].

Although a few studies have previously investigated the effects of anesthetics on MER over the past 20 years, the exact effect has not been fully elucidated. Most studies were retrospective analyses with heterogeneity in the anesthesia protocol used and the patient population, and thus, no definitive conclusions could be drawn [77]. Therefore, most of the knowledge revealed to date is derived from the case reports or small case series. During MER, background neuronal discharges and spike activity patterns are an important part of the precise localization of the target nucleus. Anesthetics have been shown to affect background activity and neuronal spike activity in a dose-dependent manner, primarily through activation of γ-aminobutyric acid (GABA) receptors. In addition, anesthetics do not have the same effect on neuronal activity in various target nucleus. Since most anesthetics enhance the inhibitory action of GABA, this difference in GABA-input of the target nucleus plays an important role [94,95].

MER from STN in PD patients was successfully obtained under sedation with low-dose anesthetics. The anesthesia techniques used during MER ranged from conscious sedation with propofol, dexmedetomidine with no airway manipulation to GA with intravenous or inhalation anesthetics. Although anesthetics have been shown to reduce the spike activity, localization of the target areas was proven possible in most studies. Nevertheless, most studies did not mention the exact effect on the background activity, degree of suppression of spike activity, and the number of trajectories used for localization [34,58,80,89].

Under desflurane inhalation, Lin et al. observed that MER could be performed with a typical neuronal firing pattern and motion-related firing of STN, and the clinical results were similar in both groups [34,96].

Our group performed MER and implantation by administering propofol and fentanyl for sedation under LA, and reported the effects of propofol and fentanyl on MER and the clinical outcome. The locations of all electrodes were positioned within the STN. The postoperative 6-months UPDRS II and III, total "off" scores, Hoehn and Yahr (H&Y) scale, Schwab-England ADL scale scores, and LEDD have been greatly improved [92,93].

Although the effects of short-acting opioid receptor agonists, such as remifentanil, on MER are not well known, some data suggest that GABAergic neurons may play a central role [76,77,97]. A few reports showed that anesthesia using propofol reduces the firing rate of basal ganglia in a few reports [95,98], while one study showed no significant difference in firing rate compared to LA when administered with propofol and fentanyl [92]. Monitored anesthesia using propofol appears to be a safe technique for DBS procedure [99]. In some studies, MER was properly performed without affecting the surgical outcome only when remifentanil administration was discontinued and propofol was carefully monitored [32,54,100]. However, the spontaneous firing patterns of STN and substantia nigra remained similar to those under LA [14,100]. Chen et al. also reported that there was no significant difference between the GA and LA groups in terms of MER trajectory, recorded STN depths, postoperative coordinates, and overall incidence of stimulation-related side effect [55]. Under remifentanil or ketamine anesthesia, no significant differences were found in number of spikes detected, mean firing rate, pause index, and burst index compared to LA [57]. However, Moll et al. observed a long interburst between abnormally long group discharges under propofol and remifentanil [89].

Benzodiazepines are direct GABA-agonists, which can completely eliminate MER and cause dyskinesia. Dexmedetomidine may be a better alternative for anxiety relief. The effect of dexmedetomidine on neural activity has not been fully elucidated, but it seems to be a reasonable option due to the non-GABA-mediated mechanism of action. Several studies to date have shown minimal effects of low-dose dexmedetomidine on MER in STN and GPi [101–104]. Some authors reported that low doses of dexmedetomidine (<0.5 µg/kg/h) did not significantly affect the quality of MER in STN or GPi [76,99,103]. Although dexmedetomidine may affect the MER result, it does not affect target localization [50].

2.2.3. Clinical Experiences of STN DBS Using MER under GA

Some authors performed STN DBS surgery on PD patients under GA and reported favorable clinical outcomes (Table 1). Hertel et al. reported that patients' daily off phases decreased from 50% to 17%, while the Unified Parkinson's Disease Rating Scale (UPDRS) III score was reduced from 43 (preoperative; medication off) to 19 (stimulation on; medication off) and 12 (stimulation on; medication on) [32]. Yamada et al. also reported that UPDRS II, III, IV on and off scores were significantly lower in the LA and GA groups at 3 months postoperatively, and the activities of daily living(ADL)s and motor symptoms, such as bradykinesia, tremor, rigidity, and axial symptoms, have improved significantly [54]. In this study, a reduction in dyskinesia duration ($p < 0.001$), disability ($p = 0.009$) and off period duration, and improvement of sleep disorders were observed. Other authors also reported significant improvement in off-medication UPDRS, levodopa-equivalent daily dose (LEDD), and quality of life [29,35]. Harries et al. reported a long-term clinical outcome of more than 5 years [49]. In their study, not only the UPDRS II and III off score, but also the total UPDRS off scores at postoperative 1 year improved significantly, and the total UPDRS score continued to improve for up to 7 years.

Previously, authors have suggested the use of bispectral analysis (BIS) of the electroencephalogram in STN DBS surgery under GA using MER. An appropriate MER signal can be easily obtained by adjusting the anesthesia depth using BIS [100,105]. BIS of 65–85 and 40–65 is recommended for sedation and GA, respectively [106]. In the case of sedation using dexmedetomidine, it has been reported that the MER signal does not differ from the nonsedated state if the BIS value is maintained below 80 [80].

2.3. Intraoperative Imaging vs. MER in STN DBS under GA

Recent meta-analysis reported that no significant difference was found in the improvement of UPDRS III score or LEDD between LA and GA cohort (Tables 2–4) [16,33,46,54,55,107]. Lefaucheur et al. reported that the rate of reduction in UPDRS III axial, gait, postural stability, and rigidity subscores tended to be greater when performed under LA compared to GA, but the difference was not statistically significant [33]. On the other hand, Chen et al. reported that the LA cohort showed greater improvement in posture and walking than the GA cohort ($p = 0.054$), while the GA cohort showed a significant decrease in cognitive function ($p = 0.017$) [55].

Some studies have used MER in STN DBS surgery under GA (mean 1.92 ± 0.68) and LA cohort (mean 2.27 ± 1.31) with respect to the maximum error of each read ($p = 0.557$) despite the varying targets [33,52,55]. Ho et al. reported that there was no significant difference between GA (mean 1.92 ± 0.68) and LA cohort (mean 2.27 ± 1.31) with respect to the maximum error of each lead ($p = 0.557$), but their study included a variety of targets [16]. The number of lead passes and the incidence of intracranial hemorrhage and infection were lower in STN DBS under GA, but treatment-related side effects based on the UPDRS IV "off" score were lower in DBS under LA (LA cohort 78.4% vs

GA cohort 59.7%, $p = 0.022$) [16,35]. However, other studies showed no difference in the UPDRS IV subscore between the GA and LA groups [24,107]. As for LEDD, some studies reported that the 6-months postoperative LEDD reduction was significantly greater in the LA group, while others showed statistically similar reductions (LA cohort 38.27%, GA cohort 49.27%, $p = 0.4447$) [26,107]. Tsai et al. reported that symptoms of the patients with PD improved after DTN DBS in both LA and GA cohorts without significant differences in LEDD and UPDRS IV scores [52].

When the long-term outcome was investigated, the authors found that the probability of side effects by stimulation and lead revision was higher in the GA cohort without MER and test stimulation [68]. On the other hand, no difference was observed in UPDRS III score, LEDD, stimulation parameters, coordination of targeting, STN recording length, and side effects in the two groups [108].

STN DBS surgery can be safely performed with a low complication rate in both LA and GA cohort, and the results of the studies to date show that there is no significant difference in complication rates between the two groups. Some authors reported that overall DBS-related complications, such as intracranial hemorrhage (GA 0.3% vs LA 1.1%) and infection (GA 0.7% vs LA 1.4%), were significantly lower in GA cohort ($p < 0.001$) [16,35]. Martin et al. reported the incidence of hardware infection is due to electrode implantation after 10 years of MRI-guided STN DBS surgery [109]. In the study, the overall infection rate of 164 iMRI-guided surgeries with 272 electrodes implanted was 3.6%, which was similar to that reported in the previous STN DBS surgery under LA. The results of a systematic review on the incidence of complications, hospitalization time, and readmission rate of patients who underwent awake and asleep STN DBS surgery were recently published, and there was no statistical difference in the complication rate, length of hospitalization, and readmission rate of LA and GA cohort [110].

The mean total cost of STN DBS surgery under GA and LA was similar at $38,850 ± $4830 in GA and $40,052 ± $6604 in LA, respectively, but the standard deviation in DBS under GA was significantly lower [111]. This indicates that there is no difference in the total cost of DBS surgery under GA and LA, but the cost fluctuation is lower due to the lower incidence of unexpected variables in DBS surgery under GA. However, there are limitations to generalizing such result, since it is a single-center experience.

Table 2. Summary data of published literature comparing clinical outcome effect of after subthalamic nucleus deep brain stimulation under general anesthesia and local anesthesia in patients with Parkinson's disease: Baseline patient characteristics

Author	Year	Study Type	Number of Patients		Age (yrs)		Disease Duration (yrs)		Follow-Up (Months)
			GA	LA	GA	LA	GA	LA	
Maltete et al. [58]	2004	Clinical	15	15	59.8 8.0	58.0 6.1	13.4 3.7	13.5 2.6	6
Yamada et al. [54]	2007	Clinical	15	10	65.2 7.0	65.6 8.6	11.1 5.0	6.8 2.4	3
Saleh et al. [26]	2015	Clinical	14	23	64.0 ± 11.9	60.6 ± 7.0	10.9 ± 3.8	11.3 ± 4.9	6
Tsai et al. [52]	2016	Clinical	8	8	49.6 ± 7.1 *	41.1 ± 10.2 *	9.3 ± 2.4	12.4 ± 9.2	6
Brodsky et al. [59]	2017	Clinical	27 (20 GPi, 7 STN)	34 (20 GPi, 14 STN)	63.7 ± 9.79	63.1 ± 7.61	NR	NR	6
Lefranc et al. [112]	2017	Clinical	13	10	62.80 ± 7.1	63.1 ± 10	12.60 ± 3.6	12.10 ± 3.5	12
Blasberg et al. [87]	2018	Clinical	48	48	65.75 ± 1.18	65.52 ± 1.13	11.65 ± 0.81	10.87 ± 0.78	6
Chen et al. [42]	2018	Clinical	41	14	64.6 ± 8.25	63.1 ± 10.1	7.5 ± 3.4	8.6 ± 4.6	6
Ho et al. [16]	2018	Meta-analysis	663	6441	58.3 ± 6.8	59.4 ± 5.2	11.0 ± 1.5	12.3 ± 2.1	12
Liu et al. [113]	2019	Meta-analysis	967	556	NR	NR	NR	NR	NR
Tsai et al. [108]	2019	Clinical	22	9	57.7 ± 7.4	49.4 ± 12.2	57.7 ± 7.4	49.4 ± 12.2	60
This study	2020	Clinical	90	56	57.43 ± 7.85	58.91 ± 8.65	11.67 ± 4.75	10.55 ± 4.89	6

Data are presented as: mean ± standard deviation GA, general anesthesia; LA, local anesthesia; GPi, Internal globus pallidus; STN, subthalamic nucleus; NR, Not reported * Age of Onset.

Table 3. Summary data of published literature comparing clinical outcome effect of after subthalamic nucleus deep brain stimulation under general anesthesia and local anesthesia in patients with Parkinson's disease: Baseline and Follow-up Unified Parkinson's Disease Rating Scale (UPDRS) III score and Levodopa equivalent daily dose (LEDD).

Author	Baseline UPDRS III		Follow-Up UPDRS III *		%UPDRS III Change			Baseline LEDD		Follow-Up LEDD		%LEDD reduction		
	GA	LA	GA	LA	GA	LA	p Value	GA	LA	GA	LA	GA	LA	p Value
Maltete et al.	47.1 ± 15.4	39.9 ± 13.9	17.0 ± 8.6	10.9 ± 7.2	63.9%	72.7%	0.07	1449 ± 398	1507 ± 465	310 ± 350	392 ± 440	78.6%	74.0%	0.06
Yamada et al.	52.4 ± 19.0	45.9 ± 17.7	14.3 ± 15.4	7.1 ± 7.0	72.7%	82.5%	No significant difference	375.7 ± 195.6	425.0 ± 171.8	303.3 ± 164.7	261.1 ± 164.0	16.6%	38.2%	NR
Saleh et al.	NR	NR	NR	NR	NR	NR	NR	2134.9 ± 1175.8	1702.7 ± 876.0	NR	NR	49.27%	38.27%	0.4447
Tsai et al.	41.7 ± 29.4	39.9 ± 16.3	NR	NR	65.7%	45.8 ± 26.2%	NR	NR	NR	NR	NR	NR	NR	NR
Brodsky et al.	42.2 ± 10.6	41.7 ± 12.5	14.8 ± 8.9 **	17.6 ± 12.26 **	35%	42.2%	0.19	NR	NR	NR	NR	NR	NR	NR
Lefranc et al.	35.92 ± 11.15	33.10 ± 5.38	18.0 ± 7.2	20.0 ± 10.47	49%	40.30%	0.336	1585.10 ± 496.40	1247.70 ± 579.80	519.17 ± 282.71	716.80 ± 320.14	Significantly greater in the GA than in the LA		0.03
Blasberg et al.	38.47 ± 1.94	34.79 ± 1.61	NR	NR	NR	NR	0.18	1070.72 ± 49.67	972.23 ± 55.15	NR	NR	NR	NR	0.008
Chen et al.	53.8 ± 16.4	53.7 ± 17.0	26.1 ± 12.0	21.6 ± 7.3	48.8%	40.3%	0.20	NR	NR	NR	NR	45 ± 12.8% (n = 444)	47 ± 26.6% (n = 3893)	0.49
Ho et al.	NR	NR	NR	NR	51.1 ± 16.6% (n = 510)	46.7 ± 27.4 ± (n = 4931)	0.494	NR	NR	NR	NR	NR	NR	0.752
Liu et al.	NR	NR	NR	NR	NR	NR	0.60	NR	NR	NR	NR	NR	NR	0.23
Tsai et al.	46.3 ± 14.4	28.6 ± 9.3	42.9 ± 17.4	24.6 ± 7.8	43.2 ± 14.1%	46.8 ± 13.8%	0.45	NR	NR	NR	NR	47.56 ± 18.98%	51.37 ± 31.73%	0.51
This study	38.11 ± 13.96	40.42 ± 15.30	21.48 ± 12.33	24.68 ± 12.51	43.6%	38.9%	0.136	1448.0 ± 546.93	1031.63 ± 451.08	483.99 ± 330.42	461.3 ± 284.65	66.6%	55.3%	<0.0001

Data are presented as: mean ± standard deviation. UPDRS, Unified Parkinson's Disease Rating Scale; LEDD, Levodopa equivalent daily dose; GA, general anesthesia; LA, local anesthesia; GPi, Internal globus pallidus; STN, subthalamic nucleus; NR, Not reported * off medication, on stimulation ** recorded as reduced score.

Table 4. Summary data of published literature comparing clinical outcome effect of after subthalamic nucleus deep brain stimulation under general anesthesia and local anesthesia in patients with Parkinson's disease: Perioperative complications.

Author	Number of MER Tracks	Overall Adverse Effects	Hemorrhage	Infection	Operation Time
Maltete et al.	NR	No adverse reaction to the use of propofol, 1 pulmonary atelectasia	NR	NR	NR
Yamada et al.	NR	NR	NR	NR	NR
Saleh et al.	NR	No significant differences	NR	NR	GA 424 ± 12 vs LA 307 ± 80, p = 0.0026
Tsai et al.	NR	No significant differences	NR	NR	NR
Brodsky et al.	NR	NR	1 small venous hemorrhage in LA, 1 small nonhemorrhagic infarct in GA	1 in GA	NR
Lefranc et al.	NR	No significant differences, p = 0.39	NR	NR	NR
Blasberg et al.	NR	No significant differences	1.00	1.00	0.31
Chen et al.	NR	NR	NR	NR	GA 266.0 ± 60.6 vs LA 260.9 ± 57.6, p = 0.78
Ho et al.	GA 1.4 ± 0.44 vs LA 2.1 ± 0.69, p = 0.006	NR	%ICH/lead: GA 0.3 ± 0.0 vs LA 1.1 ± 0.3, p < 0.001	%infection/lead GA 0.7 ± 0.0 vs LA 1.4 ± 0.0, p < 0.001	GA 253.7 ± 82.3 vs LA 272.4 ± 92.5, p = 0.748
Liu et al.	NR	0.94	0.64	NR	0.47
Tsai et al.	Significantly less in GA, p = 0.04	Similar adverse effects	NR	NR	NR
This study	NR	1 required revision due to inappropriate lead position in LA	NR	1 IPG site infection treated by antibiotics in LA	NR

MER, microelectrode recording; NR, not recorded; GA, general anesthesia; LA, local anesthesia; IPG, implantable pulse generator.

3. SNUH Experience

Our group have been implementing STN DBS under LA since 2005 initially under sedation using propofol and fentanyl from 2011 to 2014 [93], and under full GA since 2014. To determine if there is a difference in the clinical outcome of PD patients who received bilateral STN DBS under LA and GA, we compared the clinical outcomes of the consecutive 57 patients who received bilateral STN DBS under LA from 2005 to 2006 and consecutive 90 patients who received bilateral STN DBS under GA from 2014 to 2019. Because our group previously published a study on the clinical course and electrode location of patients who received bilateral STN DBS under LA [114,115], these patients were included for the comparison. After approval by the institutional review board (IRB No. 1904–015–102), we retrospectively reviewed all patient medical records and databases (unpublished data). The scales that evaluated patients were as follows: UPDRS, Hoehn and Yahr (H&Y) Staging, Schwab & England ADL, dyskinesia disability, LEDD, Short Form-36 Health Survey (SF-36), and neuropsychological tests. All clinical evaluations were performed before surgery and 6 months after surgery by experienced neurologists. Patients were evaluated in both off- and on-medication states, respectively.

STN DBS under general anesthesia was performed with maintenance of the BIS around 60-70, and MER was administered under general anesthesia. The characteristic discharges of the bilateral STN were identified using MER by LeadPoint (Medtronic, Minneapolis, MN). The permanent quadripolar electrodes were implanted along the proper trajectory to stimulate more sensorimotor region of the STN. The STNs were localized by a combination of brain MRI and intraoperative MER. We did not use an intraoperative macrostimulation technique [15]. The stereotactic frame was removed and the implantable pulse generators (IPG) (Medtronic, Minneapolis, MN, USA) were implanted in a subcutaneous pocket below both clavicles under general anesthesia in a single session. Electrical stimulation was started one day after surgery. The patients also took medications but at a reduced dose compared to their previous dose. The medications and stimulation parameters were progressively adjusted using an N'vision1programmer (Medtronic, Minneapolis, MN, USA) according to the clinical status of the patients.

Statistical analyses were performed using SPSS software (SPSS statistics 18.0; SPSS Inc.). The data for the aforementioned variables were presented as the mean ± standard deviation using unpaired Student t tests. Mann–Whitney U-test and the Wilcoxon signed-ranked test were used for categorical data comparisons as appropriate. p values < 0.05 were considered statistically significant. Table 5 represents the patient characteristics and clinical scales of LA and GA cohort before DBS surgery. At baseline before surgery, the GA cohort showed higher LEDD, Beck's Depression Inventory (BDI), and Short Form-36 (SF-36), and lower Beck Depression Inventory than the LA cohort. Table 6 shows the comparison between baseline and 6 months after DBS for each scale in LA and GA cohort. Total UPDRS and UPDRS III showed significant improvement after 6 months compared to baseline, except for LA cohort in on-medication state. H&Y stage and ADL score showed no significant change in the on-medication state in both GA and LA, and significantly decreased in the off-medication state. Dyskinesia disability and LEDD were significantly decreased in both GA and LA cohort. There was no significant change in Mini Mental State Examination (MMSE) and BDI after surgery in both groups. Physical health measured by SF-36 increased in both LA and GA cohort, and mental health showed no statistically significant increase. When analyzing the difference between the LA and GA cohort in the baseline of each item and the change after 6 months, only LEDD showed a significant difference ($p < 0.0001$). As shown in Figure 1, the degree of reduction in LEDD was greater in the GA cohort than in the LA cohort. We plotted the electrode location in each group based on the plotted position of the electrode in the axial view which is 3.5 mm below the anterior commissure(AC)-posterior commissure(PC) line in the human brain atlas of Schaltenbrand and Wahren (Figure 2). The electrode location on both sides in the LA group (n = 56) were as follows: both within STN (n = 30, 53.6%), only one within STN (n = 18, 32.1%), and both outside STN (n = 8, 14.3%). It was as follow in the GA group (n = 90): both within STN (n = 69, 76.7%), only one within STN (n = 20, 22.2%), and both outside STN (n = 1, 1.1%). There was a significant difference in the electrode location on both sides between

the two groups ($p = 0.001$). Compared to the LA cohort (Figure 2A), the GA cohort (Figure 2B) showed a higher tendency for the electrode to be located within the STN. However, it should be interpreted in consideration of the fact that our group performed DBS surgery under LA in the early days, and under GA after more experienced. As intra- or postoperative complications, one revision and one infection occurred in LA cohort. One patient required revision surgery after 2 months due to inappropriate lead location. The other patient had IPG site infection, which improved after antibiotics treatment. In our center, postoperative MRI was taken 1 month after electrode implantation, so we cannot find post-electrode edema (PEE) in most cases. As recent studies have revealed that PEE is not simply a complication due to venous congestion and has no significant relationship with the number of tracks, further studies on the occurrence pattern of PEE under GA would be required [116–119].

Table 5. Patients' characteristics and clinical measurements in patients who underwent bilateral subthalamic nucleus deep brain stimulation under local and general anesthesia.

	Medication	General Anesthesia (n = 90)	Local Anesthesia (n = 56)	*p* Value
Patient characteristics				
Age		57.43 ± 7.85	58.91 ± 8.65	0.2893
Sex				0.8110
Male		42(46.67%)	25(44.64%)	
Female		48(53.33%)	31(55.36%)	
Symptom duration		11.67 ± 4.75	10.55 ± 4.89	0.1753
Medication duration		9.82 ± 3.89	8.98 ± 3.81	0.2027
Baseline measurement				
Total UPDRS	On	31.86 ± 16.96	32.87 ± 17.76	0.7315
	Off	65.93 ± 20.42	68.53 ± 20.34	0.4569
UPDRS Part III	On	20.83 ± 10.96	21.40 ± 12.90	0.7764
	Off	38.11 ± 13.96	40.42 ± 15.30	0.3521
H & Y	On	2.36 ± 0.63	2.30 ± 0.63	0.6280
	Off	3.05 ± 0.82	3.24 ± 0.91	0.1918
ADL	On	82.89 ± 16.86	80.27 ± 15.45	0.3474
	Off	47.44 ± 23.54	50.00 ± 22.18	0.5154
Dyskinesia Disability		2.72 ± 1.31	2.21 ± 1.39	0.0294 *
LEDD (mg/day)		1448.00 ± 546.93	1031.63 ± 451.08	<0.0001 *
MMSE		27.61 ± 2.52	26.53 ± 2.76	0.0273 *
BDI		17.72 ± 10.28	19.00 ± 10.82	0.4931
SF-36 Physical health		156.25 ± 72.58	132.86 ± 61.09	0.0493 *
SF-36 Mental health		177.62 ± 80.37	150.39 ± 72.59	0.0433 *

* $p < 0.05$.

Table 6. Summary of clinical outcomes of bilateral subthalamic nucleus deep brain stimulation under local and general anesthesia.

	Medication	Anesthesia	Baseline	6 Month *	*p* Value **	*p* Value ***
Total UPDRS	On	General	31.86 ± 16.96	24.53 ± 14.95	0.004	0.205
		Local	32.87 ± 17.76	29.29 ± 14.19	0.429	
	Off	General	65.93 ± 20.42	40.32 ± 21.42	<0.001	0.120
		Local	68.53 ± 20.34	47.26 ± 17.85	<0.001	
UPDRS Part III	On	General	20.83 ± 10.96	16.20 ± 9.46	0.005	0.696
		Local	21.40 ± 12.90	16.67 ± 9.35	0.063	
	Off	General	38.11 ± 13.96	21.48 ± 12.33	<0.001	0.136
		Local	40.42 ± 15.30	24.68 ± 12.51	<0.001	
H & Y	On	General	2.36 ± 0.63	2.24 ± 0.61	0.238	0.853
		Local	2.3 ± 0.63	2.33 ± 0.68	0.959	
	Off	General	3.05 ± 0.82	2.35 ± 0.61	<0.001	0.053
		Local	3.24 ± 0.91	2.64 ± 0.72	0.002	
ADL	On	General	82.89 ± 16.86	84.80 ± 14.22	0.435	0.592
		Local	80.27 ± 15.45	82.16 ± 15.66	0.247	
	Off	General	47.44 ± 23.54	61.98 ± 25.58	<0.001	0.500
		Local	50 ± 22.18	66.92 ± 18.53	<0.001

Table 6. *Cont.*

	Medication	Anesthesia	Baseline	6 Month [*]	p Value [**]	p Value [***]
Dyskinesia Disability		General	2.72 ± 1.31	1.04 ± 1.27	<0.001	0.062
		Local	2.21 ± 1.39	0.79 ± 1.21	<0.001	
LEDD (mg/day)		General	1448.00 ± 546.93	483.99 ± 330.42	<0.001	0.000
		Local	1031.63 ± 451.08	461.3 ± 284.65	<0.001	
MMSE		General	27.61 ± 2.52	27.23 ± 2.33	0.314	0.621
		Local	26.53 ± 2.76	25.78 ± 3.71	0.493	
BDI		General	17.72 ± 10.28	16.57 ± 10.56	0.473	0.277
		Local	19 ± 10.82	19.78 ± 9.68	0.524	
SF-36 Physical health		General	156.25 ± 72.58	203.14 ± 90.03	<0.001	0.600
		Local	132.86 ± 61.09	188.34 ± 74.5	<0.001	
SF-36 Mental health		General	177.62 ± 80.37	206.88 ± 84.62	0.021	0.988
		Local	150.39 ± 72.59	181.44 ± 80.95	0.076	

* DBS on, ** between baseline and follow-up, *** between two groups: general and local anesthesia.

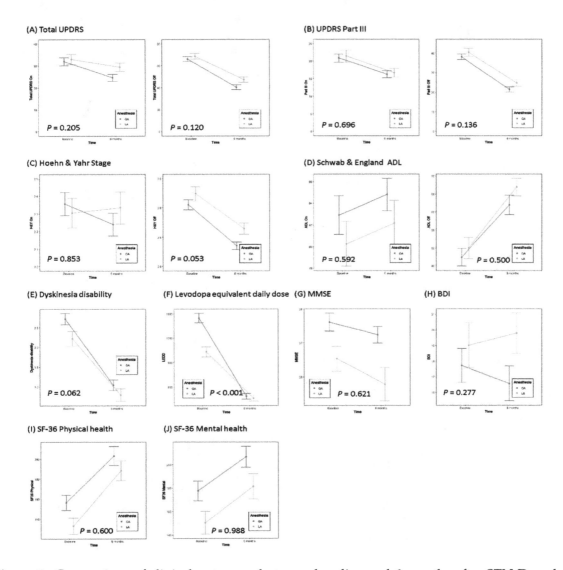

Figure 1. Comparison of clinical outcomes between baseline and 6 months after STN Deep brain stimulation (DBS) under local anesthesia (LA) and general anesthesia (GA) each cohort. (**A**) Total Unified Parkinson's Disease Rating Scale (UPDRS) and (**B**) UPDRS part III showed significant improvement after 6 months compared to baseline, except for LA cohort medication on state, there was no statistically significant difference between LA and GA cohort. (**C**) Hoehn & Yahr stage and (**D**) Schwab & England

activities of daily living (ADL) showed no significant change in the medication on state in both LA and GA cohort, and no significant difference between two cohorts. **(E)** Dyskinesia disability and **(F)** Levodopa equivalent daily dose (LEDD) were significantly decreased in both LA and GA cohort. Only LEDD showed a significant difference in the change between LA and GA cohort. **(G)** Mini Mental State Examination (MMSE) and **(H)** Beck's Depression Inventory (BDI), showed no statistically significant decrease in both LA and GA cohort. **(I)** Short form -36 (SF-36) physical health and **(J)** Short form -36 (SF-36) mental health showed no statistically significant increase in both LA and GA cohort.

Figure 2. Plotting of the electrode location based on the plotted position of the electrode in the axial view which is 3.5 mm below the anterior commissure (AC)–posterior commissure (PC) line in the human brain atlas of Schaltenbrand and Wahren. **(A)** Local anesthesia (LA) cohort, **(B)** General anesthesia (GA) cohort. Compared to LA cohort, the GA cohort showed a higher tendency for the electrode to be located within the subthalamic nucleus (STN).

4. Future Direction

Studies published to date have shown that the rationale and technology of STN DBS surgery performed under GA are accurate, and they presented similar clinical results compared to STN DBS under LA cohort. A large-scale prospective randomized controlled trial is in progress to assess the degree of the improvement of non-motor symptoms in PD patients [120].

Care should be taken when interpreting and applying the conclusion, since the STN DBS surgery under GA data reported to date have been published in large centers with considerable experiences. In general, STN DBS surgery should be performed in the most convenient way for the surgeons and center to provide the best results to the patients. Traditionally, factors, such as claustrophobia, severe off-medication symptoms, or nonspecific fear of waking during surgery, made patients choose GA. However, based on the increasingly cumulative data showing similar or better results compared to LA, a surgeon may choose STN DBS surgery under GA.

Adaptive DBS is a promising technology because it can provide more selective stimulation trigger/parameter and reduce stimulation-induced dyskinesia by suppressing beta activity when it exceeds a certain threshold level [121,122]. There is still little literature on adaptive DBS implemented under general anesthesia, and further studies for application of adaptive DBS under general anesthesia should be conducted.

There are patients who cannot undergo STN DBS surgery due to various reasons or may not benefit from STN DBS surgery. Non-invasive lesion-based therapies, such as focused ultrasound and Gamma Knife radiosurgery (GKRS), have been proposed as alternatives to DBS because of their effectiveness and safety [123–126]. The further innovative refinement of noninvasive methods of Gamma Knife radiosurgery (GKRS) and focused ultrasound may allow advanced PD patients to receive surgical treatment more conveniently and efficiently in the near future.

5. Conclusions

The number of DBS surgeries continues to increase, as indications expand and the population is aging. Currently, STN DBS surgery is performed in various ways with or without MER under LA or GA in each center. Based on the reports of previously published studies and ours, it is likely that GA does not interfere with the MER signal from STN. In addition, STN DBS under GA without intraoperative stimulation shows similar or better clinical outcome without any additional complication compared to STN DBS under LA. Although there are various pros and cons of each method in each protocol in each protocol of STN DBS under LA and under GA, the stereotype that STN DBS surgery must be performed under LA to perform intraoperative macrostimulation and MER to obtain the best clinical outcome should be changed at the moment.

In conclusion, it is suggested that, if there is no significant difference in clinical treatment effects and complications between GA and LA, it would be reasonable to implement STN DBS under GA because it can minimize unnecessary inconvenience of the patients with PD. Long-term follow-up studies with the large number of the patients would be necessary to further validate the safety and efficacy of STN DBS under GA.

Author Contributions: Conceptualization, S.H.P. and B.J.; methodology, H.-J.K.; software, Y.H.L.; validation, W.-W.L., K.H.P. and K.P.; formal analysis, H.R.P.; investigation, E.J.S.; resources, J.M.L.; data curation, Y.H.L.; writing—original draft preparation, H.R.P. and S.H.P.; writing—review and editing, H.R.P., B.J. and S.H.P.; visualization, H.-J.K.; supervision, B.J.; project administration, S.H.P.; funding acquisition, H.R.P. and S.H.P. All authors have read and agreed to the published version of the manuscript.

Acknowledgments: Yona Kim contributed to this work by English proofreading.

References

1. Han, M.; Nagele, E.; DeMarshall, C.; Acharya, N.; Nagele, R. Diagnosis of Parkinson's disease based on disease-specific autoantibody profiles in human sera. *PLoS ONE* **2012**, *7*, e32383. [CrossRef] [PubMed]
2. Benabid, A.-L.; Pollak, P.; Louveau, A.; Henry, S.; De Rougemont, J. Combined (thalamotomy and stimulation) stereotactic surgery of the VIM thalamic nucleus for bilateral Parkinson disease. *Ster. Funct. Neurosurg.* **1987**, *50*, 344–346. [CrossRef] [PubMed]
3. Fasano, A.; Daniele, A.; Albanese, A. Treatment of motor and non-motor features of Parkinson's disease with deep brain stimulation. *Lancet Neurol.* **2012**, *11*, 429–442. [CrossRef]
4. Kleiner-Fisman, G.; Herzog, J.; Fisman, D.N.; Tamma, F.; Lyons, K.E.; Pahwa, R.; Lang, A.E.; Deuschl, G. Subthalamic nucleus deep brain stimulation: Summary and meta-analysis of outcomes. *Mov. Disord.* **2006**, *21*, S290–S304. [CrossRef]
5. Kim, H.-J.; Jeon, B.S.; Paek, S.H. Nonmotor symptoms and subthalamic deep brain stimulation in Parkinson's disease. *J. Mov. Disord.* **2015**, *8*, 83. [CrossRef] [PubMed]
6. Rezai, A.R.; Kopell, B.H.; Gross, R.E.; Vitek, J.L.; Sharan, A.D.; Limousin, P.; Benabid, A.L. Deep brain stimulation for Parkinson's disease: Surgical issues. *Mov. Disord.* **2006**, *21* (Suppl. 14), S197–S218. [CrossRef]
7. Lyons, M.K.; Ziemba, K.; Evidente, V. Multichannel microelectrode recording influences final electrode placement in pallidal deep brain stimulation for Parkinson's disease: Report of twenty consecutive cases. *Turk. Neurosurg.* **2011**, *21*, 555–558. [CrossRef]
8. Kinfe, T.M.; Vesper, J. The impact of multichannel microelectrode recording (MER) in deep brain stimulation of the basal ganglia. In *Stereotactic and Functional Neurosurgery*; Springer: Berlin/Heidelberg, Germany, 2013; pp. 27–33.
9. Chen, S.-Y.; Lee, C.-C.; Lin, S.-H.; Hsin, Y.-L.; Lee, T.-W.; Yen, P.-S.; Chou, Y.-C.; Lee, C.-W.; Hsieh, W.A.; Su, C.-F. Microelectrode recording can be a good adjunct in magnetic resonance image–directed subthalamic nucleus deep brain stimulation for parkinsonism. *Surg. Neurol.* **2006**, *65*, 253–260. [CrossRef]
10. Chang, W.S.; Kim, H.Y.; Kim, J.P.; Park, Y.S.; Chung, S.S.; Chang, J.W. Bilateral subthalamic deep brain stimulation using single track microelectrode recording. *Acta Neurochir.* **2011**, *153*, 1087–1095. [CrossRef]
11. Tsai, S.-T.; Hung, H.-Y.; Lee, C.-H.; Chen, S.-Y. Letter to the Editor: Deep brain stimulation and microelectrode recording. *J. Neurosurg.* **2014**, *120*, 580. [CrossRef]
12. Machado, A.; Rezai, A.R.; Kopell, B.H.; Gross, R.E.; Sharan, A.D.; Benabid, A.L. Deep brain stimulation for Parkinson's disease: Surgical technique and perioperative management. *Mov. Disord.* **2006**, *21* (Suppl. 14), S247–S258. [CrossRef] [PubMed]
13. Priori, A.; Egidi, M.; Pesenti, A.; Rohr, M. Do intraoperative microrecordings improve subthalamic nucleus targeting in stereotactic neurosurgery for Parkinson's disease? *J. Neurosurg. Sci.* **2003**, *47*, 56. [PubMed]
14. Benazzouz, A.; Breit, S.; Koudsie, A.; Pollak, P.; Krack, P.; Benabid, A.L. Intraoperative microrecordings of the subthalamic nucleus in Parkinson's disease. *Mov. Disord. Off. J. Mov. Disord. Soc.* **2002**, *17*, S145–S149. [CrossRef] [PubMed]
15. Su, X.-L.; Luo, X.-G.; Lv, H.; Wang, J.; Ren, Y.; He, Z.-Y. Factors predicting the instant effect of motor function after subthalamic nucleus deep brain stimulation in Parkinson's disease. *Transl. Neurodegener.* **2017**, *6*, 14. [CrossRef] [PubMed]
16. Ho, A.L.; Ali, R.; Connolly, I.D.; Henderson, J.M.; Dhall, R.; Stein, S.C.; Halpern, C.H. Awake versus asleep deep brain stimulation for Parkinson's disease: A critical comparison and meta-analysis. *J. Neurol. Neurosurg. Psychiatry* **2018**, *89*, 687–691. [CrossRef]
17. Saint-Cyr, J.A.; Hoque, T.; Pereira, L.C.; Dostrovsky, J.O.; Hutchison, W.D.; Mikulis, D.J.; Abosch, A.; Sime, E.; Lang, A.E.; Lozano, A.M. Localization of clinically effective stimulating electrodes in the human subthalamic nucleus on magnetic resonance imaging. *J. Neurosurg.* **2002**, *97*, 1152–1166. [CrossRef]
18. McClelland, S., 3rd; Ford, B.; Senatus, P.B.; Winfield, L.M.; Du, Y.E.; Pullman, S.L.; Yu, Q.; Frucht, S.J.; McKhann, G.M., 2nd; Goodman, R.R. Subthalamic stimulation for Parkinson disease: Determination of electrode location necessary for clinical efficacy. *Neurosurg. Focus* **2005**, *19*, E12. [CrossRef]

19. Zonenshayn, M.; Rezai, A.R.; Mogilner, A.Y.; Beric, A.; Sterio, D.; Kelly, P.J. Comparison of anatomic and neurophysiological methods for subthalamic nucleus targeting. *Neurosurgery* **2000**, *47*, 282–292, discussion 292–284. [CrossRef]

20. Lanotte, M.M.; Rizzone, M.; Bergamasco, B.; Faccani, G.; Melcarne, A.; Lopiano, L. Deep brain stimulation of the subthalamic nucleus: Anatomical, neurophysiological, and outcome correlations with the effects of stimulation. *J. Neurol. Neurosurg. Psychiatry* **2002**, *72*, 53–58. [CrossRef]

21. Bus, S.; Pal, G.; Ouyang, B.; van den Munckhof, P.; Bot, M.; Sani, S.; Verhagen Metman, L. Accuracy of Microelectrode Trajectory Adjustments during DBS Assessed by Intraoperative CT. *Stereotact. Funct. Neurosurg.* **2018**, *96*, 231–238. [CrossRef]

22. Starr, P.A.; Martin, A.J.; Ostrem, J.L.; Talke, P.; Levesque, N.; Larson, P.S. Subthalamic nucleus deep brain stimulator placement using high-field interventional magnetic resonance imaging and a skull-mounted aiming device: Technique and application accuracy. *J. Neurosurg.* **2010**, *112*, 479–490. [CrossRef] [PubMed]

23. Foltynie, T.; Zrinzo, L.; Martinez-Torres, I.; Tripoliti, E.; Petersen, E.; Holl, E.; Aviles-Olmos, I.; Jahanshahi, M.; Hariz, M.; Limousin, P. MRI-guided STN DBS in Parkinson's disease without microelectrode recording: Efficacy and safety. *J. Neurol. Neurosurg. Psychiatry* **2011**, *82*, 358–363. [CrossRef] [PubMed]

24. Nakajima, T.; Zrinzo, L.; Foltynie, T.; Olmos, I.A.; Taylor, C.; Hariz, M.I.; Limousin, P. MRI-guided subthalamic nucleus deep brain stimulation without microelectrode recording: Can we dispense with surgery under local anaesthesia? *Stereotact. Funct. Neurosurg.* **2011**, *89*, 318–325. [CrossRef] [PubMed]

25. Ostrem, J.L.; Galifianakis, N.B.; Markun, L.C.; Grace, J.K.; Martin, A.J.; Starr, P.A.; Larson, P.S. Clinical outcomes of PD patients having bilateral STN DBS using high-field interventional MR-imaging for lead placement. *Clin. Neurol. Neurosurg.* **2013**, *115*, 708–712. [CrossRef] [PubMed]

26. Saleh, S.; Swanson, K.I.; Lake, W.B.; Sillay, K.A. Awake neurophysiologically guided versus asleep MRI-guided STN DBS for Parkinson disease: A comparison of outcomes using levodopa equivalents. *Stereotact. Funct. Neurosurg.* **2015**, *93*, 419–426. [CrossRef]

27. Ostrem, J.L.; Ziman, N.; Galifianakis, N.B.; Starr, P.A.; San Luciano, M.; Katz, M.; Racine, C.A.; Martin, A.J.; Markun, L.C.; Larson, P.S. Clinical outcomes using ClearPoint interventional MRI for deep brain stimulation lead placement in Parkinson's disease. *J. Neurosurg.* **2016**, *124*, 908–916. [CrossRef]

28. Sidiropoulos, C.; Rammo, R.; Merker, B.; Mahajan, A.; LeWitt, P.; Kaminski, P.; Womble, M.; Zec, A.; Taylor, D.; Wall, J. Intraoperative MRI for deep brain stimulation lead placement in Parkinson's disease: 1 year motor and neuropsychological outcomes. *J. Neurol.* **2016**, *263*, 1226–1231. [CrossRef]

29. Chircop, C.; Dingli, N.; Aquilina, A.; Zrinzo, L.; Aquilina, J. MRI-verified "asleep" deep brain stimulation in Malta through cross border collaboration: Clinical outcome of the first five years. *Br J. Neurosurg.* **2018**, *32*, 365–371. [CrossRef]

30. Matias, C.M.; Frizon, L.A.; Nagel, S.J.; Lobel, D.A.; Machado, A.G. Deep brain stimulation outcomes in patients implanted under general anesthesia with frame-based stereotaxy and intraoperative MRI. *J. Neurosurg.* **2018**, *129*, 1572–1578. [CrossRef]

31. Mirzadeh, Z.; Chapple, K.; Lambert, M.; Evidente, V.G.; Mahant, P.; Ospina, M.C.; Samanta, J.; Moguel-Cobos, G.; Salins, N.; Lieberman, A.; et al. Parkinson's disease outcomes after intraoperative CT-guided "asleep" deep brain stimulation in the globus pallidus internus. *J. Neurosurg.* **2016**, *124*, 902–907. [CrossRef]

32. Hertel, F.; Züchner, M.; Weimar, I.; Gemmar, P.; Noll, B.; Bettag, M.; Decker, C. Implantation of electrodes fordeep brain stimulation of the subthalamic nucleus in advanced parkinson's disease with the aid of intraoperative microrecording undergeneral anesthesia. *Neurosurgery* **2006**, *59*, E1138. [CrossRef] [PubMed]

33. Lefaucheur, J.-P.; Gurruchaga, J.-M.; Pollin, B.; Von Raison, F.; Mohsen, N.; Shin, M.; Ménard-Lefaucheur, I.; Oshino, S.; Kishima, H.; Fénelon, G. Outcome of bilateral subthalamic nucleus stimulation in the treatment of Parkinson's disease: Correlation with intra-operative multi-unit recordings but not with the type of anaesthesia. *Eur. Neurol.* **2008**, *60*, 186–199. [CrossRef] [PubMed]

34. Lin, S.H.; Chen, T.Y.; Lin, S.Z.; Shyr, M.H.; Chou, Y.C.; Hsieh, W.A.; Tsai, S.T.; Chen, S.Y. Subthalamic deep brain stimulation after anesthetic inhalation in Parkinson disease: A preliminary study. *J. Neurosurg.* **2008**, *109*, 238–244. [CrossRef] [PubMed]

35. Fluchere, F.; Witjas, T.; Eusebio, A.; Bruder, N.; Giorgi, R.; Leveque, M.; Peragut, J.C.; Azulay, J.P.; Regis, J. Controlled general anaesthesia for subthalamic nucleus stimulation in Parkinson's disease. *J. Neurol. Neurosurg. Psychiatry* **2014**, *85*, 1167–1173. [CrossRef] [PubMed]

36. Patel, N.K.; Heywood, P.; O'Sullivan, K.; Love, S.; Gill, S.S. MRI-directed subthalamic nucleus surgery for Parkinson's disease. *Stereotact. Funct. Neurosurg.* **2002**, *78*, 132–145. [CrossRef] [PubMed]

37. Burchiel, K.J.; McCartney, S.; Lee, A.; Raslan, A.M. Accuracy of deep brain stimulation electrode placement using intraoperative computed tomography without microelectrode recording. *J. Neurosurg.* **2013**, *119*, 301–306. [CrossRef]

38. Mirzadeh, Z.; Chapple, K.; Lambert, M.; Dhall, R.; Ponce, F.A. Validation of CT-MRI fusion for intraoperative assessment of stereotactic accuracy in DBS surgery. *Mov. Disord.* **2014**, *29*, 1788–1795. [CrossRef]

39. Zrinzo, L.; Foltynie, T.; Limousin, P.; Hariz, M. Image-guided and image-verified deep brain stimulation. *Mov. Disord.* **2013**, *28*, 254. [CrossRef]

40. Ferroli, P.; Franzini, A.; Marras, C.; Maccagnano, E.; D'Incerti, L.; Broggi, G. A simple method to assess accuracy of deep brain stimulation electrode placement: Pre-operative stereotactic CT+ postoperative MR image fusion. *Stereotact. Funct. Neurosurg.* **2004**, *82*, 14–19. [CrossRef]

41. Fiegele, T.; Feuchtner, G.; Sohm, F.; Bauer, R.; Anton, J.V.; Gotwald, T.; Twerdy, K.; Eisner, W. Accuracy of stereotactic electrode placement in deep brain stimulation by intraoperative computed tomography. *Park. Relat. Disord.* **2008**, *14*, 595–599. [CrossRef]

42. Chen, T.; Mirzadeh, Z.; Chapple, K.M.; Lambert, M.; Shill, H.A.; Moguel-Cobos, G.; Troster, A.I.; Dhall, R.; Ponce, F.A. Clinical outcomes following awake and asleep deep brain stimulation for Parkinson disease. *J. Neurosurg.* **2018**, *130*, 109–120. [CrossRef]

43. Ko, A.L.; Magown, P.; Ozpinar, A.; Hamzaoglu, V.; Burchiel, K.J. Asleep Deep Brain Stimulation Reduces Incidence of Intracranial Air during Electrode Implantation. *Stereotact. Funct. Neurosurg.* **2018**, *96*, 83–90. [CrossRef] [PubMed]

44. Cui, Z.; Pan, L.; Song, H.; Xu, X.; Xu, B.; Yu, X.; Ling, Z. Intraoperative MRI for optimizing electrode placement for deep brain stimulation of the subthalamic nucleus in Parkinson disease. *J. Neurosurg.* **2016**, *124*, 62–69. [CrossRef] [PubMed]

45. Chen, T.; Mirzadeh, Z.; Ponce, F.A. "Asleep" Deep Brain Stimulation Surgery: A Critical Review of the Literature. *World Neurosurg.* **2017**, *105*, 191–198. [CrossRef] [PubMed]

46. Sheshadri, V.; Rowland, N.C.; Mehta, J.; Englesakis, M.; Manninen, P.; Venkatraghavan, L. Comparison of General and Local Anesthesia for Deep Brain Stimulator Insertion: A Systematic Review. *Can. J. Neurol. Sci.* **2017**, *44*, 697–704. [CrossRef]

47. Bot, M.; van den Munckhof, P.; Bakay, R.; Stebbins, G.; Metman, L.V. Accuracy of intraoperative computed tomography during deep brain stimulation procedures: Comparison with postoperative magnetic resonance imaging. *Stereotact. Funct. Neurosurg.* **2017**, *95*, 183–188. [CrossRef]

48. Kremer, N.I.; Oterdoom, D.L.M.; van Laar, P.J.; Piña-Fuentes, D.; van Laar, T.; Drost, G.; van Hulzen, A.L.J.; van Dijk, J.M.C. Accuracy of Intraoperative Computed Tomography in Deep Brain Stimulation-A Prospective Noninferiority Study. *Neuromodul. Technol. Neural Interface* **2019**, *22*, 472–477. [CrossRef]

49. Harries, A.M.; Kausar, J.; Roberts, S.A.; Mocroft, A.P.; Hodson, J.A.; Pall, H.S.; Mitchell, R.D. Deep brain stimulation of the subthalamic nucleus for advanced Parkinson disease using general anesthesia: Long-term results. *J. Neurosurg.* **2012**, *116*, 107–113. [CrossRef]

50. Kwon, W.K.; Kim, J.H.; Lee, J.H.; Lim, B.G.; Lee, I.O.; Koh, S.B.; Kwon, T.H. Microelectrode recording (MER) findings during sleep-awake anesthesia using dexmedetomidine in deep brain stimulation surgery for Parkinson's disease. *Clin. Neurol. Neurosurg.* **2016**, *143*, 27–33. [CrossRef] [PubMed]

51. Warnke, P. Deep brain stimulation: Awake or asleep: It comes with a price either way. *J. Neurol. Neurosurg. Psychiatry* **2018**, *89*, 672. [CrossRef] [PubMed]

52. Tsai, S.-T.; Kuo, C.-C.; Chen, T.-Y.; Chen, S.-Y. Neurophysiological comparisons of subthalamic deep-brain stimulation for Parkinson's disease between patients receiving general and local anesthesia. *Tzu Chi Med. J.* **2016**, *28*, 63–67. [CrossRef] [PubMed]

53. LaHue, S.C.; Ostrem, J.L.; Galifianakis, N.B.; San Luciano, M.; Ziman, N.; Wang, S.; Racine, C.A.; Starr, P.A.; Larson, P.S.; Katz, M. Parkinson's disease patient preference and experience with various methods of DBS lead placement. *Park. Relat. Disord.* **2017**, *41*, 25–30. [CrossRef] [PubMed]

54. Yamada, K.; Goto, S.; Kuratsu, J.; Matsuzaki, K.; Tamura, T.; Nagahiro, S.; Murase, N.; Shimazu, H.; Kaji, R. Stereotactic surgery for subthalamic nucleus stimulation under general anesthesia: A retrospective evaluation of Japanese patients with Parkinson's disease. *Park. Relat. Disord.* **2007**, *13*, 101–107. [CrossRef] [PubMed]

55. Chen, S.Y.; Tsai, S.T.; Lin, S.H.; Chen, T.Y.; Hung, H.Y.; Lee, C.W.; Wang, W.H.; Chen, S.P.; Lin, S.Z. Subthalamic deep brain stimulation in Parkinson's disease under different anesthetic modalities: A comparative cohort study. *Stereotact. Funct. Neurosurg.* **2011**, *89*, 372–380. [CrossRef] [PubMed]

56. Asha, M.J.; Fisher, B.; Kausar, J.; Garratt, H.; Krovvidi, H.; Shirley, C.; White, A.; Chelvarajah, R.; Ughratdar, I.; Hodson, J.A. Subthalamic deep brain stimulation under general anesthesia and neurophysiological guidance while on dopaminergic medication: Comparative cohort study. *Acta Neurochir.* **2018**, *160*, 823–829. [CrossRef] [PubMed]

57. Lettieri, C.; Rinaldo, S.; Devigili, G.; Pauletto, G.; Verriello, L.; Budai, R.; Fadiga, L.; Oliynyk, A.; Mondani, M.; D'Auria, S.; et al. Deep brain stimulation: Subthalamic nucleus electrophysiological activity in awake and anesthetized patients. *Clin. Neurophysiol. Off. J. Int. Fed. Clin. Neurophysiol.* **2012**, *123*, 2406–2413. [CrossRef] [PubMed]

58. Maltête, D.; Navarro, S.; Welter, M.-L.; Roche, S.; Bonnet, A.-M.; Houeto, J.-L.; Mesnage, V.; Pidoux, B.; Dormont, D.; Cornu, P. Subthalamic stimulation in Parkinson disease: With or without anesthesia? *Arch. Neurol.* **2004**, *61*, 390–392. [CrossRef]

59. Brodsky, M.A.; Anderson, S.; Murchison, C.; Seier, M.; Wilhelm, J.; Vederman, A.; Burchiel, K.J. Clinical outcomes of asleep vs awake deep brain stimulation for Parkinson disease. *Neurology* **2017**, *89*, 1944–1950. [CrossRef]

60. Sharma, M.; Deogaonkar, M. Accuracy and safety of targeting using intraoperative "O-arm" during placement of deep brain stimulation electrodes without electrophysiological recordings. *J. Clin. Neurosci. Off. J. Neurosurg. Soc. Australas* **2016**, *27*, 80–86. [CrossRef]

61. Carlson, J.D.; McLeod, K.E.; McLeod, P.S.; Mark, J.B. Stereotactic Accuracy and Surgical Utility of the O-Arm in Deep Brain Stimulation Surgery. *Oper. Neurosurg. (Hagerstown)* **2017**, *13*, 96–107. [CrossRef]

62. Sillay, K.A.; Rusy, D.; Buyan-Dent, L.; Ninman, N.L.; Vigen, K.K. Wide-bore 1.5 T MRI-guided deep brain stimulation surgery: Initial experience and technique comparison. *Clin. Neurol. Neurosurg.* **2014**, *127*, 79–85. [CrossRef] [PubMed]

63. Aviles-Olmos, I.; Kefalopoulou, Z.; Tripoliti, E.; Candelario, J.; Akram, H.; Martinez-Torres, I.; Jahanshahi, M.; Foltynie, T.; Hariz, M.; Zrinzo, L. Long-term outcome of subthalamic nucleus deep brain stimulation for Parkinson's disease using an MRI-guided and MRI-verified approach. *J. Neurol. Neurosurg. Psychiatry* **2014**, *85*, 1419–1425. [CrossRef] [PubMed]

64. Chabardes, S.; Isnard, S.; Castrioto, A.; Oddoux, M.; Fraix, V.; Carlucci, L.; Payen, J.F.; Krainik, A.; Krack, P.; Larson, P. Surgical implantation of STN-DBS leads using intraoperative MRI guidance: Technique, accuracy, and clinical benefit at 1-year follow-up. *Acta Neurochir.* **2015**, *157*, 729–737. [CrossRef] [PubMed]

65. Spiegelmann, R.; Nissim, O.; Daniels, D.; Ocherashvilli, A.; Mardor, Y. Stereotactic targeting of the ventrointermediate nucleus of the thalamus by direct visualization with high-field MRI. *Stereotact. Funct. Neurosurg.* **2006**, *84*, 19–23. [CrossRef] [PubMed]

66. Lee, P.S.; Richardson, R.M. Interventional MRI-Guided Deep Brain Stimulation Lead Implantation. *Neurosurg. Clin. N. Am.* **2017**, *28*, 535–544. [CrossRef]

67. Min, H.K.; Ross, E.K.; Lee, K.H.; Dennis, K.; Han, S.R.; Jeong, J.H.; Marsh, M.P.; Striemer, B.; Felmlee, J.P.; Lujan, J.L.; et al. Subthalamic nucleus deep brain stimulation induces motor network BOLD activation: Use of a high precision MRI guided stereotactic system for nonhuman primates. *Brain Stimul.* **2014**, *7*, 603–607. [CrossRef]

68. Kochanski, R.B.; Sani, S. Awake versus Asleep Deep Brain Stimulation Surgery: Technical Considerations and Critical Review of the Literature. *Brain Sci.* **2018**, *8*, 17. [CrossRef]

69. Kamiryo, T.; Laws, E.R., Jr. Stereotactic frame-based error in magnetic-resonance-guided stereotactic procedures: A method for measurement of error and standardization of technique. *Stereotact. Funct. Neurosurg.* **1996**, *67*, 198–209. [CrossRef]

70. Ko, A.L.; Ibrahim, A.; Magown, P.; Macallum, R.; Burchiel, K.J. Factors affecting stereotactic accuracy in image-guided deep brain stimulator electrode placement. *Stereotact. Funct. Neurosurg.* **2017**, *95*, 315–324. [CrossRef]

71. Chen, T.; Mirzadeh, Z.; Chapple, K.; Lambert, M.; Dhall, R.; Ponce, F.A. "Asleep" deep brain stimulation for essential tremor. *J. Neurosurg.* **2016**, *124*, 1842–1849. [CrossRef]

72. Holloway, K.; Docef, A. A quantitative assessment of the accuracy and reliability of O-arm images for deep brain stimulation surgery. *Neurosurgery* **2013**, *72*, 47–57. [CrossRef] [PubMed]

73. Geevarghese, R.; O'Gorman Tuura, R.; Lumsden, D.E.; Samuel, M.; Ashkan, K. Registration Accuracy of CT/MRI Fusion for Localisation of Deep Brain Stimulation Electrode Position: An Imaging Study and Systematic Review. *Stereotact. Funct. Neurosurg.* **2016**, *94*, 159–163. [CrossRef] [PubMed]

74. Ivan, M.E.; Yarlagadda, J.; Saxena, A.P.; Martin, A.J.; Starr, P.A.; Sootsman, W.K.; Larson, P.S. Brain shift during bur hole-based procedures using interventional MRI. *J. Neurosurg.* **2014**, *121*, 149–160. [CrossRef] [PubMed]

75. Deuschl, G.; Schade-Brittinger, C.; Krack, P.; Volkmann, J.; Schäfer, H.; Bötzel, K.; Daniels, C.; Deutschländer, A.; Dillmann, U.; Eisner, W. A randomized trial of deep-brain stimulation for Parkinson's disease. *N. Engl. J. Med.* **2006**, *355*, 896–908. [CrossRef]

76. Erickson, K.M.; Cole, D.J. Anesthetic considerations for awake craniotomy for epilepsy. *Anesthesiol. Clin.* **2007**, *25*, 535–555, ix. [CrossRef]

77. Grant, R.; Gruenbaum, S.E.; Gerrard, J. Anaesthesia for deep brain stimulation: A review. *Curr. Opin. Anaesthesiol.* **2015**, *28*, 505. [CrossRef]

78. Khan, M.F.; Mewes, K.; Gross, R.E.; Skrinjar, O. Assessment of brain shift related to deep brain stimulation surgery. *Stereotact. Funct. Neurosurg.* **2008**, *86*, 44–53. [CrossRef]

79. Pallavaram, S.; Dawant, B.M.; Remple, M.S.; Neimat, J.S.; Kao, C.; Konrad, P.E.; D'Haese, P.F. Effect of brain shift on the creation of functional atlases for deep brain stimulation surgery. *Int. J. Comput. Assist. Radiol. Surg.* **2010**, *5*, 221–228. [CrossRef]

80. Elias, W.J.; Durieux, M.E.; Huss, D.; Frysinger, R.C. Dexmedetomidine and arousal affect subthalamic neurons. *Mov. Disord.* **2008**, *23*, 1317–1320. [CrossRef]

81. Pollak, P.; Krack, P.; Fraix, V.; Mendes, A.; Moro, E.; Chabardes, S.; Benabid, A.L. Intraoperative micro- and macrostimulation of the subthalamic nucleus in Parkinson's disease. *Mov. Disord.* **2002**, *17* (Suppl. 3), S155–S161. [CrossRef]

82. Gorgulho, A.; De Salles, A.A.; Frighetto, L.; Behnke, E. Incidence of hemorrhage associated with electrophysiological studies performed using macroelectrodes and microelectrodes in functional neurosurgery. *J. Neurosurg.* **2005**, *102*, 888–896. [CrossRef] [PubMed]

83. Binder, D.K.; Rau, G.M.; Starr, P.A. Risk factors for hemorrhage during microelectrode-guided deep brain stimulator implantation for movement disorders. *Neurosurgery* **2005**, *56*, 722–732. [CrossRef] [PubMed]

84. Vesper, J.; Haak, S.; Ostertag, C.; Nikkhah, G. Subthalamic nucleus deep brain stimulation in elderly patients–analysis of outcome and complications. *BMC Neurol.* **2007**, *7*, 7. [CrossRef] [PubMed]

85. Guridi, J.; Rodriguez-Oroz, M.C.; Lozano, A.M.; Moro, E.; Albanese, A.; Nuttin, B.; Gybels, J.; Ramos, E.; Obeso, J.A. Targeting the basal ganglia for deep brain stimulation in Parkinson's disease. *Neurology* **2000**, *55*, S21–S28.

86. Houeto, J.-L.; Welter, M.-L.; Bejjani, P.-B.; du Montcel, S.T.; Bonnet, A.-M.; Mesnage, V.; Navarro, S.; Pidoux, B.; Dormont, D.; Cornu, P. Subthalamic stimulation in Parkinson disease: Intraoperative predictive factors. *Arch. Neurol.* **2003**, *60*, 690–694. [CrossRef]

87. Blasberg, F.; Wojtecki, L.; Elben, S.; Slotty, P.J.; Vesper, J.; Schnitzler, A.; Groiss, S.J. Comparison of Awake vs. Asleep Surgery for Subthalamic Deep Brain Stimulation in Parkinson's Disease. *Neuromodulation* **2018**, *21*, 541–547. [CrossRef]

88. Castrioto, A.; Marmor, O.; Deffains, M.; Willner, D.; Linetsky, E.; Bergman, H.; Israel, Z.; Eitan, R.; Arkadir, D. Anesthesia reduces discharge rates in the human pallidum without changing the discharge rate ratio between pallidal segments. *Eur. J. Neurosci.* **2016**, *44*, 2909–2913. [CrossRef]

89. Moll, C.K.; Payer, S.; Gulberti, A.; Sharrott, A.; Zittel, S.; Boelmans, K.; Köppen, J.; Gerloff, C.; Westphal, M.; Engel, A.K. STN stimulation in general anaesthesia: Evidence beyond 'evidence-based medicine'. In *Stereotactic and Functional Neurosurgery*; Springer: Berlin/Heidelberg, Germany, 2013; pp. 19–25.

90. Sanghera, M.K.; Grossman, R.G.; Kalhorn, C.G.; Hamilton, W.J.; Ondo, W.G.; Jankovic, J. Basal ganglia neuronal discharge in primary and secondary dystonia in patients undergoing pallidotomy. *Neurosurgery* **2003**, *52*, 1358–1373. [CrossRef]

91. Tsai, S.T.; Chuang, W.Y.; Kuo, C.C.; Chao, P.C.; Chen, T.Y.; Hung, H.Y.; Chen, S.Y. Dorsolateral subthalamic neuronal activity enhanced by median nerve stimulation characterizes Parkinson's disease during deep brain stimulation with general anesthesia. *J. Neurosurg.* **2015**, *123*, 1394–1400. [CrossRef]

92. Kim, W.; Song, I.H.; Lim, Y.H.; Kim, M.-R.; Kim, Y.E.; Hwang, J.H.; Kim, I.K.; Song, S.W.; Kim, J.W.; Lee, W.-W. Influence of propofol and fentanyl on deep brain stimulation of the subthalamic nucleus. *J. Korean Med. Sci.* **2014**, *29*, 1278–1286. [CrossRef]

93. Lee, W.-W.; Ehm, G.; Yang, H.-J.; Song, I.H.; Lim, Y.H.; Kim, M.-R.; Kim, Y.E.; Hwang, J.H.; Park, H.R.; Lee, J.M. Bilateral deep brain stimulation of the subthalamic nucleus under sedation with propofol and fentanyl. *PLoS ONE* **2016**, *11*, e0152619. [CrossRef] [PubMed]

94. Galvan, A.; Wichmann, T. GABAergic circuits in the basal ganglia and movement disorders. *Prog. Brain Res.* **2007**, *160*, 287–312. [PubMed]

95. Raz, A.; Eimerl, D.; Zaidel, A.; Bergman, H.; Israel, Z. Propofol decreases neuronal population spiking activity in the subthalamic nucleus of Parkinsonian patients. *Anesth. Analg.* **2010**, *111*, 1285–1289. [CrossRef] [PubMed]

96. Lin, S.H.; Lai, H.Y.; Lo, Y.C.; Chou, C.; Chou, Y.T.; Yang, S.H.; Sun, I.; Chen, B.W.; Wang, C.F.; Liu, G.T.; et al. Decreased Power but Preserved Bursting Features of Subthalamic Neuronal Signals in Advanced Parkinson's Patients under Controlled Desflurane Inhalation Anesthesia. *Front. Neurosci.* **2017**, *11*, 701. [CrossRef] [PubMed]

97. Kouvaras, E.; Asprodini, E.K.; Asouchidou, I.; Vasilaki, A.; Kilindris, T.; Michaloudis, D.; Koukoutianou, I.; Papatheodoropoulos, C.; Kostopoulos, G. Fentanyl treatment reduces GABAergic inhibition in the CA1 area of the hippocampus 24 h after acute exposure to the drug. *Neuropharmacology* **2008**, *55*, 1172–1182. [CrossRef]

98. Hutchison, W.D.; Lang, A.E.; Dostrovsky, J.O.; Lozano, A.M. Pallidal neuronal activity: Implications for models of dystonia. *Ann. Neurol.* **2003**, *53*, 480–488. [CrossRef]

99. Khatib, R.; Ebrahim, Z.; Rezai, A.; Cata, J.P.; Boulis, N.M.; John Doyle, D.; Schurigyn, T.; Farag, E. Perioperative events during deep brain stimulation: The experience at cleveland clinic. *J. Neurosurg. Anesthesiol.* **2008**, *20*, 36–40. [CrossRef]

100. Duque, P.; Mateo, O.; Ruiz, F.; de Viloria, J.G.; Contreras, A.; Grandas, F. Intraoperative microrecording under general anaesthesia with bispectral analysis monitoring in a case of deep brain stimulation surgery for Parkinson's disease. *Eur. J. Neurol.* **2008**, *15*, e76–e77. [CrossRef]

101. Lee, J.Y.; Deogaonkar, M.; Rezai, A. Deep brain stimulation of globus pallidus internus for dystonia. *Park. Relat. Disord.* **2007**, *13*, 261–265. [CrossRef]

102. Morace, R.; De Angelis, M.; Aglialoro, E.; Maucione, G.; Cavallo, L.; Solari, D.; Modugno, N.; Santilli, M.; Esposito, V.; Aloj, F. Sedation with α2 Agonist Dexmedetomidine During Unilateral Subthalamic Nucleus Deep Brain Stimulation: A Preliminary Report. *World Neurosurg.* **2016**, *89*, 320–328. [CrossRef]

103. Rozet, I. Anesthesia for functional neurosurgery: The role of dexmedetomidine. *Curr. Opin. Anaesthesiol.* **2008**, *21*, 537–543. [CrossRef] [PubMed]

104. Sassi, M.; Zekaj, E.; Grotta, A.; Pollini, A.; Pellanda, A.; Borroni, M.; Pacchetti, C.; Menghetti, C.; Porta, M.; Servello, D. Safety in the use of dexmedetomidine (precedex) for deep brain stimulation surgery: Our experience in 23 randomized patients. *Neuromodulation* **2013**, *16*, 401–406. [CrossRef] [PubMed]

105. Hans, P.; Bonhomme, V.; Born, J.D.; Maertens de Noordhoudt, A.; Brichant, J.F.; Dewandre, P.Y. Target-controlled infusion of propofol and remifentanil combined with bispectral index monitoring for awake craniotomy. *Anaesthesia* **2000**, *55*, 255–259. [CrossRef] [PubMed]

106. Johansen, J.W.; Sebel, P.S. Development and clinical application of electroencephalographic bispectrum monitoring. *Anesthesiology* **2000**, *93*, 1336–1344. [CrossRef] [PubMed]

107. Sutcliffe, A.; Mitchell, R.; Gan, Y.; Mocroft, A.; Nightingale, P. General anaesthesia for deep brain stimulator electrode insertion in Parkinson's disease. *Acta Neurochir.* **2011**, *153*, 621–627. [CrossRef]

108. Tsai, S.-T.; Chen, T.-Y.; Lin, S.-H.; Chen, S.-Y. Five-year clinical outcomes of local versus general anesthesia deep brain stimulation for Parkinson's disease. *Parkinson's Dis.* **2019**, *2019*, 5676345. [CrossRef]

109. Martin, A.J.; Larson, P.S.; Ziman, N.; Levesque, N.; Volz, M.; Ostrem, J.L.; Starr, P.A. Deep brain stimulator implantation in a diagnostic MRI suite: Infection history over a 10-year period. *J. Neurosurg.* **2017**, *126*, 108–113. [CrossRef]

110. Chen, T.; Mirzadeh, Z.; Chapple, K.; Lambert, M.; Ponce, F.A. Complication rates, lengths of stay, and readmission rates in "awake" and "asleep" deep brain simulation. *J. Neurosurg.* **2017**, *127*, 360–369. [CrossRef]

111. Jacob, R.L.; Geddes, J.; McCartney, S.; Burchiel, K.J. Cost analysis of awake versus asleep deep brain stimulation: A single academic health center experience. *J. Neurosurg.* **2016**, *124*, 1517–1523. [CrossRef]

112. Lefranc, M.; Zouitina, Y.; Tir, M.; Merle, P.; Ouendo, M.; Constans, J.M.; Godefroy, O.; Peltier, J.; Krystkowiak, P. Asleep Robot-Assisted Surgery for the Implantation of Subthalamic Electrodes Provides the Same Clinical Improvement and Therapeutic Window as Awake Surgery. *World Neurosurg.* **2017**, *106*, 602–608. [CrossRef]

113. Liu, Z.; He, S.; Li, L. General Anesthesia versus Local Anesthesia for Deep Brain Stimulation in Parkinson's Disease: A Meta-Analysis. *Stereotact. Funct. Neurosurg.* **2019**, *97*, 381–390. [CrossRef] [PubMed]

114. Paek, S.H.; Han, J.H.; Lee, J.Y.; Kim, C.; Jeon, B.S.; Kim, D.G. Electrode position determined by fused images of preoperative and postoperative magnetic resonance imaging and surgical outcome after subthalamic nucleus deep brain stimulation. *Neurosurgery* **2008**, *63*, 925–936, discussion 936–927. [CrossRef] [PubMed]

115. Paek, S.H.; Yun, J.Y.; Song, S.W.; Kim, I.K.; Hwang, J.H.; Kim, J.W.; Kim, H.J.; Kim, H.J.; Kim, Y.E.; Lim, Y.H.; et al. The clinical impact of precise electrode positioning in STN DBS on three-year outcomes. *J. Neurol. Sci.* **2013**, *327*, 25–31. [CrossRef] [PubMed]

116. Ryu, S.I.; Romanelli, P.; Heit, G. Asymptomatic transient MRI signal changes after unilateral deep brain stimulation electrode implantation for movement disorder. *Stereotact. Funct. Neurosurg.* **2004**, *82*, 65–69. [CrossRef] [PubMed]

117. Englot, D.J.; Glastonbury, C.M.; Larson, P.S. Abnormal T2-weighted MRI signal surrounding leads in a subset of deep brain stimulation patients. *Stereotact. Funct. Neurosurg.* **2011**, *89*, 311–317. [CrossRef] [PubMed]

118. Fenoy, A.J.; Villarreal, S.J.; Schiess, M.C. Acute and subacute presentations of cerebral edema following deep brain stimulation lead implantation. *Stereotact. Funct. Neurosurg.* **2017**, *95*, 86–92. [CrossRef]

119. Deogaonkar, M.; Nazzaro, J.M.; Machado, A.; Rezai, A. Transient, symptomatic, post-operative, non-infectious hypodensity around the deep brain stimulation (DBS) electrode. *J. Clin. Neurosci.* **2011**, *18*, 910–915. [CrossRef]

120. Holewijn, R.A.; Verbaan, D.; de Bie, R.M.A.; Schuurman, P.R. General Anesthesia versus Local Anesthesia in StereotaXY (GALAXY) for Parkinson's disease: Study protocol for a randomized controlled trial. *Trials* **2017**, *18*, 417. [CrossRef]

121. Little, S.; Pogosyan, A.; Neal, S.; Zavala, B.; Zrinzo, L.; Hariz, M.; Foltynie, T.; Limousin, P.; Ashkan, K.; FitzGerald, J. Adaptive deep brain stimulation in advanced Parkinson disease. *Ann. Neurol.* **2013**, *74*, 449–457. [CrossRef]

122. Little, S.; Beudel, M.; Zrinzo, L.; Foltynie, T.; Limousin, P.; Hariz, M.; Neal, S.; Cheeran, B.; Cagnan, H.; Gratwicke, J. Bilateral adaptive deep brain stimulation is effective in Parkinson's disease. *J. Neurol. Neurosurg. Psychiatry* **2016**, *87*, 717–721. [CrossRef]

123. Higuchi, Y.; Matsuda, S.; Serizawa, T. Gamma knife radiosurgery in movement disorders: Indications and limitations. *Mov. Disord.* **2017**, *32*, 28–35. [CrossRef] [PubMed]

124. Friedman, J.H.; Epstein, M.; Sanes, J.N.; Lieberman, P.; Cullen, K.; Lindquist, C.; Daamen, M. Gamma knife pallidotomy in advanced Parkinson's disease. *Ann. Neurol.* **1996**, *39*, 535–538. [CrossRef] [PubMed]

125. Magara, A.; Bühler, R.; Moser, D.; Kowalski, M.; Pourtehrani, P.; Jeanmonod, D. First experience with MR-guided focused ultrasound in the treatment of Parkinson's disease. *J. Ther. Ultrasound* **2014**, *2*, 11. [CrossRef] [PubMed]

126. Martínez-Fernández, R.; Rodríguez-Rojas, R.; Del Álamo, M.; Hernández-Fernández, F.; Pineda-Pardo, J.A.; Dileone, M.; Alonso-Frech, F.; Foffani, G.; Obeso, I.; Gasca-Salas, C. Focused ultrasound subthalamotomy in patients with asymmetric Parkinson's disease: A pilot study. *Lancet Neurol.* **2018**, *17*, 54–63. [CrossRef]

## 8

Effectiveness, Timing and Procedural Aspects of Cognitive Behavioral Therapy after Deep Brain Stimulation for Therapy-Resistant Obsessive Compulsive Disorder

Meltem Görmezoğlu [1,2], Tim Bouwens van der Vlis [2], Koen Schruers [3,4], Linda Ackermans [2,4], Mircea Polosan [5] and Albert F.G. Leentjens [3,4,*]

[1] Department of Psychiatry, Ondokuz Mayıs University, 55270 Samsun, Turkey; gormezoglumeltem@gmail.com

[2] Department of Neurosurgery, Maastricht University Medical Centre, 6229 Maastricht, The Netherlands; tim.bouwens@mumc.nl (T.B.v.d.V.); linda.ackermans@mumc.nl (L.A.)

[3] Department of Psychiatry and Neuropsychology, Maastricht University Medical Center, 6229 Maastricht, The Netherlands; koen.schruers@maastrichtuniversity.nl

[4] School of Mental Health and Neuroscience, Maastricht University, 6229 Maastricht, The Netherlands

[5] Grenoble Institute of Neurosciences, University of Grenoble Alpes, 38058 Grenoble, France; MPolosan@chu-grenoble.fr

[*] Correspondence: a.leentjens@maastrichtuniversity.nl

Abstract: *Background and aim:* Deep brain stimulation (DBS) is an effective treatment for patients with severe therapy-resistant obsessive-compulsive disorder (OCD). After initiating DBS many patients still require medication and/or behavioral therapy to deal with persisting symptoms and habitual behaviors. The clinical practice of administering postoperative cognitive behavioral therapy (CBT) varies widely, and there are no clinical guidelines for this add-on therapy. The aim of this review is to assess the efficacy, timing and procedural aspects of postoperative CBT in OCD patients treated with DBS. *Method:* Systematic review of literature. *Results:* The search yielded 5 original studies, one case series and three reviews. Only two clinical trials have explicitly focused on the effectiveness of CBT added to DBS in patients with therapy-resistant OCD. These two studies both showed effectiveness of CBT. However, they had a distinctly different design, very small sample sizes and different ways of administering the therapy. Therefore, no firm conclusions can be drawn or recommendations made for administering CBT after DBS for therapy-resistant OCD. *Conclusion:* The effectiveness, timing and procedural aspects of CBT added to DBS in therapy-resistant OCD have hardly been studied. Preliminary evidence indicates that CBT has an added effect in OCD patients being treated with DBS. Since the overall treatment effect is the combined result of DBS, medication and CBT, future trials should be designed in such a way that they allow quantification of the effects of these add-on therapies in OCD patients treated with DBS. Only in this way information can be gathered that contributes to the development of an algorithm and clinical guidelines for concomittant therapies to optimize treatment effects in OCD patients being treated with DBS.

Keywords: deep brain stimulation; obsessive compulsive disorder; cognitive behavioral therapy

---

1. Introduction

Obsessive-compulsive disorder (OCD) is a chronic psychiatric disorder characterized by the presence of obsessions and/or compulsions. Its prevalence varies from 0.8% to 3% in the adult population [1]. The World Health Organization lists OCD as the 11th most common cause of secondary disability, accounting for 2.2% of the total years lived with disability [2]. Cognitive behavioral therapy (CBT), including exposure and response prevention (ERP), as well as pharmacotherapy with serotonergic medication, are the main forms of treatment for OCD. The effectiveness of CBT as treatment for OCD has been established in multiple studies [3,4]. However, its acceptability is limited: as much as 16% to 30% of patients offered CBT drops out during treatment [4,5]. Serotonergic medication, as well as augmentation with atypical antipsychotics, were shown to be effective, and the combination of medication and CBT is even more effective [6,7]. However, a large percentage of OCD patients show only a partial response, or are refractory to psychotherapy and pharmacotherapy. In severe therapy-resistant cases, deep brain stimulation (DBS) may be an option. Although the target and stimulation characteristics may vary across studies and clinics, DBS is generally considered safe and effective for the treatment of therapy-resistant OCD [8]. DBS received approval as treatment for OCD by the European Comission (EC) in 2009, and in the same year it was approved as a Humanitarian Device Exemption by the U.S. Food and Drug Administration (FDA).

After DBS, patients often still need medication, and CBT is often offered because it is considered useful in the treatment of remaining obsessive and compulsive symptoms, in dealing with behavior that has become habitual and persists even when the urge has subsided, and in helping to adjust to the new situation and new expectancies. In addition, CBT provides the patient with new coping styles and problem solving skills that may be important to prevent relapse and contribute to the long-term efficacy of DBS. Whereas guidelines for CBT in OCD have suggested offering CBT after DBS, clinical practice varies widely across institutions and often depends on local possibilities and traditions [9,10]. A more uniform and evidence-based approach may be beneficial for patients.

Up until now, the added effect of CBT to DBS for OCD has not been reviewed. The aim of this systematic review is to assess the literature on efficacy, timing and procedural aspects of postoperative CBT in patients being treated with DBS for therapy-resistant OCD, and to formulate clinical recommendations for future research and for offering CBT after DBS.

2. Methods

A systematic review of studies catalogued in PubMed was performed following the Preferred Reporting Items for Systematic Reviews and Meta-Analyses (PRISMA) guidelines (www.prisma-statement.org). The search was done over the full time span up until 17 April 2020. Only papers in English were included. We used the following broad Booleian search strategy: "(deep brain stimulation) AND (obsessive compulsive disorder) AND ((exposure and response prevention) OR (behavioral therapy) OR (cognitive behavioral therapy))". Given the limited yield of a narrower, exploratory search, all papers that addressed any form of postoperative CBT in patients receiving DBS for therapy-resistant OCD were included. This not only comprised clinical trials, cohort studies, case series and case studies, but also systematic and narrative reviews on DBS for OCD and position papers if they also commented on CBT after DBS. Reference lists of the included studies were checked for additional papers. The Evidence Project risk of bias tool was used to assess the quality of the included studies (not being reviews) [11]. Two authors rated the quality (MG and AL) and discrepancies were resolved by consensus. Due to the very limited yield of our search, no minimum quality score was applied for inclusion. The effectiveness of CBT added to DBS was quantified by looking at the changes in scores on the Yale–Brown Obsessive Compulsive Scale (Y-BOCS) before and after CBT. Although the initial intention was to perform a meta-analysis, this was not possible because of the limited number of included studies that, in addition, used different indication criteria and different forms and ways of delivery of CBT. Timing and procedural aspects of CBT in the studies are reported in a descriptive way.

3. Results

3.1. Literature Search

The search yielded 181 papers. One additional paper was added after checking the reference lists of included papers [12]. Based on the title and/or abstract, 154 of these were excluded because of the following reasons: animal studies ($n = 14$), not referring to OCD ($n = 61$), not referring to DBS ($n = 15$), not referring to CBT ($n = 28$), not in English ($n = 10$) and other reasons (including the absence of an abstract) ($n = 17$). The remaining 28 papers were read in full. An additional 19 of these were excluded due to the following reasons: not referring to CBT ($n = 11$), not referring to DBS ($n = 1$) and other reasons ($n = 7$). Eventually, 9 papers were included in the review: three randomized controlled trials (RCTs) [13–15], one cohort study [16], one case series [12], one qualitative study [17], one systematic review [18] and 2 narrative reviews [19,20]. These reviews were focused on the efficacy of DBS for OCD and not on the efficacy of CBT after DBS for OCD. Two of the included papers were based on the same RCT [13,14] (see Figure 1 for a PRISMA flowchart). The quality assessment of these studies are displayed in supplementary Table S1. The included systematic and narrative reviews are not discussed in the 'results' section since they did not include other relevant papers than the ones discussed below.

Figure 1. PRISMA flow diagramme. Abbreviations: OCD = obsessive compulsive disorder; DBS = deep brain stimulation; BT = behavioral therapy.

3.2. Description of Included Studies

The first RCT, by Denys et al. (2010) was a double-blind, sham–controlled, clinical trial of DBS of the nucleus accumbens (NA) that included 16 therapy resistant OCD patients [13]. In this study, refractoriness was defined as no or insufficient response to treatment with at least 2 different selective serotonin reuptake inhibitors (SSRIs) at maximum dosage for at least 12 weeks, treatment with clomipramine hydrochloride for at least 12 weeks with adequacy of treatment established by plasma levels, one augmentation trial with an atypical antipsychotic for 8 weeks in combination with an selective serotonin reuptake inhibitor, and at least 16 sessions of CBT [13].

Design: The study had 3 sequential treatment phases: an initial open phase, starting immediately after electrode implantation and lasting for 8 months, in which stimulation parameters were optimized and CBT was started. DBS was administered per protocol, with restricted stimulation settings at 90 μs, 130 Hz and a maximum stimulation intensity of 5.0 V. The effects of DBS were assessed with the Y-BOCS for obsessions and compulsions, with the Hamilton Anxiety Rating Scale (HAMA) for anxiety symptoms, and with the Hamilton Depression Scale (HAMD) for depression. After this open phase, a 1-month, double blind, sham-controlled phase started in which patients were randomly allocated to 2 periods of 2 weeks with the stimulators blindly turned 'on' (active stimulation) or 'off' (sham stimulation). CBT was continued throughout this phase. The double-blind phase was followed by a 12-month maintenance phase in which the stimulator was turned on for all patients and settings adjusted as required. Patients were allowed to use psychopharmacological medication during the trial.

Effectiveness: Stimulation in the initial open phase resulted in a mean decrease of 46% in Y-BOCS score from 33.7 (baseline) to 18.0 points; a mean decrease of 52% on the HAMA score from 20.9 (baseline) to 10.1 points, and a mean decrease of 46% in HAMD scores from 19.5 (baseline) to 10.5 points. Without stimulation, the improvement gained with the addition of CBT disappeared rapidly, suggesting that efficacy of CBT depends on stimulation. In this double-blind phase, the mean difference in Y-BOCS score between the active and sham condition after correction for period effects was 8.3 ($p = 0.04$). The mean difference in HAMA scores was 12.1 ($p = 0.1$) and the difference in HAMD scores was 11.3 ($p = 0.01$). It was reported that CBT was particularly effective in decreasing compulsions and avoidance behavior.

Mantione et al. (2014) performed a secondary analysis of this same RCT that was aimed at quantifying the added treatment effect of CBT after DBS, as well as to discuss the methodology of the CBT programme used (see above) [11]. The average decrease on the Y-BOCS after optimization of stimulation settings was 25%. With the addition of 24 weeks of CBT to ongoing DBS treatment, there was an additional 22% decrease of total Y-BOCS score ($p = 0.021$), without any additional effects on the HAMA or HAMD scores. The number of responders after CBT increased from 6 to 9 out of 16.

Timing: CBT was added when three conditions were fulfilled: an initial and substantial decrease (on average 6 points) in Y-BOCS score had to be obtained, there had to be no further decrease in Y-BOCS during three consecutive visits (which was usually after 8 weeks of stimulation), and it had to be observed that patients avoided resisting their compulsions or avoided anxiety-provoking exposure situations.

Procedural aspects: The CBT program consisted of 24 weekly individual face-to-face sessions of 60 min each. The protocolized treatment started with an extensive evaluation of the patient's motivation. Once motivation was established, therapy started with ERP and gradually introduced more cognitive elements at later stages [14,21].

Tyaghi et al. (2019) performed a randomized, double-blind counterbalanced comparison of DBS of the anteromedian subthalamic nucleus (STN) and ventral capsule/ventral striatal (VC/VS) stimulation in 6 patients [12]. In this study, treatment resistance was defined as no sustained benefit from treatment with at least two SSRIs for a minimum of 12 weeks at optimal doses, augmentation of SSRI treatment with an antipsychotic or extension of the SSRI dose beyond recommended limits, and at least two trials of CBT with a minimum of 10 sessions, of which one as inpatient.

Design: the study consisted of two phases: an initial randomized phase of 12 weeks with stimulation of either the STN or the VC/VS, followed by an open phase in which both targets were stimulated. Stimulation was started after a mapping session at 60 μs and 130 Hz, without restrictions for stimulation intensity and also allowing stimulation of different contact points, both monopolar and bipolar. Next, there were two additional 12-week open phases: in the first one stimulation settings were optimized using data from previous phases. In the second phase, CBT was added to optimized DBS using the combined VC/VS and STN targets.

Effectiveness: Psychopharmacological treatment was allowed and kept constant during the trial. Overall, the score on the Y-BOCS reduced by 60%, from 36.2 at baseline to 14.3 when optimal stimulation settings were administered. Adding in-patient CBT resulted in an additional decline of the Y-BOCS score by 35% to 9.3 ($p = 0.09$; total decline from baseline 74%). Although obsessions and compulsions improved significantly from baseline to optimal stimulation, there was no statistically significant added improvement after CBT. Scores on the Montgomery–Asberg Depression Rating Scale (MADRS) declined from 28 at baseline to 13 during optimal stimulation settings and further reduced to 7 after CBT (information from the authors). The authors conclude that there is no further improvement in obsessions and compulsions due to CBT after optimal stimulation settings, and that this reflects a 'floor effect' of DBS on OCD. With 'floor effect' they intend to say that no further improvement of OCD symptoms would be possible after optimization of stimulation settings.

Timing: CBT was started standard after 24 weeks

Procedural aspects: CBT, including ERP, was applied in an inpatient unit while optimal stimulation settings were maintained.

Greenberg et al. (2006) report on the long-term (>3 years) follow-up of 10 therapy-resistant OCD patients being treated with VC/VS DBS [16].

Effectiveness: The average Y-BOCS score declined by 35% from 34.6 preoperatively to 22.3 after three years of DBS. All pharmacotherapy was allowed, but kept constant up to three months after the start of DBS treatment. The information provided in the paper does not allow to calculate the added effect of behaviour therapy to DBS on OCD symptoms. Clinically, the authors describe a 'notably enhanced motivation to engage in goal directed activities' during DBS, which also included enhanced motivation for CBT, which all patients had attempted unsuccessfully before the procedure. They consider that this increased motivation may have been a key factor in the patients' clinical progress.

Timing: If patients had had behavior therapy immediately prior to DBS, this was allowed to continue after the start of DBS; if behavior therapy was newly indicated, it was allowed to start only six months after the start of DBS. No details on the number of patients that received behavioral therapy postoperatively is given, nor details about the type, frequency, duration and way of delivery of the behavioral therapy.

Procedural aspects: There is no information on procedural aspects.

Abelson et al. (2005) reported a case series of 4 therapy resistant OCD patients being treated with DBS of the anterior limb of the internal capsula, with the tip of the electrode adjacent to the nucleus accumbens [12]. After operation, a 12-week double-blind testing stage was followed by an open-ended, open stimulation phase, with efforts to optimize results by adjusting stimulation settings and by pharmacotherapy and CBT. No further details on the effectiveness, timing and procedural aspects of CBT is given.

The qualitative study by van Westen et al. (2019) reports on the results of interviews with 8 professionals involved in DBS treatment of OCD patients, as well as experiences from embedded patient observation of the author [17]. These professionals identified the process in which patients become increasingly engaged in their process of improvement as an important predictor of effect. As the patient changes, new possibilities emerge, one of which is renewed treatment with CBT, to reduce remaining symptoms and expand healthy behavioral repertoires [17].

4. Discussion

Whereas it is a common practice to offer patients with therapy-resistant OCD treated with DBS a course of CBT after their operation, its effectiveness, timing and procedural aspects, such as the preferred way of delivery of such therapy, has hardly been studied. In spite of the fact that the importance of post-operative CBT is stressed by various authors [18–20], only two trials have specifically focussed on CBT added to DBS [13–15].

4.1. Effectiveness

The two studies that assessed the effects of CBT added on to DBS both support its effectiveness. In the study by Denys et al., CBT was responsible for significant additional reduction of 22% on the Y-BOCS after optimal stimulation settings were achieved [14]. In the study by Tyagi et al., there was a trend for an additional improvement of 35% on the Y-BOCS ($p = 0.09$). Whereas this was not statistically significant, there is a clear trend towards significance for this finding and it constitutes a clinically relevant improvement. In our opinion the lack of a statistical significance may well be due to a power problem because of the very low number of included patients ($n = 6$). So contrary to the authors, who present this as a negative outcome, we consider this study in support of postoperative CBT.

In theory, the effectiveness of CBT may also depend on the preoperative cognitive state of the patient, as well as on the potential cognitive side effects of DBS. Whereas in patients with Parkinson's disease, cognitive side effects of DBS—especially of the subthalamic nucleus—have been associated with reduced processing speed and working memory [22], there is little evidence of any detrimental effect of DBS—of any target—on the cognitive performance of OCD patients [23]. Studies that do report on neuropsychological measures report no relevant change in cognitive performance after DBS [24], and in one case even an improvement in cognitive flexibility for STN DBS but not for VC/VS DBS [15]. None of the included papers report on problems administering CBT due to cognitive side effects.

There has been some discussion on whether the effects of CBT may depend on the DBS target. Mantione et al. suggest that the effect of CBT in their study may be specific to stimulation of the NA, since NA DBS has a profound effect on anxiety and depression, as opposed to, e.g., DBS of the STN, which reduces compulsions without significant effects on mood and anxiety [11]. However, in the study by Tyagi et al., the additional improvement in patients with STN and VC/VS DBS is in the same range, if not larger than in the study by Mantione et al. [15]. Based on these scarce data, we expect CBT to be effective as add-on treatment to DBS in therapy-resistant OCD patients, irrespective of the stimulation target. However, only further studies comparing the effectiveness of CBT in OCD patients with different DBS stimulation targets can reveal a potential target related effect of CBT.

4.2. Timing

The same two studies used different criteria for starting CBT. Denys et al. started CBT after partial response, defined as a substantial reduction of on average 6 points on the Y-BOCS, without further decrease during three consecutive visits [13,14]. In the study by Tyagi, CBT was started after 36 weeks in every patient, irrespective of the amount of improvement achieved by DBS [15]. In clinical practice the question of when to best start CBT is an important one. It does not seem sensible to start CBT immediately postoperatively after electrode implantation and activating the DBS system. The mental state of the patient has not changed yet, and because of that there is no reason to expect that treatments that were ineffective before DBS would now be effective. It also makes no sense to start CBT if the response to DBS is very large, since there may not be any relevant treatment goals left to work towards. The best time to start CBT is probably when there is a partial response to DBS. The altered mental state of the patient, with not only some reduction in obsessive-compulsive behavior, but usually also reduced anxiety and improved mood, provides a different starting position for CBT, and the patient may be more able and motivated to comply with therapy, as was also described by Greenberg et al., and by Van Westen et al. in their qualitative study [16,17]. The question then is when to start CBT in case of partial response? Some clinicians routinely start after a certain period (e.g., after 8 or 12 weeks). Other clinicians start CBT when it is assumed that optimal stimulation settings have been achieved. Whereas this may be preferable in a research context, in order to separate the differential contribution of DBS and CBT to the response, clinically this is debatable. On one hand, reaching optimal stimulation settings may take a long time in many patients, which would lead to an unacceptable delay for therapy and loss of momentum; on the other hand, these patients have already experienced non-effective CBT and it is important to spare them another failure because of starting CBT to soon, as this would decrease their motivation for another attempt when stimulation parameters are optimal. One option is to assess the "readiness" for CBT, as mentioned above. Another option may be to look for improvement of cognitive measures that may increase the likelihood of successful CBT. A recent intervention study showed that the effect of VC/VS DBS is explained in part by enhancement of cognitive control by the prefrontal cortex. In this study, DBS improved the patients' performance on a cognitive control task and increases theta (5–8 Hz) oscillations in both medial and lateral PFC, which predicts the clinical outcome [25]. Perhaps such indicators could be made to clinical use and help to indicate the best time to start CBT after DBS.

4.3. Procedural Aspects

In the study by Denys et al., CBT/ERP consisted of 24 weekly individual face-to-face sessions of 60 min each, administered on an outpatient basis. Tyagi et al. provided CBT/ERP for 12 weeks on an in-patient basis in a neuropsychiatry unit. In both studies, the therapy was provided by the DBS clinic. This may be feasible in a research setting, but in routine clinical practice this will be more difficult to ask from patients once the DBS settings are optimized, given the distance that many of them will have to travel to the DBS clinic. Because of this, therapy is often organized in the region where the patient lives. However, whereas many behavioral therapists from local or regional psychiatric services may have experience in treating OCD patients, few will have experience treating OCD patients with DBS. In-patient treatment is one option to let patients benefit from the expertise of therapists of the DBS clinic, but this will be costly and may not be more effective than out-patient treatment. Another way of letting patients benefit from therapists with DBS experience is to explore novel ways of administering therapy, such as by telephone, videoconferencing or online.

In addition, other indications for CBT in the peri-operative period should also be considered. CBT could be administered with different objectives and if necessary, a different procedural approach. It could for instance already be started pre-operatively with the intent to enhance motivation for change post-operatively. Such pre-operative intervention has not been studied yet. Additionally, the content of the cognitive aspects of therapy could be adapted to address some issues specific to DBS, such as specific psychoeducational purposes related to DBS and preoccupation with stimulation settings. Moreover, after substantial improvement, low frequency long term continuation therapy may be helpful in preventing relapse.

4.4. Synthesis and Recommendations

Only two studies specifically address postoperative CBT. These used different stimulation targets and stimulation protocols, as well as different approaches to administering the therapy. Both studies suffer from a number of limitations, most importantly a small sample size, and the lack of a control condition for the CBT. In addition, the focus is strongly on obsessive and compulsive symptoms, whereas a focus on quality of life and general (social) functioning may be more important to the patient [26]. The other included studies mention postoperative CBT, but do not provide any details on effectiveness, timing and procedure.

DBS is not a stand-alone treatment for therapy-resistant OCD. After their operation, many patients continue to take medication for OCD, and/or receive some form of psychotherapy to deal with remaining symptoms or problems adjusting to the new situation. The overall treatment effect is the resultant of the DBS plus adjunctive therapies, and studies into the effectiveness of DBS should also take these concurrent treatments into account.

From a clinical point of view, there is a need for an evidence based algorithm for applying concommittant therapies, both psychotherapy as well as pharmacotherapy. As far as psychotherapy is concerned, there should be clear criteria as to when to start psychotherapy and the module should be adjusted to patients being treated with DBS. In our opinion, CBT should be started after a predefined level of clinical response to DBS, which is open for dicussion. The CBT module should address issues specific to DBS patients such as a changed personal identity due to being dependent on a device for symptom control and well-being, preoccupation with stimulation settings, and having to adjust to 'real life' after a long time of therapy-resistance and severe obsessive-compulsive behaviors that rendered typical family life, social contacts or employments unfeasible [27]. In order to let patients benefit from the experience of CBT therapists working in DBS clinics, other ways of administering CBT such as by telephone, videoconferencing or online, should also be developed and evaluated.

From a research point of view, future studies into the efficacy of DBS for OCD should follow a design that also allows the evaluation of the added effect of these concurrent treatments, and helps determining the place of these concurrent treatments in a treatment algorithm of OCD patients after DBS. This implies that there should be a control condition for CBT in order to assess the placebo response of CBT treatment. It also implies that sample size should be large enough to allow evaluation of the added treatment effects of CBT. Since it is unlikely that the required sample sizes will be achieved within a reasonable amount of time in a single DBS center, multicenter studies should be initiated. It is essential that collaborating centers not only protocolize their CBT treatment, but also that they align their clinical practice with respect to DBS with respect to stimulation target, strategies to optimalize stimulation parameters and follow-up assessments. This would require a closer collaboration between DBS clinics on both a national and international level.

5. Conclusions

Preliminary findings show that postoperative CBT is effective as an add-on treatment to DBS in patients with therapy-resistent OCD. Further studies are necessary to establish the place of CBT after DBS. These studies should have larger sample sizes and designs that are adequate to quantify the added effects of both CBT as well as pharmacotherapy. In order to let patients benefit optimally from the experience and expertise of behavioral therapists working in DBS clinics, novel ways of administering CBT, such as administered by telephone, videoconferencing or online, should also be studied.

Author Contributions: Conceptualization, A.F.G.L.; methodology, A.F.G.L.; formal analysis, M.G.; writing—original draft preparation, M.G.; writing—review and editing, T.B.v.d.V., K.S., L.A., M.P.; supervision, A.F.G.L. All authors have read and agreed to the published version of the manuscript.

References

1. Heyman, I.; Mataix-Cols, D.; Fineberg, N.A. Obsessive-compulsive disorder. *BMJ* **2006**, *333*, 424–429. [CrossRef] [PubMed]
2. Vos, S.P.; Flaxman, A.D.; Naghavi, M.; Lozano, R.; Michaud, C.; Ezzati, M.; Shibuya, K.; Salomon, J.A.; Abdalla, S.; Aboyans, V.; et al. Years lived with disability (YLD) for 1160 sequelae 289 diseases and injuries 1990–210: A systematic analysis for the Global Burden of Disease Study 2010. *Lancet* **2012**, *380*, 2163–2196. [CrossRef]
3. Law, C.; Boisseau, C.L. Exposure and Response Prevention in the Treatment of Obsessive-Compulsive Disorder: Current Perspectives. *Psychol. Res. Behav. Manag.* **2019**, *12*, 1167–1174. [CrossRef] [PubMed]

4.   Olatunji, B.O.; Davis, M.L.; Powers, M.B.; Smits, J.A. Cognitive-behavioral therapy for obsessive-compulsive disorder: A meta-analysis of treatment outcome and moderators. *J. Psychiatr. Res.* **2013**, *47*, 33–41. [CrossRef]

5.   Leeuwerik, T.; Cavanagh, K.; Strauss, C. Patient adherence to cognitive behavioural therapy for obsessive-compulsive disorder: A systematic review and meta-analysis. *J. Anxiety Disord.* **2019**, *68*, 102135. [CrossRef]

6.   Romanelli, R.J.; Wu, F.M.; Gamba, R.; Mojtabai, R.; Segal, J.B. Behavioral therapy and serotonin reuptake inhibitor pharmacotherapy in the treatment of obsessive-compulsive disorder: A systematic review and meta-analysis of head-to-head randomized controlled trials. *Depress. Anxiety* **2014**, *31*, 641–652. [CrossRef]

7.   Denys, D. Pharmacotherapy of obsessive-compulsive disorder and obsessive-compulsive spectrum disorders. *Psychiatr. Clin. N. Am.* **2006**, *29*, 553–584. [CrossRef]

8.   Kisely, S.; Hall, K.; Siskind, D.; Frater, J.; Olson, S.; Crompton, D. Deep brain stimulation for obsessive-compulsive disorder: A systematic review and meta-analysis. *Psychol. Med.* **2014**, *44*, 3533–3542. [CrossRef]

9.   Abramowitz, J.S. *Understanding and Treating Obsessive-Compulsive Disorder: A Cognitive Behavioral Approach*; Lawrence Erlbaum Associates Publisher: Mahwah, NJ, USA, 2006.

10.   Brakoulias, V.; Starcevic, V.; Albert, U.; Arumugham, S.S.; Bailey, B.E.; Belloch, A.; Borda, T.; Dell'Osso, L.; Elias, J.A.; Falkenstein, M.J.; et al. Treatments used for obsessive-compulsive disorder: An international perspective. *Hum. Psychopharmacol.* **2019**, *34*, e2686. [CrossRef]

11.   Kennedy, C.E.; Fonner, V.A.; Armstrong, K.A.; Denison, J.A.; Yeh, P.T.; O'Reilly, K.R.; Sweat, M.D. The Evidence Project risk of bias tool: Assessing study rigor for both randomized and non-randomized intervention studies. *Syst. Rev.* **2019**, *8*, 3. [CrossRef]

12.   Abelson, J.L.; Curtis, G.C.; Sagher, O.; Albucher, R.C.; Harrigan, M.; Taylor, S.F.; Martis, B.; Giordani, B. Deep brain stimulation for refractory obsessive-compulsive disorder. *Biol. Psychiatry* **2005**, *57*, 510–516. [CrossRef] [PubMed]

13.   Denys, D.; Mantione, M.; Figee, M.; Van Den Munckhof, P.; Koerselman, F.; Westenberg, H.; Bosch, A.; Schuurman, R. Deep brain stimulation of the nucleus accumbens for treatment-refractory obsessive-compulsive disorder. *Arch. Gen. Psychiatry* **2010**, *67*, 1061–1068. [CrossRef]

14.   Mantione, M.; Nieman, D.H.; Figee, M.; Denys, D. Cognitive-behavioural therapy augments the effects of deep brain stimulation in obsessive-compulsive disorder. *Psychol. Med.* **2014**, *44*, 3515–3522. [CrossRef] [PubMed]

15.   Tyagi, H.; Apergis-Schoute, A.M.; Akram, H.; Foltynie, T.; Limousin, P.; Drummond, L.M.; Fineberg, N.A.; Matthews, K.; Jahanshahi, M.; Robbins, T.W.; et al. A Randomized Trial Directly Comparing Ventral Capsule and Anteromedial Subthalamic Nucleus Stimulation in Obsessive-Compulsive Disorder: Clinical and Imaging Evidence for Dissociable Effects. *Biol. Psychiatr.* **2019**, *85*, 726–734. [CrossRef] [PubMed]

16.   Greenberg, B.D.; Malone, D.A.; Friehs, G.M.; Rezai, A.R.; Kubu, C.S.; Malloy, P.F.; Salloway, S.P.; Okun, M.S.; Goodman, W.K.; Rasmussen, S.A. Three-year outcomes in deep brain stimulation for highly resistant obsessive-compulsive disorder. *Neuropsychopharmacology* **2006**, *31*, 2384–2393. [CrossRef] [PubMed]

17.   Van Westen, M.; Rietveld, E.; Denys, D. Effective Deep Brain Stimulation for Obsessive-Compulsive Disorder Requires Clinical Expertise. *Front. Psychol.* **2019**, *10*, 2294. [CrossRef] [PubMed]

18.   Guzick, A.; Hunt, P.J.; Bijanki, K.R.; Schneider, S.C.; Sheth, S.A.; Goodman, W.K.; Storch, E.A. Improving long term patient outcomes from deep brain stimulation for treatment-refractory obsessive-compulsive disorder. *Expert Rev. Neurother.* **2020**, *20*, 95–107. [CrossRef] [PubMed]

19.   Tastevin, M.; Spatola, G.; Régis, J.; Lançon, C.; Richieri, R. Deep brain stimulation in the treatment of obsessive-compulsive disorder: Current perspectives. *Neuropsychiatr. Dis. Treat.* **2019**, *15*, 1259–1272. [CrossRef] [PubMed]

20.   Bais, M.; Figee, M.; Denys, D. Neuromodulation in obsessive-compulsive disorder. *Psychiatr. Clin. N. Am.* **2014**, *37*, 393–413. [CrossRef]

21.   Verbraak, M.J.P.M.; Hoogduin, C.A.L.; Methorst, G.J.; Arts, W.J.J.M.; Hansen, A.M.D.; Keijsers, G.P.J. Protocollaire behandeling van patiënten met een obsessieve-compulsieve stoornis: Exposure, responspreventie en cognitieve therapie. In *Protocollaire Behandelingen in de Ambulante Geestelijke Gezondheidszorg I*; Keijsers, G.P.J., van Minnen, A., Hoogduin, C.A.L., Eds.; Bohn Stafleu Van Loghum: Houten, The Netherlands, 2004; pp. 63–97.

22.   Rughani, A.; Schwalb, J.M.; Sidiropoulos, C.; Pilitsis, J.; Ramirez-Zamora, A.; Sweet, J.A.; Mittal, S.; Espay, A.J.;
      Martinez, J.G.; Abosch, A.; et al. Congress of Neurological Surgeons Systematic Review and Evidence-Based
      Guideline on Subthalamic Nucleus and Globus Pallidus Internus Deep Brain Stimulation for the Treatment
      of Patients With Parkinson's Disease: Executive Summary. *Neurosurgery* **2018**, *82*, 753–756. [CrossRef]
23.   Vicheva, P.; Butler, M.; Shotbolt, P. Deep Brain Stimulation for Obsessive-Compulsive Disorder: A Systematic
      Review of Randomised Controlled Trials. *Neurosci. Biobehav. Rev.* **2020**, *109*, 129–138. [CrossRef] [PubMed]
24.   Mallet, L.; Polosan, M.; Jaafari, N.; Baup, N.; Welter, M.-L.; Fontaine, D.; Tezenas du Montcel, S.; Yelnik, J.;
      Chereau, I.; Arbus, C.; et al. Subthalamic nucleus stimulation in severe obsessive-compulsive disorder.
      N. Engl. J. Med. **2008**, *359*, 2121–2134. [CrossRef] [PubMed]
25.   Widge, A.S.; Zorowitz, S.; Basu, I.; Paulk, A.C.; Cash, S.S.; Eskandar, E.N.; Deckerbach, T.; Miller, E.K.;
      Dougherty, D.D. Deep brain stimulation of the internal capsule enhances human cognitive control and
      prefrontal cortex function. *Nat. Commun.* **2019**, *10*, 1536. [CrossRef]
26.   Ooms, P.; Mantione, M.; Figee, M.; Schuurman, P.R.; van den Munckhof, P.; Denys, D. Deep brain stimulation
      for obsessive-compulsive disorders: Long-term analysis of quality of life. *J. Neurol. Neurosurg. Psychiatr.*
      2014, *85*, 153–158. [CrossRef] [PubMed]
27.   Horstkötter, D.; de Wert, G. Ethical considerations. In *Fundamentals and Clinics of Deep Brain Stimulation*;
      Temel, Y., Leentjens, A.F.G., de Bie, R.M.A., Chabardes, S., Fasasno, A., Eds.; Springer Nature: Cham,
      Switzerland, 2020; pp. 145–159.

Methodological Considerations for Neuroimaging in Deep Brain Stimulation of the Subthalamic Nucleus in Parkinson's Disease Patients

Bethany R. Isaacs [1,2,*], **Max C. Keuken** [3], **Anneke Alkemade** [1], **Yasin Temel** [2], **Pierre-Louis Bazin** [1,4] and **Birte U. Forstmann** [1]

[1] Integrative Model-based Cognitive Neuroscience Research Unit, University of Amsterdam, 1018 WS Amsterdam, The Netherlands; jmalkemade@gmail.com (A.A.); pilou.bazin@uva.nl (P.-L.B.); buforstmann@gmail.com (B.U.F.)

[2] Department of Experimental Neurosurgery, Maastricht University Medical Center, 6202 AZ Maastricht, The Netherlands; y.temel@mumc.nl

[3] Municipality of Amsterdam, Services & Data, Cluster Social, 1000 AE Amsterdam, The Netherlands; mckeuken@gmail.com

[4] Max Planck Institute for Human Cognitive and Brain Sciences, D-04103 Leipzig, Germany

[*] Correspondence: broseisaacs@gmail.com

Abstract: Deep brain stimulation (DBS) of the subthalamic nucleus is a neurosurgical intervention for Parkinson's disease patients who no longer appropriately respond to drug treatments. A small fraction of patients will fail to respond to DBS, develop psychiatric and cognitive side-effects, or incur surgery-related complications such as infections and hemorrhagic events. In these cases, DBS may require recalibration, reimplantation, or removal. These negative responses to treatment can partly be attributed to suboptimal pre-operative planning procedures via direct targeting through low-field and low-resolution magnetic resonance imaging (MRI). One solution for increasing the success and efficacy of DBS is to optimize preoperative planning procedures via sophisticated neuroimaging techniques such as high-resolution MRI and higher field strengths to improve visualization of DBS targets and vasculature. We discuss targeting approaches, MRI acquisition, parameters, and post-acquisition analyses. Additionally, we highlight a number of approaches including the use of ultra-high field (UHF) MRI to overcome limitations of standard settings. There is a trade-off between spatial resolution, motion artifacts, and acquisition time, which could potentially be dissolved through the use of UHF-MRI. Image registration, correction, and post-processing techniques may require combined expertise of traditional radiologists, clinicians, and fundamental researchers. The optimization of pre-operative planning with MRI can therefore be best achieved through direct collaboration between researchers and clinicians.

Keywords: Parkinson's disease; magnetic resonance imaging; deep brain stimulation; ultra-high field

1. Introduction

Longevity is increasing and consequently triggering a surge in age-related, multimorbid neurodegenerative diseases [1,2]. One of these diseases is Parkinson's disease (PD). PD is the second most common neurodegenerative disorder worldwide and typically occurs after 50 years of age [3]. This is a multi-systems disease primarily characterized by symptoms that affect movement control, such as bradykinesia, tremor, rigidity, postural instability, and gait difficulties [3].

Drug treatments for PD are symptomatic in nature and function to replace the dopamine deficiency within the brain that occurs due to loss of nigrostriatal dopamine neurons [4–6]. While dopaminergic medications relieve the motor-related symptoms of PD, they do not address non-motor symptoms, further complications, or disease progression [6]. Moreover, drug therapy in PD is associated with side effects that include but are not limited to nausea and vomiting, sleep disorders, hallucinations, and delusions. Furthermore, as the disease progresses, initially beneficial drug treatments become less effective in about 40% of patients. At this stage, the therapeutic window begins to narrow and the medication may wear off faster, resulting in the re-emergence or worsening of motor fluctuations [7,8]. Chronic drug treatment and disease progression are also associated with levodopa-induced dyskinesias, which refer to involuntary, uncontrolled movements that occur when medications are most effective [7–9]. Increasing the dosages in response to reduced durability of levodopa or dopamine agonists is not always feasible. Alternative treatments such as device-aided therapies may then be considered.

The next step for a subset of patients is neurosurgery intervention by means of deep brain stimulation (DBS) of the subthalamic nucleus (STN) [10–13]. The STN is a small, glutamatergic, biconvex structure with a high iron content that is located within the subcortex [14,15]. DBS involves the implantation of electrodes that emit persistent high frequency stimulation in this nucleus [11–13]. The STN is a viable target for DBS as it modulates output of both the indirect and hyper-direct cortico-basal pathways, whose functions are assumed to suppress undesirable motor behavior and inappropriate movements, respectively [16,17]. In PD, dopaminergic degradation of the substantia nigra (SN) is thought to result in inhibition of direct pathways, as well as disinhibition of indirect and hyper-direct pathways. Collectively, this leads to the functional disinhibition of output to motor-related areas of the cortex, which is thought to produce impaired movement and reduced movement control [16]. However the exact mechanisms underlying DBS are still poorly understood, although the general consensus is that DBS results in a functional normalization of pathologically overactive circuits [17–19].

While DBS may ameliorate between 60 to 90% of the motor-related symptoms of PD, it can produce neuropsychiatric side effects and emotional or associative disturbances, with side effects ranging from hypomania; apathy; hallucinations; and, as well as general changes in moral competency, personality and reckless behavior [20–23]. A fraction of patients will fail to exhibit a long-term clinical benefit in the reduction of parkinsonian symptoms [24,25]. Revisions or removals of the DBS system occur in between 15 and 34% of operated patients, 17% of which are attributed solely to electrode misplacement [26,27]. Additional risks can arise from the surgery itself, with implantation posing a 15% risk of "minor and reversible problems", and a 2–3% risk of fatal or hemorrhagic events, infection, lead fracture, and dislocation [28]. Between 2013 and 2017, there were 711 bilateral DBS placement surgeries in The Netherlands, a subset of which were suffering from PD. Of those 711 surgeries, 169 patients required the DBS system to be either replaced or removed entirely [29]. These side effects and adverse outcomes can partially be attributed to suboptimal placement of the DBS lead, which is dependent on the accuracy of the preoperative planning procedures [30,31].

2. Using MRI to Target the STN in PD for DBS

As noted, the success of DBS treatment is partly determined by the accuracy of targeting the STN. Further, targeting is dependent on stereotaxic precision, neuroimaging methods, and electrophysiological mappings [32]. Identification of the STN can be achieved in two ways: indirectly or directly. Indirect targeting refers to identification of the DBS target via application of reformatted anatomical atlases, formulae coordinates, and distances from anatomical landmarks. These standard targets can be applied to a patient's individual magnetic resonance imaging (MRI), or can be used as a coordinate for navigation with a stereotaxic reference system (see next paragraph). Additionally, intra-operative microelectrode recordings, macrostimulation, and intraoperative behavioral feedback are commonly used for verification with indirect targeting [32,33]. Direct targeting refers to visualization of the STN on patient-specific MRI images [34,35].

For indirect targeting, the most common landmarks are the mid-way point between the anterior and posterior commissure (AC and PC, respectively), which are visualized and marked on a T1-weighted

(T1w) MRI, computer tomography (CT), or ventriculography [33,36]. The native brain is commonly realigned to the AC-PC with a Euclidean transform [37,38]. This transform provides an augmented matrix with a 3D homogenous coordinate system, allowing for application of formulae coordinates and distances. The standardized STN coordinates are defined as 12 mm lateral, 4 mm posterior, and 5 mm inferior to the mid commissural point [39]. Some centers may utilize their own reference points, such as the top of the red nucleus [40–42].

Direct targeting with patient-specific MRI is generally preferred as the STN is known to shift with both age and disease, as well as vary in size, shape, and location across individuals [43–47]. Clinical MRI typically visualizes the STN using T2-weighted (T2w) images, which present the nucleus as a hypointense region relative to surrounding tissue. The optimal part of the STN is considered to be the ventral dorsolateral portion, also termed the somatosensory region, and is assumed to have direct connections with pre-motor cortical areas [48]. As with indirect targeting, direct targeting also incorporates AC-PC alignment, which provides the common reference system required for frame-based stereotaxic surgeries. Additionally, AC-PC alignment allows for comparisons between planned target location, actual target location, and postoperative verification. Therefore, clinical identification of the STN is usually achieved with a combination of both direct and indirect targeting methods.

The presence of extreme side effects and lack of clinical effect that can occur with DBS may arise from either direct or indirect targeting. One method for increasing the success and efficacy of DBS is to optimize preoperative planning procedures via neuroimaging techniques. For instance, advanced MRI can be used to increase visualization and understanding of anatomy, connectivity, and functioning of the STN. This information can then be used to inform on optimal electrode placement on a patient-specific basis.

The goal of this paper is to explain the current procedures for structural target identification of the STN for DBS in PD using MRI. We identify limitations that may contribute to suboptimal identification of the STN and provide alternatives for optimizing MRI in order to visualize the STN. The organization of topics is as follows: field strength; current procedures for intra and post-operative verification with microelectrode recordings; SAR limitations; shimming and magnetic field corrections; sequence types and contrasts; voxel sizes; motion correction; registration and image fusion; quantitative maps; complications unrelated to pre-operative planning; and conclusions. The suggestions are presented with the underlying expectation that more accurate visualization can translate into targeting and implantation with increased precision.

3. Field Strength

Pre-operative MRIs are obtained to both visualize the DBS target and to assess for potential comorbidity and identify venous architecture to ensure a safe entry route for surgery. The quality of MRI is dependent on a large number of factors. One of these factors is the signal-to-noise ratio (SNR), which is strongly influenced by field strength (Tesla or T for short) (see Figure 1) [24,49,50]. SNR can be defined as the difference in signal intensity, effectively determining the amount of signal that represents the true anatomy compared to noise and random variation [51,52]. Low-field MRIs such as 1.5 or 3 T are routinely used for DBS targeting. However, recently, an ultra-high field (UHF) 7 T MRI system has been approved for medical neuroimaging [53]. Compared to 7 T, 1.5 and 3 T MRI tend to suffer from both inherently lower SNR and low contrast-to-noise (CNR). CNR reflects the difference in SNR between different tissue types, which is therefore essential for specificity [54,55]. Moreover, the STN is an inherently difficult structure to visualize as it is a small structure located within a very deep and dense portion of the basal ganglia and is surrounded by structures containing similar chemical compositions. This is exemplified by vast inconsistencies in observed volumetric measures, size, and location estimates of subcortical nuclei reported at low field strengths [44–46].

DBS Target

Figure 1. Visualizing deep brain stimulation (DBS) targets with different magnetic resonance imaging (MRI) field strengths (adapted from [24] illustrating DBS targets across field strengths, requiring different contrasts. We obtained 1.5 T images from a 52-year-old male Parkinson's disease patient at the Maastricht University Medical Center (MUMC). Clinical 3 T and 7 T images were obtained from a from 57-year-old male Parkinson's disease patient at the Maastricht University Medical Center (MUMC), and the optimized 3 T images were obtained from a healthy male age-matched subject at the Spinoza Center for Neuroimaging, Amsterdam. All images are shown in the axial plane and are present in their native space with no post-processing to replicate the visualization of each nucleus as performed on neurosurgical planning software. The T1 contrasts show the anterior thalamic nucleus and nucleus accumbens at all field strengths. The subthalamic nucleus and globus pallidus (GP) are shown with a T2 contrast at 1.5 T and clinical 3 T scan. Note that in the 7 T contrast, the medial medullary lamina is visible, allowing us to distinguish between the internal and external segment of the GP. For optimized 3 T and 7 T, the STN and GP are shown with a T2* contrast. The acquisition times (TA) for each scan are included to highlight the fact that optimized 3 T can provide high-quality images similar to those at 7 T but take nearly twice as long to obtain. While the STN and GP are visible in both 3 T images, the contrast and sharpness of borders increases at 7 T.

The quality of the magnetic field is also determined by magnetic field gradients. MRI gradients are characterized by the change in the magnetic field as a function of distance. The MRI gradient arises from gradient coils, which are a set of electromagnetic components within the scanner that are used to control the magnetic field [56,57]. Weaker gradients arising from lower magnetic fields cause g-factor penalties, whereby an inhomogeneous B1 field causes artificial signal differences and noise amplification in tissues further from the coil in the subcortex at 3 T compared with 7 T MRI [58,59]. SNR is therefore lower in subcortical structures relative to the cortex due to the larger distance between the center of the brain and receiver coil elements. These differences are amplified at low field compared to UHF [60–62].

However, SNR scales supra-linearly with the static magnetic field, with up to a sixfold increase at 7 T compared to 3 T MRI [54,55]. This means that UHF-MRI can provide better quality images at a higher spatial resolution, increased contrast, and shorter acquisition times [51,63,64]. Reduced acquisition is essential, as clinical radiologists are often under strict time pressures that are intrinsically linked to value-based healthcare systems and cost-effectiveness rather than scientific value [65]. Numerous empirical studies and reviews have noted the advantages of utilizing UHF-MRI in clinical settings, performing direct comparisons between low- and high-field strengths for visualizing finer details of smaller nuclei, which are common targets for DBS [34,52,66–70].

Developments in array coil designs and parallel imaging techniques have resulted in the possibility to measure specific portions of tissue simultaneously. The simultaneous measurement increases SNR by a factor of 3 to 10 when compared to standard volume coils used at clinical field strengths, which are unable to selectively excite separate portions of tissue [60,63]. This is discussed in more detail later in the paper.

Importantly, there are caveats with regards to the implementation of UHF-MRI. Firstly, the Siemens 7 T MAGNETOM Terra is the only UHF-MR system to have obtained Food and Drug Administration (FDA) 510(k) clearance for clinical neuroradiology, and other applications of 7 T MRI are therefore considered experimental. Expense and accessibility is among the most important and most time-limiting factors in implementing UHF-MRI into clinical settings; less than one hundred 7 T systems exist worldwide, making up about 0.2% of all MRI systems [24,71]. Moreover, increased specific absorption rates (SAR), field inhomogeneities, local signal intensity variations, and signal dropout are factors that can reduce the benefits of 7 T MRI when not properly accounted for [72]. These can be countered with optimized shimming and pre-processing techniques such as bias field correction. However, these techniques require expertise that is not typically available within clinical settings [73–75].

4. Current Procedures for Intra- and Post-Operative Verification with Microelectrode Recordings

Current standard practices within The Netherlands includes both pre-operative planning with neuroimaging methods and intra-operative verification with microelectrode recordings (MER). In this case, once the target has been decided, the DBS system will be implanted in two steps. First, the surgeon will create a burr hole in the skull on both hemispheres. If microelectrode recordings (MER) are used, the MER leads will be inserted into predefined coordinates. In 0.5 to 2 mm intervals from around 10 mm above the target coordinate, MER will start recording activity through macrostimulation. Multiple MERs may be placed into the STN at around 2 mm apart within the anterior, posterior, central, medial, and lateral portions. The MER lead that outputs consistent oscillations of beta bursts that are indicative of STN activity will be selected for test stimulation and subsequent implantation. If the patient is awake, additional intraoperative behavioral testing may be performed to assess the therapeutic effect of specific stimulation programs. Once the target has been verified via intra-operative neuroimaging (CT or ultra-low field MRI), the leads will be permanently implanted and then connected to a cortical grid and a stimulator will be inserted under the chest [76–79].

Not all centers use pre-operative CT or MRI and instead rely on standard coordinates with MER verification (and vice versa). There are reports that suggest MER significantly improves DBS outcomes [80], and that MER fails to show any significant benefit compared to direct targeting [81]. Moreover, there remains a mismatch of around 20% in the planned target coordinate based on MRI, compared to the actual optimal location identified with MER when using 1.5 and 3 T [82,83]. Further, the use of intra-operative ultra-low field MRI for identification of the test leads during surgery has shown to be as effective as MER in improving post-operative motor symptoms [84]. Moreover, while not a strictly scientific issue, the application of MER more than doubles the cost of a bilateral STN surgery [85]. See [86] for an extensive overview on comparisons between MER and MRI for STN identification in PD.

Lastly, post-operative management requires the identification of optimal stimulation parameters. These parameters can vary per patient, and some patients may require DBS in combination with medication. Microlesioning effects and acute foreign body reactions can impact the homeostasis of

STN function and lead to a misinterpretation of DBS efficacy. Therefore the patient should ideally be assessed several times at different stages after the surgery [87]. Baseline motor function is initially obtained after total withdrawal of dopaminergic medication [88]. Axial motor symptoms such as bradykinesia, rigidity, stability, gait, posture, and dysarthria are assessed with rating scales such as the Unified Parkinson's Disease Rating Scale Part 3 (UPDRS, III) or Movement Disorders Society (MDS)-UPDRS [79,89]. As the DBS lead consists of multiple contact points, each point is tested separately through monopolar stimulation, beginning with a standard frequency of 130 Hz and pulse width of 60 μs [90]. Amplitudes are varied in a step-wise manner and the lowest amplitude that results in the highest suppression of clinical symptoms with the absence of sustained adverse effects will be chosen as the optimal stimulation parameters [27]. More in-depth literature on practices for post-operative verification, stimulation programming, and care can be found in [91–93] and the references therein.

5. SAR Limitations

SAR refers to the amount of energy deposited into the body due to the radio frequency (RF) pulses applied with MRI sequences. RF pulses are emitted via electrical currents through coils, being used to generate the B1 field [74]. RF deposition can result in tissue heating, and to ensure that the absorbed energy does not induce local thermal damage, there are SAR limitations based on the region of interest, with the amount of SAR depending on tissue type [94,95]. However, field inhomogeneities increase with field strength, as the RF wavelength scales according to the size of the object being imaged, which then reduces its ability to penetrate the brain with a uniform power [96,97]. In the case of UHF-MRI, stronger gradients are required to magnetize tissues in the middle of the brain and to create a homogenous field, which results in higher SAR. Therefore, the safety limits are reached sooner at UHF than with lower field. Moreover, SAR can vary person to person due to individual differences in anatomy. This means that scan acquisition can require real-time parameter adaptation. Maintaining a low SAR can be achieved by increasing the repetition time (TR), reducing the flip angle (FA), or by reducing the number of acquired slices. Unfortunately, introducing these parameter changes to MR sequences can negatively affect the quality of the scan [98,99]. This invites an ethical debate as to whether future FDA-approved sequences and image pre-processing methods at UHF would allow for such real-time deviations in a clinical protocol where SAR limitations are reached and sequence amendments are required.

Further, there are more absolute and relative contraindications at UHF including pacemakers, surgical implants and prosthesis, and foreign bodies, even if they are not metallic or comprised of diamagnetic materials due to potential local heating and subsequent torque and increased SAR. Moreover, in our experience, many DBS candidates may not be scanned due to site-specific criteria. For instance, while a non-metallic or non-paramagnetic dental bridge is not listed as a contraindication, the guidelines for the 7 T site at some locations required such patients to be excluded. Even more contraindications exist at 7 T, including circulatory and clotting disorders, which makes UHF-MRI less compatible with a larger portion of the elderly population, including the majority of PD DBS patients [100]. Therefore, optimizing 3 T remains a viable option where UHF-MRI cannot be applied. However, while 3 T may theoretically be optimized to allow for increased visualization of subcortical nuclei, it is essential to remember that acquisition times will be much longer than that of an analogous 7 T sequence [24,101–103]; this concept will be discussed throughout the paper.

6. Shimming and Magnetic Field Corrections

Shimming refers to the process of homogenizing either the main magnetic field (B0) or the radiofrequency field (B1). Inhomogeneity of the B0 field occurs when materials with different magnetic properties and susceptibility enter the bore, resulting in image distortion and signal loss. For example, the interface between brain tissue and air arising from the sinuses can cause artifacts within the frontal and temporal areas. These brain–air interface-induced artifacts can result in large shifts in the observed anatomical locations of nearby brain structures and cortical surfaces [104]. While post-processing techniques exist to correct some of these erroneous signals, they cannot control for complete signal loss and dropout. Therefore, the field needs to be shimmed prior to the acquisition of the main MRI scan.

Shimming the B0 field can occur passively by strategically placing ferromagnetic sheets within the bore itself to form the distribution of the magnetic field toward a more uniform state [105] or by using patient-related inserts such as an intra-oral pyrolytic carbon plate [106]. This process is useful for removing field imperfections related to hardware, although is not generally utilized in clinical practice as it is laborious, inflexible, and temperature-dependent. More commonly, the field can be actively shimmed, which uses currents within the MRI system to generate corrective magnetic fields in areas showing inhomogeneous signals [105].

Active shimming is limited by the ability to model and reproduce the distortions that occur within the field. Shimming is generally based on the principles of spherical harmonics (SH), which use orthonormal equations to index changes in signal waveforms representative of field inhomogeneity. The mapping and the correction of the inhomogeneity is achieved by superimposing the magnetic field with an opposing corrective field equal to and a reversal of the polarity within a spatial distribution deemed erroneous by the SH coefficients [107,108].

The order of SH is dependent on the number of dedicated current-driven coils. Traditional clinical and low-field MR systems will employ lower-order shimming methods mainly due to cost and space restraints [57]. Low-order shims primarily utilize linear terms including addition, scaling, and rotation of the SH coefficients to model the magnetic field. Linear SH coefficients function to resemble and compensate large-scale, shallow magnetic field components that can be corrected with a current offset applied with a standard gradient coil. This is typically achieved automatically with the use of a pre-scan B0 map. More local changes can be compensated for with dynamic shimming. However, this is most commonly used for multi-slice MR, which is prone to additional eddy current distortions and requires dedicated amplifier hardware. Further, the optimal shim method will depend on the desired contrast [109]. Ideally, each sequence should require an additional shim.

As field inhomogeneities increase with field strength, higher order harmonics are therefore required for UHF. Higher order SH allows for correcting more complex-shaped inhomogeneities by incorporating an additional non-linear quadratic field variation that allows for modelling the bending of curves in space. This requires supplementary dedicated shim coils, which can counter-intuitively induce additional distortions in the middle of the brain. Despite efforts to harmonize parameters, shimming is often site- and field-dependent, and manual iterative shimming is not always possible due to time constraints and/or limited expertise.

Additional B1 mapping is essential for accurate quantitative measures of signal intensities within the correct geometric space. Inhomogeneous B1 fields can result in distorted flip angles (FAs). FAs index the amount of net magnetization rotation experienced during the application of an RF pulse. If FAs are incorrectly calculated, geometric distortions occur, which reduces the accuracy in T1 and T2 values. B1 mapping allows for the correction of FA values prior to acquiring a structural scan. Primary B1+ mapping methods can be incorporated into sequence acquisition. This is most commonly achieved with the double angle method (DAM), which estimates local FAs from the ratio of two images obtained with different FA values. An additional 3D multi-shot method can be incorporated, which uses non-selective excitation to minimize inhomogeneous spin excitation across slices. Alternatively, spoiled gradient echo (GRE) sequences with variable FAs (VFA) and actual FA imaging (AFI) are commonly employed, which sample multiple T1 values to simulate signal differences across tissues [110–113].

Pre-processing of gradient non linearities (GNL) and intensity non-uniformity with retrospective image-based interpolation is also possible. Corrections for GNL are rarely accomplished in clinical settings but are commonplace for research-based applications. The magnitude of GNL increases with distance from the isocenter and can cause the visualization of structures to shift by up to 5 mm, which is detrimental for preoperative planning [114]. Correcting for GNL can be achieved by incorporating a low-pass filter to remove smooth spatially varying functions. Other GNL correction schemes include surface fitting and feature matching that rely on intensity-based methods. Intensity-based methods assume that different tissue intensities do not vary significantly unless they are subject to an erroneous bias field, where variations within one area can be corrected from the field of another spatial location within the image. Alternatively, histogram-based methods use a priori knowledge and manual input of known intensity and gradient probability distributions to correct images. B1 corrections can be achieved offline via image pre-processing steps with the FMRIB Software Library (FSL), Statistical Parametric Mapping (SPM), or Advanced Normalization Tools (ANTs) [115–118]. However, these methods must be considered experimental and their use in image correction for MRI in pre-operative planning is not currently FDA-approved.

7. Sequence Types and Contrasts

7.1. T1

As discussed, accurate DBS implantation requires careful trajectory planning and identification of vasculature to limit the risk of hemorrhagic complications. Visualization of larger venous architecture is most commonly achieved with an anatomical T1w scan with added gadolinium [119,120]. In its most basic form, T1w can be viewed as an anatomical scan that approximates the appearance of macroscopic tissues. T1w will visualize white matter as hyperintense; fluid, e.g., cerebral spinal fluid (CSF) as hypointense; and grey matter at intermediate intensity. A T1w contrast is achieved with a short echo time (TE) and repetition time (TR) and is a function of the longitudinal relaxation time, referring to the time it takes excited protons to return to their equilibrium subsequent to the application of an RF pulse. T1 is more sensitive to fat and fluid and therefore provides excellent differentiation between grey and white matter. Additional intravenous contrast agents will cause the recovery of the longitudinal magnetization of blood to quicken and therefore increase further contrast between veins and white matter [121–123]. For visualization of venous architecture, some centers may use any or a combination of T1w structural imaging, or they may use post-processing techniques such as susceptibility weighted imaging (SWI) and venography, which can be created from GRE-based sequences with flow compensation, or time-of-flight angiography. These types of sequences apply multiple RF pulses with short TRs to over-saturate static tissues and therefore suppress their signal, causing moving components such as blood to appear more hyperintense [124–126]. T1w MRI can also be used to rule out co-morbidities such as oedema, tumors, or other brain pathologies. See Figure 2 for an example of different contrasts.

7.2. T2

T2w images visualize grey matter as intermediate intensity and white matter as hypointense, although deep grey matter structures can appear even darker depending on the ferromagnetism of their tissue composition. As mentioned, visualization of STN is traditionally achieved with T2w sequences [127–129]. T2w MRI represents transverse relaxation, referring to the amount of time it takes excited protons to lose phase coherence. This dephasing is a tissue-specific process and takes longer for areas with high paramagnetic metal deposition such as iron. As the STN is iron-rich, the contrast is increased, and the nucleus appears hypointense compared to white matter tracts and surrounding grey matter structures. Typically, T2w contrasts within the clinic will come from fast-spin echo sequences that have both a long TE and TR, which are relatively immune to magnetic susceptibility artifacts. However, there is no general consensus as to the optimal sequence required for prime STN imaging. Theoretically, various sequences can achieve the same weighting but vary significantly in terms of their ability to accurately visualize the STN [130]. Moreover, the type of sequence will depend on the field strength, and contrasts are not always analogous across, for instance, 3 and 7 T [131]. Similarly, different MRI vendors will supply similar contrasts via sequences and sequence parameters with different names, making it difficult to draw comparisons between them [50,132,133].

7.3. T2* and Susceptibility-Based Contrasts

Traditional clinical T2w sequences suffer from low signal and contrast. An alternative contrast that can be used to image the STN directly comes from 3D gradient echo (GRE) sequences, which can be used to create T2* images. Typically, GRE sequences will include a low FA, long TEs, and long TRs. Moreover, gradients are applied to initiate dephasing, as opposed to an RF pulse in traditional spin echo sequences [109,134]. These gradients do not refocus field inhomogeneities such as RF pulses do. Therefore the T2* contrast arising from GRE reflects magnetic field inhomogeneities caused by the dephasing of neighboring areas that occurs at different rates, and further interact with the signal of adjacent voxels [135]. As GRE sequences assess macroscopic intervoxel and microscopic intravoxel magnetic susceptibilities, it is important to adapt sequence parameters according to the tissue of interest [136]. The tissue characteristics of the STN undergo PD-specific changes, such as dopaminergic denervation and excessive iron deposit, which require adjusted parameters such as TE for optimal contrast [137,138]. Similarly, iron increases with normal aging requires different adaptations to TEs [139]. GRE sequences also incorporate multiple echoes to account for differences in magnetic susceptibility across tissues. Further, susceptibility effects are stronger for smaller voxel sizes as the dephasing is reduced [135]. This makes T2* imaging more appropriate for higher field strength MR, as smaller voxel sizes can be achieved with faster acquisition times [130,140]. These T2* images can be further processed to create quantitative maps that will be discussed in later sections.

Alternatively, susceptibility weighted images (SWI) can be created from T2*-based sequences by independently processing magnitude and phase images. Magnitude images reflect the overall MR signal, and their corresponding phase image contains information about field inhomogeneity, differences in local precession frequencies, and motion [141]. Phase images were largely discarded before the implementation of SWI as they require complex unwrapping, referring to the extraction of their original numerical range, which is constrained in the outputted image to $[-\pi, +\pi]$ [142]. However, phase can be used to visualize information that would otherwise be barely visible in magnitude images. Small structures result in field variations with high spatial frequencies, which can be used to enhance contrast by applying a high pass filter. The resulting SWI image is the product of multiplying the phase mask with the magnitude image [142–144]. It remains somewhat controversial to what extent SWI signal increases from 1.5 T to 3 T MRI. Moreover there is little evidence for increased accuracy for SWI at 3 T compared to classic T2 imaging [145]. However, SWI is significantly more accurate compared to traditional contrasts at higher field strengths [146–148]. GRE-based sequences and T2* contrasts can provide more detail regarding the shape, surface, and location of the STN compared to standard T2w spin echo-based sequences. This could translate to more accurate DBS targeting if it were used for preoperative planning. Improvements can refer to a smaller deviation between planned and actual lead location, a reduction in reimplantation or removal requirements, increased clinical efficacy, or decrease in associated side effects. However, the use of T2* contrasts and UHF-MRI remains widely debated and requires further validation [37,70,144,148–150].

We attempted to use a T2*-based UHF-MRI with a GRE-ASPIRE sequence [151] on a 7 T Siemens MAGNETOM system (Siemens Healthcare, Erlangen, Germany) for STN DBS planning in PD patients. The 7 T T2* scan consisted of a partial volume covering the subcortex, obtained with multiple echoes (TE1–4 = 2.47, 6.75, 13.50, 20.75) and 0.5 mm isotropic voxel sizes in just under 8 min. This was overlaid with a 3 T T2w turbo field echo sequence obtained on a 3 Tesla Phillips Ingenia system, with a single TE of 80 ms and voxel sizes of $0.45 \times 0.45 \times 2$ mm, and an acquisition time of around 6 min. When merging the 3 T and 7 T data, the STN appeared elongated along the posterior direction on 7 T. The optimal target coordinate appeared more superior, posterior, and lateral on the 7 T image than the optimal coordinate on 3 T. Here, the 7 T coordinate was used as the posterior test site sampled with MER was used as a target for DBS surgery. Typical STN activity was not observed, although intraoperative behavioral testing revealed that patients would exhibit a beneficial clinical effect. Such a finding may be explained by the fact that the test electrode was instead stimulating white matter fibers exciting the STN, such as the fasciculus lenticularis or medial fiber bundles. It is, however, unclear as to whether this discrepancy in optimal STN coordinate is due to errors in registration across field strength, smoothing factors and interpolation automatically applied by the pre-operative planning system that reduced the resolution of the 7 T data, magnetic field inhomogeneity, or geometric distortions of the T2* image. The issues regarding image correction and manipulation are discussed in later sections. It is entirely plausible that the discrepancy in optimal target location across field strength was due to human error, and the operating surgeons perhaps were not used to interpreting the high-resolution susceptibility-based images. Therefore, factors other than contrast and sequence type can influence the usability and accuracy of susceptibility-based imaging for neurosurgical applications.

It is important to note that the sequences described in this specific instance are not standardized across centers, and scanner vendors, field strengths, contrasts, and sequence parameters, even within the same sequence type, will differ across DBS centers and research institutes. This makes a direct comparison across the quality and replicability of MRI scans very difficult, and unless systems are harmonized, interpretations should be site-specific. See [86,130] for a comprehensive review on sequences used for imaging the STN.

7.4. Multi-Contrast MRI

Multi-contrast sequences may offer a novel alternative for eliminating the requirement of registration and resampling of separate scans while simultaneously reducing scan acquisition time (Figure 2) [152]. A recently developed multiparametric imaging sequence is the Multi Echo (ME) MP2RAGE, which is largely unaffected by B1 inhomogeneities [153–160]. This allows for the acquisition of T2*-based contrasts from which subsequent SWI and quantitative susceptibility maps (QSM) can be created in the same space as the T1 images [158,160]. Other benefits of multiple contrasts is that they contain complimentary information that can be used to jointly denoise and improve the SNR of the acquired images [161–163].

Figure 2. Multi-contrast imaging. The top row shows MP2RAGE T1-weighted, T1, T2*, and R2* maps and a quantitative susceptibility map (QSM) image obtained at 7 T within a single multi echo (ME) MP2RAGE sequence. Below are a 3 T T1-weighted map, a T2* map, and a QSM image, where each T1 and T2* were obtained with different sequences but were optimized to provide a contrast comparable to those obtainable at 7 T but without the inversions required for creating T1 maps. Both the 3 and 7 T images came from the same subject and are shown in the axial plane. The contrast and visibility of subcortical structures is indeed comparable across field strengths [164].

8. Voxel Sizes

Clinical T2w images often incorporate anisotropic voxel sizes with large slice thickness in the z direction. This allows for higher in-plane resolution along the axial plane, which is primarily used for targeting (Figure 3) [145,149]. Voxel sizes will typically range between 0.45 × 0.45 × 2 mm and 1 × 1 × 3 mm. Lower resolution allows for shorter acquisition times of around 5 min, simultaneously limiting the effect of artifacts due to subject movement. However, anisotropic voxels suffer from partial voluming effects (PVE), which refer to the blurring of signals across voxels, resulting in averaging different tissue types and reducing specificity [165]. PVE are especially problematic for small structures such as the STN. Volume estimates are commonly used as an index of scan quality, and have shown consistent deviations of more than 50% from ground truths when slice thicknesses were three times the size of the alternate planes [166]. Moreover, anisotropic voxels will decrease the accuracy of resampling to super resolutions, which is an automatically incorporated step of pre-operative planning systems [167].

Figure 3. The effects of voxel geometry on the visualization of subcortical structures (adapted from [164]). Figure 3 shows clinical 3 T T2-weighted (T2w) with 0.45 × 0.45 × 2.0 mm voxel sizes, optimized 3 T T2* with 1.0 × 1.0 × 1.0 mm voxel sizes, and 7 T T2* maps with 0.64 × 0.64 × 0.7 mm voxel sizes. All images are acquired from a single subject and are shown at approximately the same anatomical level. The subthalamic nucleus (STN) and substantia nigra (SN) are shown at sagittal, coronal, and axial planes, with the red nucleus (RN) also highlighted in the axial plane. The anisotropic nature of the sagittal and coronal planes on the clinical 3 T do not allow for identification of any structure.

As spatial resolution is dependent on voxel size; smaller voxels should allow for more detailed and finer grained visualization of smaller structures. Voxel sizes can be reduced by increasing the acquisition matrix, reducing slice thickness, or decreasing the field of view. However, these factors can each negatively affect the SNR. The loss of SNR can be compensated by simply including more repetitions per sequence, which is an issue for PD populations as it necessitates an increase in acquisition time and requires the patient to be still. However this is often not possible for patients with movement disorders [166]. The loss of SNR caused by decreasing voxel sizes at lower fields can be counteracted through the use of UHF-MRI [130].

When targets in clinical MRI are verified with MER, the large slice thickness means that the spatial resolution is penalized along the z-axis. Therefore the depth of the electrode cannot be optimally planned and electrophysiological samplings are conducted to identify the ideal electrode placement [32,38,40]. This testing often requires that the patient is awake and endures behavioral assessments, which are stressful and physically demanding, prolong the time of the surgery, and can increase the risk of infection or hemorrhaging [168–170]. If smaller voxels can increase spatial resolution, three-dimensional anatomical accuracy, and tissue specificity, the requirement for intraoperative microelectrode recordings, multiple test electrode implantations, and awake behavioral testing could be eliminated, ultimately increasing patient comfort and reducing operation time.

However, voxels with a sub millimeter isotropic resolution used purely for identification of DBS targets, rather than for instance venous architecture, may not directly improve targeting accuracy. This is because the spatial resolution of stereotaxic coordinate systems is around 1.2 mm and chronically implanted conventional DBS electrodes are larger than 1 mm [171]. In addition, segmented DBS leads with directional steering may offer increased spatial resolution when recording local field potentials compared to traditional omnidirectional contacts [172,173]. Further, the development of microscale DBS contacts via multiresolution electrodes would allow for finer control of the stimulation volume and more precise targeting of smaller regions, matching the order and spatial resolution of submillimeter resolution MRI [174].

9. Motion Correction

Generally, clinical imaging for preoperative planning for DBS does not correct for motion, and the scans do not tend to incorporate acceleration methods such as parallel imaging. Accurate imaging requires the subject to remain still. If a patient scan exhibits severe motion artifacts, the scan is simply run again. MR images can be distorted by multiple sources of motion arising from breathing, cardiac movement, blood flow, pulsation of cerebrospinal fluid, and patient movement [104]. This can cause distortions in the image such as ghosting, signal loss, and blurring, as well as Gibb's and chemical shift artifacts [175]. Such artifacts can mask or simulate pathological effects [104]. Motion artifacts are particularly prevalent when imaging patients with movement disorders but can be controlled for in a number of ways such as timing medication to be most optimal during the time of scanning or administering additional sedatives during the scan. Moreover, the head and neck should be supported with pads to improve patient comfort, which will also limit movement.

The most logical method of limiting motion artifacts is to decrease the acquisition time. Sequence paraments can be manipulated to shorten the acquisition time by obtaining larger voxel sizes, a partial field of view (FOV), incorporating simultaneous multi slice 3D imaging and parallel imaging techniques, signal averaging, or obtaining multi contrast images. To correctly utilize these potential solutions, each factor should be considered relative to one another. For instance, partial FOVs can induce aliasing, fold over artifacts, and reduce the SNR, which can, to a certain extent, be countered by isolating the excitation to a localized region by using either multiple pulses, signal averaging, or fat suppression methods. Contrary to this, it may increase the effects of field inhomogeneity, but be combated with factors such as spatial pre-saturation. Such issues highlight the dynamic nature and interplay of sequence parameters and hardware, which can be largely overcome through the use of stronger field strengths such as 7 T.

Parallel imaging (PI) is a reconstruction technique rather than a sequence commonly employed to accelerate acquisition time [176]. Magnetic resonance (MR) images are not directly collected but are instead stored in a Cartesian grid, representing a spatial frequency domain known as k-space. K-space data is collected via superimposing spatially varying magnetic field gradients onto the main magnetic field [55,177]. Generalized auto-calibrating partially parallel acquisition (GRAPPA) methods speed up acquisition n time under-sampling each line of k-space in the phase-encoding direction. Additionally, partial FOVs are collected independently, corrected, and then reconstructed within the frequency domain [178–180]. Alternatively, sensitive encoding methods (SENSE or ASSET) can shorten scan times, and these methods occur in the image domain where data are obtained using multiple independent receiver channels where each coil is sensitive to a specific volume of tissue, which is then unfolded and recombined to form the MR image [177]. However, PI methods are associated with a number of artifacts including ghosting, speckling, wrap around, and g factor penalties and ought to be used with caution [181–183].

Motion correction can be conducted prospectively in real time by updating the image geometry during the scan, or retrospectively by post-acquisition registration techniques and manipulations during image reconstructions [184]. Additional hardware is required for prospective methods that are implemented within the scanner itself. In this case, fiducials can be attached to the patient's head, which assesses the extent of movement and adjusts the gradients accordingly. Alternatively, you can employ optical tracking or reflective markers, which are linked to a camera inside the bore. Motion correction is then achieved by either re-registration slice-by-slice during the scan, adjusting first order shims, and/or varying the gradient system online [185,186]. As discussed, motion artifacts do not have to come from patient movement but can arise on a much smaller scale at the proton level. Protons in blood, for example, exhibit a non-static magnetic field due to the variation of gradients in space. That is, they can miss rephasing pulses and therefore decay in signal before it can be read out by the scanner, especially for spin echo sequences that are used for obtaining T2w images [187]. This phenomenon is known as flow-related dephasing and results in artifactual phase shifts and signal distortion. In some instances, this can be useful, for example in angiography sequences, the negative effect is larger in sequences with longer TEs, such as those required for accurately imaging the STN. Adding in flow compensation or gradient moment nulling, which applies additional gradient pulses prior to the signal readout to compensate for signal decay, can compensate for this dephasing [188,189]. However, this is a computationally heavy process and is largely only suitable for partial FOVs. Alternatively, the sequence may be synchronized so that the acquisition occurs in time with the cardiac or respiratory cycle, which is known as cardiac gating and simultaneously requires pulse recordings or electrocardiograms [104].

10. Registration and Image Fusion

Using MRI to visualize deep brain structures such as the STN for DBS is a multi-stage process that involves the acquisition of multiple separate contrasts that require registration to a common, patient-specific native space. For pre-operative planning, at least two sets of image registrations are required: (i) anatomical T2 to T1 and (ii) pre-registered anatomical T1 and T2 to stereotaxic space defined by the CT or MRI including the coordinate frame. In this section, we focus on registration and fusion of MRI. For literature including alternative imaging modalities such as CT and ventriculography, see [190,191].

Image registration refers to the process of aligning a moving source image onto a fixed target through an estimated mapping between the pair of images. While the exact parameters incorporated within pre-operative planning systems are mostly proprietary, the general process will require a rigid registration, defined by six parameters: translation and rotations along the x-, y-, and z-axes. This refers to the spatial transformation of how a voxel can move from one space to another [192]. Transformations also require additional parameters such as interpolation and cost function. Interpolation refers to the process of re-gridding voxels from the source image to the target, an essential procedure as each pixel within the transformed image may not represent a whole integer within the target image. This is especially true when T2w images consist of anisotropic voxel sizes and the T1 images are isotropic. Therefore, the goal of interpolation is to piece back together the voxels that have been moved. Clinical neuroimaging traditionally employs the simplest intensity-based methods such as nearest neighbor interpolation, also known as point sampling, which assumes that similar values in different images are closer together and therefore constitute the same location [193,194]. Cost functions are used to assess the suitability of a given transform. This can be achieved with either similarity metrics such as mutual information, which compares, on the basis of pixel intensities, the differences between the transformed source and target image [195]. These registration steps are all conducted automatically within pre-operative planning systems, with the only manual alterations relating to viewing criteria such as brightness and intensity. This is suboptimal, as registrations often need tweaking and optimizing, and it becomes challenging to suggest exact methods for optimizing registrations with regards to pre-operative planning systems as it remains unclear as to what exact parameters are employed.

Linear within-subject registrations typically employ intensity-based similarity metrics, matching images on the basis of intensities or intensity distributions. Intensity methods can be optimized to incorporate local patches that account for textures and geometric information that are missed when assessing for global identical intensities. An example is boundary-based registration, which forms the basis of intra-subject registration of T2 to T1 images within the Human Connectome Project minimal processing pipeline [196,197]. Registrations could be optimized to include an additional affine transform that incorporates scaling or sheering [198]. Alternatively, deformable registrations via attribute matching and mutual saliency (DRAMMS) can be achieved. DRAMMS applies confidence weightings for matching voxels across contrast and will relax deformation in local regions where contrast-specific tissues are mutually exclusive to image type. DRAMMS has proven useful in accounting for pathology, subcortical structures, and cortical thinning, which are all factors to consider when imaging PD patients [199].

Further, no quality or standardized evaluation for registration accuracy currently exists in clinical neuroimaging beyond subjective visual assessment. This is problematic as it becomes unclear as to whether the initial rigid body transforms are an accurate spatial representation of individual anatomy, which, if erroneous, could result in targeting errors and DBS lead placement. The gold standard of accuracy is instead dependent on the stereotaxic frame, which is an extrinsic marker and does not include information directly related to the MR image.

Medical imaging often incorporates automated image fusion, which refers to the process of aligning, resampling, smoothing, and combining the information of multiple images into a more informative and descriptive output; for instance, by combining T1 and T2 into a single image. Fusion occurs after registration with the goal of interpolating and smoothing MRI images to make them more visually appealing, which can theoretically recover a signal within the data despite the noise [200]. However, smoothing and resampling voxel sizes will reduce anatomical variability and location accuracy as they can include signal from neighboring structures, leading to an erroneous increase in the size of the nucleus and PVEs [166,201]. Such smoothing methods may not be compatible with quantitative images such as T2* maps and QSM, as these images represent distinct signal intensities of specific voxels that are outside the predefined values of the planning system. In effect, this could be a simple viewing error, rather than a total incompatibility.

11. Quantitative Maps

Broadly speaking, MR contrasts are driven by how much T1 or T2 signal contributes to the image. These T1w or T2w images are qualitative in nature and fail to accurately assess tissue parameters such as recovery or relaxation time. However, certain sequences allow for parametric mapping (quantitative MRI or qMRI), where the intensities within each pixel are proportional to the T1 or T2. These values can be used to quantify intrinsic, biologically meaningful tissue information [202]. Additionally, qMRI allows for direct comparison across time, across subjects, and across scanners or sites, which is essential for the development of neuroscientific research and its application to the clinical situation [203]. Moreover, quantitative measures can aid identification and visualization of target structures with an objective approach and can minimize human error resulting from subjective interpretation. qMRI can only be made from specific sequences that comply with the principles of differential weightings, which incorporate an inversion or saturation recovery parameter with multiple inversion times or spoiled gradient echo sequences with variable flip angles [204]. However, in our experience, quantitative sequences at 3 T take at least twice as long as weighted MRI sequences used in clinical settings.

As mentioned, quantitative maps are used to index anatomical composition. For instance, the observed relaxation of T1 is extremely fast in myelinated white matter. The inverse of longitudinal relaxation rates, known as R1 [205], is thought to be linearly related to myelin concentrations [206,207]. T1 maps have been utilized clinically, for example, with quantifying perfusion; imaging hemorrhages and infarctions; evaluating contrast uptake; monitoring of tumors, gliosis, and multiple sclerosis lesions [205,208,209]. Quantitative T1 maps will usually require post-processing, most commonly achieved with the look-up table method, which functions to relate pixelwise T1 values within the native map with predefined and validated intensity values [159]. The automated creation of these T1 parametric maps can be built into the sequence at a cost of both time and capacity. Further post-processing is often required and relies on expertise that is again typically not available within a standard clinical setting [160,210].

For DBS of the STN, T2* maps can be used to improve visualization of the STN because iron content causes the T2* relaxation time to shorten, which for the STN at 7 T is around 15 ms [61,211]. A frequently used method to create T2* maps is done by fitting an exponential decay curve to the signal intensities per pixel from each of the multiple echoes obtained from a GRE sequence [212]. Moreover, the pixel intensities of reciprocal T2* maps (R2*) are proportional to iron load, with STN R2* values hovering around 67 s^{-1} (1/15 ms) at 7 T [155,213–216]. Alternatively, T2* images can be post-processed to create quantitative susceptibility maps (QSM), which quantify a tissue's magnetic susceptibility distribution on the basis of its perturbation of the magnetic field [213]. They are similar to SWI in that they are made from the separate magnitude and phase images of a GRE sequence, but they comprise multiple echoes and allow for quantitative measures rather than weightings. QSM requires initial phase unwrapping, background field extraction, and calculation of locally generated phase offsets, which refer to the fact that the phase of a single voxel can be expressed as either positive of negative, depending on its orientation relative to the magnetic field [214]. These phase-offsets are then deconvolved, typically with a dipole kernel, from which the underlying tissue susceptibility can be extracted per voxel, independently of surrounding voxels [215]. Moreover, QSMs are preferred over SWI, as SWI is limited by the non-local orientation-dependent effects of phase, which means that the same tissues can appear with different intensities on the basis of their location, whereas QSM solves this problem by convolving dipole fields [216,217]. Background removal methods based on principles of sophisticated harmonic artifact reduction for phase data (SHARP, also known as spherical mean value (SMV) filtering) and projection onto dipole fields (PDF) are commonly employed. SHARP is based on a theory similar to shimming, in that static magnetic fields and the corresponding phase maps are represented by harmonic functions. In regions of inhomogeneous susceptibility, the field will be non-harmonic, and background fields that are harmonic are eliminated from the phase data by subtraction [213,218]. The PDF method removes background fields by comparing the magnetic fields of dipoles inside a region of interest with those directly outside [219,220]. Alternatively, Laplacian boundary values can be used, which are based on a finite difference scheme [221]. However, quantifying an arbitrary distribution of susceptibility from the phase signal is challenging and poses an inverse problem whereby effects are first calculated from which parameters or causes are then determined, resulting in a noise amplification of the ensuing signal. The inversion problem can be solved with calculation of susceptibility through multiple orientation sampling (COSMOS). However, this method requires the acquisition of multiple head orientations, which is time-consuming and impractical for clinical use [222,223]. Morphology-enabled dipole inversion, or MEDI, will match the boundaries of each dipole with those observed in the T2*-weighted magnitude images [222]. Quantitative susceptibility and residual mapping (QUASAR) accounts for biophysical frequency contributions, which acknowledges that the notion that the local Larmor frequency is affected by the static field perturbations related to tissue susceptibility, as well as the magnetic field, chemical shifts, directional alignment of axons, and energy exchange between water and macromolecules [224]. Alternatively, some algorithms solve the entire equation within a single step by incorporating SHARP principles with simultaneous total generalized variation (TGV)-regularized dipole inversion [225,226]. Similarly phase removal using the Laplacian operator (HARPERELLA) simultaneously combines phase unwrapping and background removal [227]. These methods comprise tool boxes that are largely available in Matlab or Python (see [228] and the references therein).

The clinical potential of QSM lies in its sensitivity to variations in iron stored in ferritin and hemosiderin, lipids and calcium, levels of differential oxygenation-saturation present in venous blood, and identification of sub millimeter white matter microstructure [229–231]. Further, QSM has been shown to be superior to T2* in parcellations of the STN, which could translate into better visualization and targeting for DBS [223,228,232]. T2 relaxometry has been shown to predict motor outcome in some PD patients with STN DBS, where patients who have low T2 values may fail to show a clinical benefit [233]. It is possible that this can be explained by the fact that patients with low T2 relaxometry will have less contrast between the STN and the surrounding tissue, hindering the accurate visualization and targeting of the structure, which could be solved by employing QSM. However, QSM obtained during a scanning session is still experimental and under development. Further, there are many competing post-processing methods for creating QSM images, which makes translation challenging.

12. Complications Unrelated to Pre-Operative Planning

Lastly, we would like to mention that while this paper specifically refers to suboptimal placement of DBS leads due to the limitations of neuroimaging, negative outcomes of DBS application can arise independently of planning procedures and surgical expertise. For example, neurosurgery has been linked to brain deformation and shift, changes in cerebral spinal fluid volume, and intracranial pressure, which may induce spatial variability both during the surgery and cause a shift in the implanted lead location during recovery [27,234]. Similarly, DBS surgeries are associated with infection (mostly found in the chest and connector) [235]; reactive gliosis and gliotic scarring [236]; hemorrhage either during the surgery or delayed (in less than 5%) [237]; and, although rare, cerebral pneumocephalus [238]. In all these cases, the DBS system may require reimplantation, replacement, or removal.

13. Conclusions

In this paper, we have discussed some of the differences in current clinical MRI practices with optimized and UHF-MRI methods commonly employed in research environments. Clinical MRI hinges on weighted imaging with anisotropic voxel sizes and maintaining short acquisition, therefore being limited in signal and resolution. These current clinical practices are FDA-approved and are therefore deemed acceptable for neurosurgical purposes. However, the presence of side effects and non-responding patients nonetheless exist. Optimized 3 T and UHF-MRI tend to incorporate isotropic high-resolution imaging with quantitative and susceptibility-based contrasts for better visualization of deep brain structures, which, however, require more complex pre-processing and longer scan durations. The limitations incurred regarding reduced signal in clinical MRI and increased acquisition time with optimized 3 T can be largely overcome with the use of UHF-MRI. However, many of the image registration, correction, and post-processing techniques will typically require expertise that is outside the realm of traditional clinical settings. Importantly, the use of UHF-MRI and alternative contrasts such as QSM can only be implemented once pre-operative planning systems allow for their compatibility, which will require further FDA approval, not only for the MRI system but also for specific sequences. Additional approval for clinical use may be required for pre- and post-processing, such as the algorithms used for registration or calculation of quantitative maps.

We therefore propose that where UHF-MRI is not accessible, higher quality imaging can be obtained with optimized 3 T, although this will take longer than is perhaps clinically feasible for patients with severe movement disorders. Continued direct collaboration and combined efforts between fundamental neuroscience researchers and clinicians will be essential for the development of optimized 3 T and UHF-MRI in the pre-operative planning process for DBS of the STN in PD. Multi-site clinical trials can facilitate the optimization and validation of certain sequences. Sequences with identical parameters should be compared on identical MRI systems and different sites to ensure harmonization and reliability, as well as to validate the desired sequences. Rates of deviations between planned and actual target locations should be compared across vendors and systems as well as across sequences. Similarly, access agreements to work-in-progress protocols from MR vendors would facilitate the development and optimization of sequences, and would open access to underling algorithms and adjustable parameters within to pre-operative planning software vendors (e.g., Medtronic, St. Judes, Brainlab, Abott, Nextim, and Boston Scientific).

Of note, while this paper focused specifically on the STN as the most popular target for DBS in PD, alternative targets also exist (for example, see Figure 1). Some centers have long preferred the internal segment of the globus pallidus, and more recent research is being conducted on the suitability of alternate areas such as the ventral intermediate nucleus or the pedunculopontine nucleus for DBS targets. For a more in-depth review, please see [10,239,240] and the references therein.

Author Contributions: Conceptualization, B.R.I., M.C.K., A.A., Y.T., P.-L.B., and B.U.F.; validation, B.R.I., M.C.K., A.A., Y.T., P.-L.B., and B.U.F.; investigation, B.R.I., M.C.K., A.A., Y.T., P.-L.B., and B.U.F.; resources, Y.T. and B.U.F.; data curation, X.X.; writing—original draft preparation, B.R.I., M.C.K., and B.U.F.; writing—review and editing, B.R.I., M.C.K., A.A., Y.T., P.-L.B., and B.U.F.; visualization, B.R.I. and A.A.; supervision, B.U.F. and P.-L.B.; project administration, B.R.I. and M.C.K. All authors have read and agreed to the published version of the manuscript.

References

1. Van Oostrom, S.H.; Gijsen, R.; Stirbu, I.; Korevaar, J.C.; Schellevis, F.G.; Picavet, H.S.J.; Hoeymans, N. Time trends in prevalence of chronic diseases and multimorbidity not only due to Aging: Data from general practices and health Surveys. *PLoS ONE* **2016**, *11*, e0160264. [CrossRef] [PubMed]

2. Rossi, A.; Berger, K.; Chen, H.; Leslie, D.L.; Mailman, R.B.; Huang, X. Projection of the prevalence of Parkinson's disease in the coming decades: Revisited. *Mov. Disord.* **2018**, *33*, 156–159. [CrossRef] [PubMed]

3. Sveinbjornsdottir, S. The clinical symptoms of Parkinson's disease. *J. Neurochem.* **2016**, *139*, 318–324. [CrossRef] [PubMed]

4. Evans, A.H.; Lees, A.J. Dopamine dysregulation syndrome in Parkinson's disease. *Curr. Opin. Neurol.* **2004**, *17*, 393–398. [CrossRef] [PubMed]

5. Olanow, C.W.; Obeso, J.A.; Stocchi, F. Continuous dopamine-receptor treatment of Parkinson's disease: Scientific rationale and clinical implications. *Lancet Neurol.* **2006**, *5*, 677–687. [CrossRef]

6. Lang, A.E.; Obeso, J.A. Challenges in Parkinson's disease: Restoration of the nigrostriatal dopamine system is not enough. *Lancet Neurol.* **2004**, *3*, 309–316. [CrossRef]

7. Ahlskog, J.E.; Muenter, M.D. Frequency of levodopa-related dyskinesias and motor fluctuations as estimated from the cumulative literature. *Mov. Disord.* **2001**, *16*, 448–458. [CrossRef]

8. Holloway, R.; Shoulson, I.; Kieburtz, K. Pramipexole vs. Levodopa as initial treatment for Parkinson disease: A randomized controlled trial. *J. Am. Med. Assoc.* **2000**, *284*, 1931–1938. [CrossRef]

9. Ahlskog, J.E. Medical Treatment of later-stage motor problems of Parkinson disease. *Mayo. Clin. Proc.* **1999**, *74*, 1239–1254. [CrossRef]

10. Odekerken, V.J.; Boel, J.A.; Schmand, B.A.; De Haan, R.J.; Figee, M.; Munckhof, P.V.D.; Schuurman, P.R.; De Bie, R.M.; For the NSTAPS study group; Bour, L. GPi vs. STN deep brain stimulation for Parkinson disease. *Neurology* **2016**, *86*, 755–761. [CrossRef]

11. Benabid, A.L.; Chabardes, S.; Mitrofanis, J.; Pollak, P. Deep brain stimulation of the subthalamic nucleus for the treatment of Parkinson's disease. *Lancet Neurol.* **2009**, *8*, 67–81. [CrossRef]

12. Limousin, P.; Krack, P.; Pollak, P.; Benazzouz, A.; Ardouin, C.; Hoffmann, D.; Benabid, A.L. Electrical stimulation of the subthalamic nucleus in advanced Parkinson's disease. *N. Engl. J. Med.* **2002**, *339*, 1105–1111. [CrossRef] [PubMed]

13. Limousin, P.; Pollak, P.; Benazzouz, A.; Hoffmann, D.; Le Bas, J.F.; Perret, J.; Benabid, A.L.; Broussolle, E. Effect on parkinsonian signs and symptoms of bilateral subthalamic nucleus stimulation. *Lancet* **1995**, *345*, 91–95. [CrossRef]

14. De Hollander, G.; Keuken, M.C.; Bazin, P.L.; Weiss, M.; Neumann, J.; Reimann, K.; Wähnert, M.; Turner, R.; Forstmann, B.U.; Schäfer, A. A gradual increase of iron toward the medial-inferior tip of the subthalamic nucleus. *Hum. Brain Mapp.* **2014**, *35*, 4440–4449. [CrossRef] [PubMed]

15. Alkemade, A.; De Hollander, G.; Miletic, S.; Keuken, M.C.; Balesar, R.; De Boer, O.; Swaab, D.F.; Forstmann, B.U. The functional microscopic neuroanatomy of the human subthalamic nucleus. *Brain Struct. Funct.* **2019**, *224*, 3213–3227. [CrossRef]

16. Chiken, S.; Nambu, A. Mechanism of deep brain stimulation. *Neuroscientist* **2016**, *22*, 313–322. [CrossRef]

17. Stefani, A.; Cerroni, R.; Mazzone, P.; Liguori, C.; Di Giovanni, G.; Pierantozzi, M.; Galati, S. Mechanisms of action underlying the efficacy of deep brain stimulation of the subthalamic nucleus in Parkinson's disease: Central role of disease severity. *Eur. J. Neurosci.* **2018**, *49*, 805–816. [CrossRef] [PubMed]

18. Petsko, G.A. The coming epidemic of neurologic disorders: What science is—And should be—Doing about it. *Daedalus* **2012**, *141*, 98–107. [CrossRef]

19. Bosco, D.A.; Lavoie, M.J.; Petsko, G.A.; Ringe, D. Proteostasis and movement disorders: Parkinson's disease and amyotrophic lateral sclerosis. *Cold Spring Harb. Perspect. Biol.* **2011**, *3*, a007500. [CrossRef]

20. Weaver, F.M.; Follett, K.; Stern, M.; Hur, K.; Harris, C.; Marks, W.J.; Rothlind, J.; Sagher, O.; Reda, D.; Moy, C.S.; et al. Bilateral deep brain stimulation vs. best medical therapy for patients with advanced parkinson disease. A randomized controlled Trial. *JAMA* **2009**, *301*, 63–73. [CrossRef]

21. Obeso, J.A.; Olanow, C.W.; Rodriguez-Oroz, M.C.; Krack, P.; Kumar, R.; Lang, A.E. Deep-brain stimulation of the subthalamic nucleus or the pars interna of the globus pallidus in Parkinson's disease. *N. Engl. J. Med.* **2001**, *345*, 956–963. [CrossRef] [PubMed]

22. Deuschl, G.; Schade-Brittinger, C.; Krack, P.; Volkmann, J.; Schafer, H.; Bötzel, K.; Daniels, C.; Deutschländer, A.; Dillmann, U.; Eisner, W.; et al. A randomized trial of deep-brain stimulation for Parkinson's disease. *N. Engl. J. Med.* **2006**, *355*, 896–908. [CrossRef]

23. Cyron, D. Mental side effects of deep brain stimulation (DBS) for movement disorders: The futility of denial. *Front. Integr. Neurosci.* **2016**, *10*, 17. [CrossRef] [PubMed]

24. Forstmann, B.U.; Isaacs, B.R.; Temel, Y. Ultra high field MRI-guided deep brain stimulation. *Trends Biotechnol.* **2017**, *35*, 904–907. [CrossRef] [PubMed]

25. Temel, Y.; Blokland, A.; Steinbusch, H.W.M.; Visser-Vandewalle, V. The functional role of the subthalamic nucleus in cognitive and limbic circuits. *Prog Neurobiol.* **2005**, *76*, 393–413. [CrossRef] [PubMed]

26. Rolston, J.D.; Englot, D.J.; Starr, P.A.; Larson, P.S. An unexpectedly high rate of revisions and removals in deep brain stimulation surgery: Analysis of multiple databases. *Park Relat Disord.* **2016**, *33*, 72–77. [CrossRef]

27. Hartmann, C.J.; Fliegen, S.; Groiss, S.J.; Wojtecki, L.; Schnitzler, A. An update on best practice of deep brain stimulation in Parkinson's disease. *Ther Adv Neurol Disord.* **2019**, *12*, 175628641983809. [CrossRef]

28. Fenoy, A.J.; Simpson, R.K. Risks of common complications in deep brain stimulation surgery: Management and avoidance—Clinical article. *J Neurosurg.* **2014**, *120*, 132–139. [CrossRef]

29. DIS Open Data. Available online: https://www.opendisdata.nl/ (accessed on 24 February 2020).

30. Kloc, M.; Kosutzka, Z.; Steno, J.; Valkovic, P. Prevalent placement error of deep brain stimulation electrode in movement disorders (technical considerations). *Bratislava Med. J.* **2017**, *118*, 647–653. [CrossRef]

31. Nagy, A.M.; Tolleson, C.M. Rescue procedures after suboptimal deep brain stimulation outcomes in common movement disorders. *Brain Sci.* **2016**, *6*, 46. [CrossRef]

32. Tonge, M.; Kocabicak, E.; Ackermans, L.; Kuijf, M.; Temel, Y. Final electrode position in subthalamic nucleus deep brain stimulation surgery: A comparison of indirect and direct targeting methods. *Turk Neurosurg.* **2016**, *26*, 900–903. [CrossRef] [PubMed]

33. Tu, P.H.; Liu, Z.H.; Chen, C.C.; Lin, W.Y.; Bowes, A.L.; Lu, C.S.; Lee, S.-T. Indirect targeting of subthalamic deep brain stimulation guided by stereotactic computed tomography and microelectrode recordings in patients with Parkinson's disease. *Front Hum Neurosci.* **2018**, *12*, 470. [CrossRef] [PubMed]

34. Cho, Z.H.; Min, H.K.; Oh, S.H.; Han, J.Y.; Park, C.W.; Chi, J.G.; Kim, Y.B.; Paek, S.H.; Lozano, A.M.; Lee, K.H. Direct visualization of deep brain stimulation targets in Parkinson disease with the use of 7-tesla magnetic resonance imaging. *J Neurosurg.* **2010**, *113*, 639–647. [CrossRef]

35. Machado, A.; Rezai, A.R.; Kopell, B.H.; Gross, R.E.; Sharan, A.D.; Benabid, A.-L. Deep brain stimulation for Parkinson's disease: Surgical technique and perioperative management. *Mov Disord.* **2006**, *21*, 247–258. [CrossRef] [PubMed]

36. Landi, A.; Grimaldi, M.; Antonini, A.; Parolin, M.; Marina, Z.A. MRI indirect stereotactic targeting for deep brain stimulation in Parkinson's disease. *J. Neurosurg. Sci.* **2003**, *47*, 26–32.

37. Duchin, Y.; Shamir, R.R.; Patriat, R.; Kim, J.; Vitek, J.L.; Sapiro, G.; Harel, N. Patient-specific anatomical model for deep brain stimulation based on 7 Tesla MRI. Toft M, ed. *PLoS ONE* **2018**, *13*, e0201469. [CrossRef]

38. Rabie, A.; Metman, L.V.; Slavin, K.V. Using "Functional" target coordinates of the subthalamic nucleus to assess the indirect and direct methods of the preoperative planning: Do the anatomical and functional targets coincide? *Brain Sci.* **2016**, *6*, 65. [CrossRef]

39. Starr, P.A. Placement of deep brain stimulators into the subthalamic nucleus or Globus pallidus internus: Technical approach. *Stereotact Funct Neurosurg.* **2002**, *79*, 118–145. [CrossRef]

40. Andrade-Souza, Y.M.; Schwalb, J.M.; Hamani, C.; Eltahawy, H.; Hoque, T.; Saint-Cyr, J.; Lozano, A.M. Comparison of three methods of targeting the subthalamic nucleus for chronic stimulation in Parkinson's disease. *Neurosurgery* **2005**, *56*, 360–368. [CrossRef]

41. Bejjani, B.P.; Dormont, D.; Pidoux, B.; Yelnik, J.; Damier, P.; Arnulf, I.; Bonnet, A.-M.; Marsault, C.; Agid, Y.; Philippon, J.; et al. Bilateral subthalamic stimulation for Parkinson's disease by using three-dimensional stereotactic magnetic resonance imaging and electrophysiological guidance. *J Neurosurg* **2000**, *92*, 615–625. [CrossRef]

42. Pallavaram, S.; D'Haese, P.F.; Lake, W.; Konrad, P.E.; Dawant, B.M.; Neimat, J.S. Fully automated targeting using nonrigid image registration matches accuracy and exceeds precision of best manual approaches to subthalamic deep brain stimulation targeting in parkinson disease. *Neurosurgery* **2015**, *76*, 756–763. [CrossRef] [PubMed]

43. Ashkan, K.; Blomstedt, P.; Zrinzo, L.; Tisch, S.; Yousry, T.; Limousin-Dowsey, P.; Hariz, M.I. Variability of the subthalamic nucleus: The case for direct MRI guided targeting. *Br. J. Neurosurg.* **2007**, *21*, 197–200. [CrossRef] [PubMed]

44. Isaacs, B.R.; Trutti, A.C.; Pelzer, E.; Tittgemeyer, M.; Temel, Y.; Forstmann, B.U.; Keuken, M.C. Cortico-basal white matter alterations occurring in Parkinson's disease. *PLoS ONE* **2019**, *14*, e0214343. [CrossRef] [PubMed]

45. Kaya, M.O.; Ozturk, S.; Ercan, I.; Gonen, M.; Kocabicak, E.; Erol, F.S. Statistical shape analysis of subthalamic nucleus in patients with Parkinson disease. *World Neurosurg.* **2019**, *126*, e835–e841. [CrossRef]

46. Keuken, M.C.; Bazin, P.L.; Crown, L.; Hootsmans, J.; Laufer, A.; Müller-Axt, C.; Sier, R.; Van Der Putten, E.; Schäfer, A.; Turner, R.; et al. Quantifying inter-individual anatomical variability in the subcortex using 7 T structural MRI. *NeuroImage* **2014**, *94*, 40–46. [CrossRef]

47. Xiao, Y.; Jannin, P.; D'Albis, T.; Guizard, N.; Haegelen, C.; Lalys, F.; Verin, M.; Collins, D.L. Investigation of morphometric variability of subthalamic nucleus, red nucleus, and substantia nigra in advanced Parkinson's disease patients using automatic segmentation and PCA-based analysis. *Hum. Brain Mapp.* **2014**, *35*, 4330–4344. [CrossRef]

48. Welter, M.L.; Schüpbach, M.; Czernecki, V.; Karachi, C.; Fernandez-Vidal, S.; Golmard, J.L.; Serra, G.; Navarro, S.; Welaratne, A.; Hartmann, A.; et al. Optimal target localization for subthalamic stimulation in patients with Parkinson disease. *Neurology* **2014**, *82*, 1352–1361. [CrossRef]

49. Rutt, B.K.; Lee, D.H. The impact of field strength on image quality in MRI. *J. Magn. Reson. Imaging* **1996**, *6*, 57–62. [CrossRef]

50. McRobbie, D.W.; Moore, E.A.; Graves, M.J. *Prince MR. MRI From Picture to Proton*; Cambridge University Press: Cambridge, UK, 2006.

51. Edelstein, W.A.; Glover, G.H.; Hardy, C.J.; Redington, R.W. The intrinsic signal-to-noise ratio in NMR imaging. *Magn. Reson. Med.* **1986**, *3*, 604–618. [CrossRef]

52. Springer, E.; Dymerska, B.; Cardoso, P.L.; Robinson, S.; Weisstanner, C.; Wiest, R.; Schmitt, B.; Trattnig, S. Comparison of Routine Brain Imaging at 3 T and 7 T. *Investig. Radiol.* **2016**, *51*, 469–482. [CrossRef]

53. U.S. Food and Drug Administration. *FDA Clears First 7T Magnetic Resonance Imaging Device. FDA News Release.* Available online: https://www.fda.gov/news-events/press-announcements/fda-clears-first-7t-magnetic-resonance-imaging-device (accessed on 3 February 2020).

54. Pohmann, R.; Speck, O.; Scheffler, K. Signal-to-noise ratio and MR tissue parameters in human brain imaging at 3, 7, and 9.4 tesla using current receive coil arrays. *Magn. Reson. Med.* **2015**, *75*, 801–809. [CrossRef] [PubMed]

55. De Zwart, J.A.; Ledden, P.J.; Kellman, P.; Van Gelderen, P.; Duyn, J.H. Design of a SENSE-optimized high-sensitivity MRI receive coil for brain imaging. *Magn. Reson. Med.* **2002**, *47*, 1218–1227. [CrossRef] [PubMed]

56. Turner, R. Gradient coil design: A review of methods. *Magn. Reson. Imaging* **1993**, *11*, 903–920. [CrossRef]

57. Winkler, S.A.; Schmitt, F.; Landes, H.; De Bever, J.; Wade, T.; Alejski, A.; Rutt, B.K. Gradient and shim technologies for Ultra High Field MRI. *NeuroImage* **2018**, *168*, 59–70. [CrossRef] [PubMed]

58. Hendriks, A.D.; Luijten, P.R.; Klomp, D.W.J.; Petridou, N. Potential acceleration performance of a 256-channel whole-brain receive array at 7 T. *Magn. Reson. Med.* **2019**, *81*, 1659–1670. [CrossRef]

59. Setsompop, K.; Gagoski, B.A.; Polimeni, J.R.; Witzel, T.; Wedeen, V.J.; Wald, L.L. Blipped-controlled aliasing in parallel imaging for simultaneous multislice echo planar imaging with reduced g -factor penalty. *Magn. Reson. Med.* **2011**, *67*, 1210–1224. [CrossRef]

60. Wiggins, G.C.; Polimeni, J.R.; Potthast, A.; Schmitt, M.; Alagappan, V.; Wald, L.L. 96-Channel receive-only head coil for 3 Tesla: Design optimization and evaluation. *Magn. Reson. Med.* **2009**, *62*, 754–762. [CrossRef]

61. De Hollander, G.; Keuken, M.C.; Van Der Zwaag, W.; Forstmann, B.U.; Trampel, R. Comparing functional MRI protocols for small, iron-rich basal ganglia nuclei such as the subthalamic nucleus at 7 T and 3 T. *Hum. Brain Mapp.* **2017**, *38*, 3226–3248. [CrossRef]

62. Forstmann, B.U.; De Hollander, G.; Van Maanen, L.; Alkemade, A.; Keuken, M.C. Towards a mechanistic understanding of the human subcortex. *Nat. Rev. Neurosci.* **2016**, *18*, 57–65. [CrossRef]

63. Duyn, J.H. The future of ultra-high field MRI and fMRI for study of the human brain. *NeuroImage* **2012**, *62*, 1241–1248. [CrossRef]

64. Van Der Zwaag, W.; Schäfer, A.; Marques, J.P.; Turner, R.; Trampel, R. Recent applications of UHF-MRI in the study of human brain function and structure: A review. *NMR Biomed.* **2015**, *29*, 1274–1288. [CrossRef] [PubMed]

65. Van Beek, E.J.R.; Kuhl, C.; Anzai, Y.; Desmond, P.; Ehman, R.L.; Gong, Q.; Gold, G.; Gulani, V.; Hall-Craggs, M.A.; Leiner, T.; et al. Value of MRI in medicine: More than just another test? *J. Magn. Reson. Imaging* **2018**, *49*, e14–e25. [CrossRef] [PubMed]

66. Beisteiner, R.; Robinson, S.; Wurnig, M.; Hilbert, M.; Merksa, K.; Rath, J.; Höllinger, I.; Klinger, N.; Marosi, C.; Trattnig, S.; et al. Clinical fMRI: Evidence for a 7T benefit over 3T. *NeuroImage* **2011**, *57*, 1015–1021. [CrossRef] [PubMed]

67. Cho, Z.H.; Kim, Y.B.; Han, J.Y.; Min, H.K.; Kim, K.N.; Choi, S.H.; Veklerov, E.; Shepp, L.A. New brain atlas—Mapping the human brain in vivo with 7.0 T MRI and comparison with postmortem histology: Will these images change modern medicine? *Int. J. Imaging Syst. Technol.* **2008**, *18*, 2–8. [CrossRef]

68. Duchin, Y.; Abosch, A.; Yacoub, E.; Sapiro, G.; Harel, N. Feasibility of using ultra-high field (7 T) MRI for clinical surgical targeting. *PLoS ONE* **2012**, *7*, e37328. [CrossRef]

69. Kraff, O.; Fischer, A.; Nagel, A.M.; Mönninghoff, C.; Ladd, M.E. MRI at 7 tesla and above: Demonstrated and potential capabilities. *J. Magn. Reson. Imaging* **2014**, *41*, 13–33. [CrossRef]

70. Plantinga, B.R.; Temel, Y.; Duchin, Y.; Uludag, K.; Patriat, R.; Roebroeck, A.; Kuijf, M.; Jahanshahi, A.; Romenij, B.T.H.; Vitek, J.; et al. Individualized parcellation of the subthalamic nucleus in patients with Parkinson's disease with 7T MRI. *NeuroImage* **2018**, *168*, 403–411. [CrossRef]

71. Straub, S.; Zaiss, M. Pros and cons of ultra-high-field MRI/MRS for human application. *Prog. Nucl. Magn. Reson. Spectrosc.* **2018**, *109*, 1–50. [CrossRef]

72. Truong, T.-K.; Chakeres, D.W.; Beversdorf, D.Q.; Scharre, D.; Schmalbrock, P. Effects of static and radiofrequency magnetic field inhomogeneity in ultra-high field magnetic resonance imaging. *Magn. Reson. Imaging* **2006**, *24*, 103–112. [CrossRef]

73. Stockmann, J.P.; Witzel, T.; Keil, B.; Polimeni, J.R.; Mareyam, A.; Lapierre, C.; Setsompop, K.; Wald, L.L. A 32-channel combined RF and B0 shim array for 3T brain imaging. *Magn. Reson. Med.* **2016**, *75*, 441–451. [CrossRef]

74. Mao, W.; Smith, M.B.; Collins, C. Exploring the limits of RF shimming for high-field MRI of the human head. *Magn. Reson. Med.* **2006**, *56*, 918–922. [CrossRef] [PubMed]

75. Available online: https://www.ismrm.org/20/program_files/DP13-02.htm (accessed on 3 February 2020).

76. Anderson, W.S.; Lenz, F.A. Surgery Insight: Deep brain stimulation for movement disorders. *Nat. Clin. Pr. Neurol.* **2006**, *2*, 310–320. [CrossRef] [PubMed]

77. Ashkan, K.; Wallace, B.; Bell, B.A.; Benabid, A.L. Deep brain stimulation of the subthalamic nucleus in Parkinson's disease 1993-2003: Where are we 10 years on? *Br. J. Neurosurg.* **2004**, *18*, 19–34. [CrossRef] [PubMed]

78. Gielen, F.L.H. Deep brain stimulation: Current practice and challenges for the future. In Proceedings of the First International IEEE EMBS Conference on Neural Engineering, Capri Island, Italy, 20–22 March 2003. [CrossRef]

79. Aviles-Olmos, I.; Kefalopoulou, Z.; Tripoliti, E.; Candelario, J.; Akram, H.; Martinez-Torres, I.; Jahanshahi, M.; Foltynie, T.; Hariz, M.; Zrinzo, L.; et al. Long-term outcome of subthalamic nucleus deep brain stimulation for Parkinson's disease using an MRI-guided and MRI-verified approach. *J. Neurol. Neurosurg. Psychiatry* **2014**, *85*, 1419–1425. [CrossRef]

80. Chen, S.Y.; Lee, C.C.; Lin, S.H.; Hsin, Y.L.; Lee, T.W.; Yen, P.S.; Chou, Y.C.; Lee, C.W.; Hsieh, W.A.; Su, C.F.; et al. Microelectrode recording can be a good adjunct in magnetic resonance image–directed subthalamic nucleus deep brain stimulation for parkinsonism. *Surg. Neurol.* **2006**, *65*, 253–260. [CrossRef]

81. Patel, N.K.; Heywood, P.; O'Sullivan, K.; Love, S.; Gill, S.S. MRI-directed subthalamic nucleus surgery for Parkinson's disease. *Ster. Funct. Neurosurg.* **2002**, *78*, 132–145. [CrossRef]

82. Lozano, C.S.; Ranjan, M.; Boutet, A.; Xu, D.S.; Kucharczyk, W.; Fasano, A.; Lozano, A.M. Imaging alone versus microelectrode recording–guided targeting of the STN in patients with Parkinson's disease. *J. Neurosurg.* **2019**, *130*, 1847–1852. [CrossRef]

83. Frequin, H.L.; Bot, M.; Dilai, J.; Scholten, M.N.; Postma, M.; Bour, L.J.; Contarino, M.F.; De Bie, R.M.; Schuurman, P.R.; Munckhof, P.V.D. Relative contribution of magnetic resonance imaging, microelectrode recordings, and awake test stimulation in final lead placement during deep brain stimulation surgery of the subthalamic nucleus in Parkinson's disease. *Ster. Funct. Neurosurg.* **2020**, *98*, 118–128. [CrossRef]

84. Ostrem, J.L.; Galifianakis, N.B.; Markun, L.C.; Grace, J.K.; Martin, A.J.; Starr, P.A.; Larson, P.S. Clinical outcomes of PD patients having bilateral STN DBS using high-field interventional MR-imaging for lead placement. *Clin. Neurol. Neurosurg.* **2013**, *115*, 708–712. [CrossRef]

85. McClelland, S. A cost analysis of intraoperative microelectrode recording during subthalamic stimulation for Parkinson's disease. *Mov. Disord.* **2011**, *26*, 1422–1427. [CrossRef]

86. Habets, J.; Isaacs, B.; Vinke, S.; Kubben, P. Controversies in deep brain stimulation surgery: Micro-electrode recordings. In *Evidence for Neurosurgery*; Springer: Cham, Switzerland, 2019; pp. 97–109. [CrossRef]

87. Tykocki, T.; Nauman, P.; Koziara, H.; Mandat, T. Microlesion effect as a predictor of the effectiveness of subthalamic deep brain stimulation for Parkinson's disease. *Ster. Funct. Neurosurg.* **2013**, *91*, 12–17. [CrossRef] [PubMed]

88. Slotty, P.; Wille, C.; Kinfe, T.M.; Vesper, J. Continuous perioperative apomorphine in deep brain stimulation surgery for Parkinson's disease. *Br. J. Neurosurg.* **2013**, *28*, 378–382. [CrossRef] [PubMed]

89. Kleiner-Fisman, G.; Herzog, J.; Kleiner-Fisman, G.; Tamma, F.; Lyons, K.E.; Pahwa, R.; Lang, A.E.; Deuschl, G. Subthalamic nucleus deep brain stimulation: Summary and meta-analysis of outcomes. *Mov. Disord.* **2006**, *21* (Suppl. S14), S290–S304. [CrossRef]

90. Moro, E.; Esselink, R.J.; Xie, J.; Hommel, M.; Benabid, A.L.; Pollak, P. The impact on Parkinson's disease of electrical parameter settings in STN stimulation. *Neurology* **2002**, *59*, 706–713. [CrossRef] [PubMed]

91. Esselink, R.A.J.; Kuijf, M.L. Organization of Care for Patients Treated by Deep Brain Stimulation. In *Fundamentals and Clinics of Deep Brain Stimulation*; Springer: Cham, Switzerland, 2020; pp. 161–168. [CrossRef]

92. Aubignat, M.; Lefranc, M.; Tir, M.; Krystkowiak, P. Deep brain stimulation programming in Parkinson's disease: Introduction of current issues and perspectives. *Rev. Neurol.* **2020**. [CrossRef]

93. De Oliveira Godeiro, C.; Moro, E.; Montgomery, E.B. Programming: General aspects. In *Fundamentals and Clinics of Deep Brain Stimulation*; Springer: Cham, Switzerland, 2020. [CrossRef]

94. Food and Drug Administration. Guidance for the Submission of Premarket Notifications for Magnetic Resonance Diagnostic Devices. Available online: https://www.fda.gov/regulatory-information/search-fda-guidance-documents/submission-premarket-notifications-magnetic-resonance-diagnostic-devices (accessed on 3 February 2020).

95. International Electrochemical Commission. *Medical Electrical Equipment: Part 2-33. Particular Requirements for the Safety of Magnetic Resonance Equipment for Medical Diagnosis*; IEC—International Electrotechnical Commission: Geneva, Switzerland, 2010.

96. Vaughan, J.; Garwood, M.; Collins, C.; Liu, W.; DelaBarre, L.; Adriany, G.; Andersen, P.; Merkle, H.; Goebel, R.; Smith, M.; et al. 7T vs. 4T: RF power, homogeneity, and signal-to-noise comparison in head images. *Magn. Reson. Med.* **2001**, *46*, 24–30. [CrossRef]

97. Balchandani, P.; Naidich, T.P. Ultra-high-field MR neuroimaging. *Am. J. Neuroradiol.* **2015**, *36*, 1204–1215. [CrossRef]

98. Bergen, B.V.D.; Berg, C.V.D.; Bartels, L.W.; Lagendijk, J.J.W. 7 T body MRI:B1shimming with simultaneous SAR reduction. *Phys. Med. Biol.* **2007**, *52*, 5429–5441. [CrossRef]

99. Allison, J.; Yanasak, N. What MRI sequences produce the highest specific absorption rate (SAR), and is there something we should be doing to reduce the SAR during standard examinations? *Am. J. Roentgenol.* **2015**, *205*, W140. [CrossRef]

100. Ghadimi, M.; Sapra, A. *Magnetic Resonance Imaging (MRI), Contraindications*; StatPearls Publishing: Treasure Island, FL, USA, 2019.

101. Horn, A.; Reich, M.; Vorwerk, J.; Li, N.; Wenzel, G.; Fang, Q.; Schmitz-Hübsch, T.; Nickl, R.; Kupsch, A.; Volkmann, J.; et al. Connectivity Predicts deep brain stimulation outcome in Parkinson disease. *Ann. Neurol.* **2017**, *82*, 67–78. [CrossRef]

102. Schmitz, B.L.; Aschoff, A.J.; Hoffmann, M.H.K.; Grön, G. Advantages and pitfalls in 3T MR brain imaging: A pictorial review. *Am. J. Neuroradiol.* **2006**, *26*, 2229–2237.

103. Marques, J.P.; Simonis, F.; Webb, A.G. Low-field MRI: An MR physics perspective. *J. Magn. Reson. Imaging* **2019**, *49*, 1528–1542. [CrossRef] [PubMed]

104. Bekiesińska-Figatowska, M. Artifacts in magnetic resonance imaging. *Pol. J. Radiol.* **2015**, *80*, 93–106. [CrossRef]

105. Wachowicz, K. Evaluation of active and passive shimming in magnetic resonance imaging. *Res. Rep. Nucl. Med.* **2014**, *4*, 1. [CrossRef]

106. Wilson, J.L.; Jenkinson, M.; Jezzard, P. Optimization of static field homogeneity in human brain using diamagnetic passive shims. *Magn. Reson. Med.* **2002**, *48*, 906–914. [CrossRef]

107. Golay, M.J.E. Field homogenizing coils for nuclear spin resonance instrumentation. *Rev. Sci. Instruments* **1958**, *29*, 313–315. [CrossRef]

108. Roméo, F.; Hoult, D.I. Magnet field profiling: Analysis and correcting coil design. *Magn. Reson. Med.* **1984**, *1*, 44–65. [CrossRef]

109. Bitar, R.; Leung, G.; Perng, R.; Tadros, S.; Moody, A.R.; Sarrazin, J.; McGregor, C.; Christakis, M.; Symons, S.; Nelson, A.; et al. MR Pulse sequences: What every radiologist wants to know but is afraid to ask. *Radiographics* **2006**, *26*, 513–537. [CrossRef]

110. Cheng, H.L.M.; Wright, G.A. Rapid high-resolutionT1 mapping by variable flip angles: Accurate and precise measurements in the presence of radiofrequency field inhomogeneity. *Magn. Reson. Med.* **2006**, *55*, 566–574. [CrossRef]

111. Hurley, S.A.; Yarnykh, V.L.; Johnson, K.M.; Field, A.S.; Alexander, A.L.; Samsonov, A. Simultaneous variable flip angle-actual flip angle imaging method for improved accuracy and precision of three-dimensional T1 and B1 measurements. *Magn. Reson. Med.* **2012**, *68*, 54–64. [CrossRef]

112. Yarnykh, V.L. Optimal radiofrequency and gradient spoiling for improved accuracy of T1 and B1 measurements using fast steady-state techniques. *Magn. Reson. Med.* **2010**, *63*, 1610–1626. [CrossRef]

113. Eggenschwiler, F.; Kober, T.; Magill, A.W.; Gruetter, R.; Marques, J.P. SA2RAGE: A new sequence for fast B1+-mapping. *Magn. Reson. Med.* **2011**, *67*, 1609–1619. [CrossRef] [PubMed]

114. Karger, C.P.; Höss, A.; Bendl, R.; Canda, V.; Schad, L. Accuracy of device-specific 2D and 3D image distortion correction algorithms for magnetic resonance imaging of the head provided by a manufacturer. *Phys. Med. Biol.* **2006**, *51*, N253–N261. [CrossRef] [PubMed]

115. Tustison, N.J.; Avants, B.B.; Cook, P.A.; Zheng, Y.; Egan, A.; Yushkevich, P.A.; Gee, J.C. N4ITK: Improved N3 bias correction. *IEEE Trans. Med. Imaging* **2010**, *29*, 1310–1320. [CrossRef] [PubMed]

116. Zhang, Y.; Brady, M.; Smith, S.M. Segmentation of brain MR images through a hidden Markov random field model and the expectation-maximization algorithm. *IEEE Trans. Med. Imaging* **2001**, *20*, 45–57. [CrossRef] [PubMed]

117. Sled, J.G.; Zijdenbos, A.; Evans, A. A nonparametric method for automatic correction of intensity nonuniformity in MRI data. *IEEE Trans. Med. Imaging* **1998**, *17*, 87–97. [CrossRef]

118. Ganzetti, M.; Wenderoth, N.; Mantini, D. Quantitative evaluation of intensity inhomogeneity correction methods for structural MR brain images. *Neuroinformatics* **2016**, *14*, 5–21. [CrossRef]

119. Delgado, A.; Van Westen, D.; Nilsson, M.; Knutsson, L.; Sundgren, P.C.; Larsson, E.M.; Delgado, A.F. Diagnostic value of alternative techniques to gadolinium-based contrast agents in MR neuroimaging-a comprehensive overview. *Insights Imaging* **2019**, *10*, 84. [CrossRef]

120. Oliveira, I.S.; Hedgire, S.S.; Li, W.; Ganguli, S.; Prabhakar, A.M. Blood pool contrast agents for venous magnetic resonance imaging. *Cardiovasc. Diagn. Ther.* **2016**, *6*, 508–518. [CrossRef]

121. Bloem, J.L.; Reijnierse, M.; Huizinga, T.W.J.; Van Der Helm-Van Mil, A.H.M. MR signal intensity: Staying on the bright side in MR image interpretation. *RMD Open* **2018**, *4*, e000728. [CrossRef]

122. Vymazal, J.; Hajek, M.; Patronas, N.; Giedd, J.N.; Bulte, J.W.; Baumgarner, C.; Brooks, R.A. The quantitative relation between T1-weighted and T2-weighted MRI of normal gray matter and iron concentration. *J. Magn. Reason. Imaging* **1995**, *5*, 554–560. [CrossRef]

123. Barral, J.K.; Gudmundson, E.; Stikov, N.; Etezadi-Amoli, M.; Stoica, P.; Nishimura, D.G. A robust methodology for in vivo T1 mapping. *Magn. Reson. Med.* **2010**, *64*, 1057–1067. [CrossRef]

124. Beriault, S.; Sadikot, A.F.; Alsubaie, F.; Drouin, S.; Collins, D.L.; Pike, G.B. Neuronavigation using susceptibility-weighted venography: Application to deep brain stimulation and comparison with gadolinium contrast: Technical note. *J. Neurosurg.* **2014**, *121*, 131–141. [CrossRef] [PubMed]

125. Ko, S.B.; Kim, S.H.; Kim, N.E.; Roh, J.K. Visualization of venous systems by time-of-flight magnetic resonance angiography. *J. Neuroimaging* **2006**, *16*, 353–356. [CrossRef] [PubMed]

126. Barnes, S.R.; Haacke, E.M. Susceptibility-weighted imaging: Clinical angiographic applications. *Magn. Reson. Imaging Clin. N. Am.* **2009**, *17*, 47–61. [CrossRef]

127. Dormont, D.; Ricciardi, K.G.; Tandé, D.; Parain, K.; Menuel, C.; Galanaud, D.; Navarro, S.; Cornu, P.; Agid, Y.; Yelnik, J. Is the subthalamic nucleus hypointense on T2-weighted images? A correlation study using MR imaging and stereotactic atlas data. *Am. J. Neuroradiol.* **2004**, *25*, 1516–1523.

128. Aquino, D.; Bizzi, A.; Grisoli, M.; Garavaglia, B.; Bruzzone, M.G.; Nardocci, N.; Savoiardo, M.; Chiapparini, L. Age-related iron deposition in the basal ganglia: Quantitative analysis in healthy subjects. *Radiology* **2009**, *252*, 165–172. [CrossRef]

129. Drayer, B.P. Basal ganglia: Significance of signal hypointensity on T2-weighted MR images. *Radiology* **1989**, *173*, 311–312. [CrossRef]

130. Keuken, M.C.; Isaacs, B.R.; Trampel, R.; Van Der Zwaag, W.; Forstmann, B.U. Visualizing the human subcortex using ultra-high field magnetic resonance imaging. *Brain Topogr.* **2018**, *31*, 513–545. [CrossRef]

131. Marques, J.P.; Norris, D.G. How to choose the right MR sequence for your research question at 7 T and above? *NeuroImage* **2018**, *168*, 119–140. [CrossRef]

132. Chavhan, G.B.; Babyn, P.S.; Jankharia, B.; Cheng, H.-L.M.; Shroff, M. Steady-state MR imaging sequences: Physics, classification, and clinical applications. *Radiographics* **2008**, *28*, 1147–1160. [CrossRef] [PubMed]

133. Hargreaves, B. Rapid gradient-echo imaging. *J. Magn. Reson. Imaging* **2012**, *36*, 1300–1313. [CrossRef] [PubMed]

134. Tang, M.Y.; Chen, T.W.; Zhang, X.M.; Huang, X.H. GRE T2*-weighted MRI: Principles and clinical applications. *BioMed Res. Int.* **2014**, *2014*, 312142. [CrossRef]

135. Chavhan, G.B.; Babyn, P.S.; Thomas, B.; Shroff, M.M.; Haacke, E.M. Principles, techniques, and applications of T2*-based MR imaging and its special applications. *Radiographics* **2009**, *29*, 1433–1449. [CrossRef] [PubMed]

136. Haacke, E.M.; Tkach, J.A.; Parrish, T.B. Reduction of T2* dephasing in gradient field-echo imaging. *Radiology* **1989**, *170*, 457–462. [CrossRef] [PubMed]

137. Pyatigorskaya, N.; Gallea, C.; Garcia-Lorenzo, D.; Vidailhet, M.; Lehéricy, S. A review of the use of magnetic resonance imaging in Parkinson's disease. *Ther. Adv. Neurol. Disord.* **2013**, *7*, 206–220. [CrossRef]

138. Kosta, P.; Argyropoulou, M.I.; Markoula, S.; Konitsiotis, S. MRI evaluation of the basal ganglia size and iron content in patients with Parkinson's disease. *J. Neurol.* **2006**, *253*, 26–32. [CrossRef] [PubMed]

139. Keuken, M.C.; Bazin, P.-L.; Schäfer, A.; Neumann, J.; Turner, R.; Forstmann, B.U. Ultra-high 7T MRI of structural age-related changes of the subthalamic nucleus. *J. Neurosci.* **2013**, *33*, 4896–4900. [CrossRef] [PubMed]

140. Abosch, A.; Yacoub, E.; Ugurbil, K.; Harel, N. An assessment of current brain targets for deep brain stimulation surgery with susceptibility-weighted imaging at 7 tesla. *Neurosurgery* **2010**, *67*, 1745–1756. [CrossRef]

141. Haacke, E.M.; Mittal, S.; Wu, Z.; Neelavalli, J.; Cheng, Y.C. Susceptibility-weighted imaging: Technical aspects and clinical applications, part 1. *Am. J. Neuroradiol.* **2008**, *30*, 19–30. [CrossRef]

142. Ishimori, Y.; Monma, M.; Kohno, Y. Artifact reduction of susceptibility-weighted imaging using a short-echo phase mask. *Acta Radiol.* **2009**, *50*, 1027–1034. [CrossRef]

143. Rauscher, A.; Sedlacik, J.; Barth, M.; Mentzel, H.-J.; Reichenbach, J.R. Magnetic susceptibility-weighted MR phase imaging of the human brain. *Am. J. Neuroradiol.* **2005**, *26*, 736–742. [PubMed]

144. Elolf, E.; Bockermann, V.; Gringel, T.; Knauth, M.; Dechent, P.; Helms, G. Improved visibility of the subthalamic nucleus on high-resolution stereotactic MR imaging by added susceptibility (T2*) contrast using multiple gradient echoes. *Am. J. Neuroradiol.* **2007**, *28*, 1093–1094. [CrossRef] [PubMed]

145. Bot, M.; Verhagen, O.; Caan, M.; Potters, W.; Dilai, J.; Odekerken, V.; Dijk, J.; De Bie, R.; Schuurman, R.; Munckhof, P.V.D. Defining the dorsal STN border using 7.0-Tesla MRI: A comparison to microelectrode recordings and lower field strength MRI. *Brain Stimul.* **2019**, *97*, 587. [CrossRef]

146. O'Gorman, R.; Shmueli, K.; Ashkan, K.; Samuel, M.; Lythgoe, D.J.; Shahidiani, A.; Wastling, S.J.; Footman, M.; Selway, R.P.; Jarosz, J. Optimal MRI methods for direct stereotactic targeting of the subthalamic nucleus and globus pallidus. *Eur. Radiol.* **2011**, *21*, 130–136. [CrossRef] [PubMed]

147. Keuken, M.C.; Schäfer, A.; Forstmann, B.U. Can we rely on susceptibility-weighted imaging (SWI) for subthalamic nucleus identification in deep brain stimulation surgery? *Neurosurgery* **2016**, *79*, e945–e946. [CrossRef]

148. Bot, M.; Bour, L.; De Bie, R.; Contarino, M.F.; Schuurman, R.; Munckhof, P.V.D. Can we rely on susceptibility-weighted imaging (SWI) for subthalamic nucleus identification in deep brain stimulation surgery? *Neurosurgery* **2016**, *78*, 353–359. [CrossRef]

149. Bus, S.; Munckhof, P.V.D.; Bot, M.; Pal, G.; Ouyang, B.; Sani, S.; Metman, L.V. Borders of STN determined by MRI versus the electrophysiological STN. A comparison using intraoperative CT. *Acta Neurochir.* **2018**, *160*, 373–383. [CrossRef]

150. Vertinsky, A.; Coenen, V.; Lang, D.J.; Kolind, S.; Honey, C.; Li, D.; Rauscher, A. Localization of the subthalamic nucleus: Optimization with susceptibility-weighted phase MR imaging. *Am. J. Neuroradiol.* **2009**, *30*, 1717–1724. [CrossRef]

151. Eckstein, K.; Dymerska, B.; Bachrata, B.; Bogner, W.; Poljanc, K.; Trattnig, S.; Robinson, S. Computationally efficient combination of multi-channel phase data from multi-echo acquisitions (ASPIRE). *Magn. Reson. Med.* **2018**, *79*, 2996–3006. [CrossRef]

152. Weiskopf, N.; Mohammadi, S.; Lutti, A.; Callaghan, M.F. Advances in MRI-based computational neuroanatomy: From morphometry to in-vivo histology. *Curr. Opin. Neurol.* **2015**, *28*, 313–322. [CrossRef] [PubMed]

153. Shin, W.; Shin, T.; Oh, S.-H.; Lowe, M.J. CNR improvement of MP2RAGE from slice encoding directional acceleration. *Magn. Reson. Imaging* **2016**, *34*, 779–784. [CrossRef] [PubMed]

154. Tsialios, P.; Thrippleton, M.; Pernet, C. Evaluation of MRI sequences for quantitative T1 brain mapping. *bioRxiv* **2017**, *931*, 195859. [CrossRef]

155. Sun, H.; Cleary, J.O.; Glarin, R.; Kolbe, S.C.; Ordidge, R.J.; Moffat, B.A.; Pike, G.B. Extracting more for less: Multi-echo MP2RAGE for simultaneous T1-weighted imaging, T1 mapping, R2* mapping, SWI, and QSM from a single acquisition. *Magn. Reson. Med.* **2020**, *83*, 1178–1191. [CrossRef] [PubMed]

156. Choi, U.S.; Kawaguchi, H.; Matsuoka, Y.; Kober, T.; Kida, I. Brain tissue segmentation based on MP2RAGE multi-contrast images in 7 T MRI. *PLoS ONE* **2019**, *14*, e0210803. [CrossRef]

157. Kerl, H.U.; Gerigk, L.; Pechlivanis, I.; Al-Zghloul, M.; Groden, C.; Nolte, I. The subthalamic nucleus at 3.0 Tesla: Choice of optimal sequence and orientation for deep brain stimulation using a standard installation protocol: Clinical article. *J. Neurosurg.* **2012**, *117*, 1155–1165. [CrossRef]

158. Marques, J.P.; Kober, T.; Krueger, G.; Van Der Zwaag, W.; Van De Moortele, P.F.; Gruetter, R. MP2RAGE, a self bias-field corrected sequence for improved segmentation and T1-mapping at high field. *NeuroImage* **2010**, *49*, 1271–1281. [CrossRef]

159. Metere, R.; Kober, T.; Möller, H.E.; Schäfer, A. Simultaneous quantitative MRI mapping of T1, T2* and magnetic susceptibility with multi-echo MP2RAGE. *PLoS ONE* **2017**, *12*, e0169265. [CrossRef]

160. Bazin, P.L.; Alkemade, A.; Van Der Zwaag, W.; Caan, M.; Mulder, M.; Forstmann, B.U. Denoising high-field multi-dimensional MRI with local complex PCA. *Front. Neurosci.* **2019**, *13*, 1066. [CrossRef]

161. Visser, E.; Keuken, M.C.; Douaud, G.; Gaura, V.; Bachoud-Lévi, A.C.; Rémy, P.; Forstmann, B.U.; Jenkinson, M. Automatic segmentation of the striatum and globus pallidus using MIST: Multimodal image segmentation tool. *NeuroImage* **2016**, *125*, 479–497. [CrossRef]

162. Visser, E.; Keuken, M.C.; Forstmann, B.U.; Jenkinson, M. Automated segmentation of the substantia nigra, subthalamic nucleus and red nucleus in 7 T data at young and old age. *NeuroImage* **2016**, *139*, 324–336. [CrossRef] [PubMed]

163. Isaacs, B.R.; Mulder, M.J.; Groot, J.; Van Berendonk, N.; Lute, N.; Bazin, P.L.; Forstmann, B. 3 versus 7 Tesla MRI for parcellations of subcortical brain structures. *bioRxiv* **2020**. under review.

164. Somasundaram, K.; Kalavathi, P. Analysis of imaging artifacts in MR brain images. *Orient J. Comput. Sci. Technol.* **2012**, *5*, 135–141.

165. Mulder, M.J.; Keuken, M.C.; Bazin, P.L.; Alkemade, A.; Forstmann, B.U. Size and shape matter: The impact of voxel geometry on the identification of small nuclei. *PLoS ONE* **2019**, *14*, e0215382. [CrossRef]

166. Van Reeth, E.; Tham, I.W.K.; Tan, C.H.; Poh, C.L. Super-resolution in magnetic resonance imaging: A review. *Concepts Magn. Reson. Part. A* **2012**, *40A*, 306–325. [CrossRef]

167. Chen, S.Y.; Tsai, S.T.; Li, S.H. Controversial issues in deep brain stimulation in Parkinson's disease. *Towar. New Ther. Park. Dis.* **2011**, *2*, 1–20. [CrossRef]

168. Chen, T.; Mirzadeh, Z.; Chapple, K.M.; Lambert, M.; Shill, H.A.; Moguel-Cobos, G.; Tröster, A.I.; Dhall, R.; Ponce, F.A. Clinical outcomes following awake and asleep deep brain stimulation for Parkinson disease. *J. Neurosurg.* **2018**, *130*, 109–120. [CrossRef]

169. Hardaway, F.A.; Raslan, A.M.; Burchiel, K.J. Deep brain stimulation-related infections: Analysis of rates, timing, and Seasonality. *Neurosurgery* **2017**, *83*, 540–547. [CrossRef]

170. Pouratian, N. *Stereotactic and Functional Neurosurgery: Principles and Applications*; Springer: Cham, Switzerland, 2020.

171. Aman, J.E.; Johnson, L.; Sanabria, D.E.; Wang, J.; Patriat, R.; Hill, M.; Marshall, E.; MacKinnon, C.D.; Cooper, S.E.; Schrock, L.E.; et al. Directional deep brain stimulation leads reveal spatially distinct oscillatory activity in the globus pallidus internus of Parkinson's disease patients. *Neurobiol. Dis.* **2020**, *139*, 104819. [CrossRef]

172. Tinkhauser, G.; Pogosyan, A.; Debove, I.; Nowacki, A.; Shah, S.A.; Seidel, K.; Tan, H.; Brittain, J.S.; Petermann, K.; Di Biase, L.; et al. Directional local field potentials: A tool to optimize deep brain stimulation. *Mov. Disord.* **2017**, *33*, 159–164. [CrossRef]

173. Anderson, D.N.; Anderson, C.; Lanka, N.; Sharma, R.; Butson, C.R.; Baker, B.W.; Dorval, A.D. The μDBS: Multiresolution, directional deep brain stimulation for improved targeting of small diameter fibers. *Front. Neurosci.* **2019**, *13*, 1152. [CrossRef] [PubMed]

174. Budrys, T.; Veikutis, V.; Lukosevicius, S.; Gleizniene, R.; Monastyreckiene, E.; Kulakienė, I. Artifacts in magnetic resonance imaging: How it can really affect diagnostic image quality and confuse clinical diagnosis? *J. Vibroengineering* **2018**, *20*, 1202–1213. [CrossRef]

175. Brau, A. New Parallel Imaging Method Enhances Imaging Speed and Accuracy. *A GE Healthc MR Publ.* **2007**, 36–38.

176. Deshmane, A.; Gulani, V.; Griswold, M.A.; Seiberlich, N. Parallel MR imaging. *J. Magn. Reson. Imaging* **2012**, *36*, 55–72. [CrossRef]

177. Brau, A.C.; Beatty, P.J.; Skare, S.; Bammer, R. Comparison of reconstruction accuracy and efficiency among autocalibrating data-driven parallel imaging methods. *Magn. Reson. Med.* **2008**, *59*, 382–395. [CrossRef] [PubMed]

178. Blaimer, M.; Breuer, F.; Mueller, M.; Heidemann, R.; Griswold, M.A.; Jakob, P. SMASH, SENSE, PILS, GRAPPA. How to Choose the Optimal Method. *Top. Magn. Reson. Imaging* **2004**, *15*, 223–236. [CrossRef] [PubMed]

179. Griswold, M.A.; Fromm, M.; Heidemann, R.; Nittka, M.; Jellus, V.; Wang, J.; Kiefer, B.; Haase, A. Generalized autocalibrating partially parallel acquisitions (GRAPPA). *Magn. Reson. Med.* **2002**, *47*, 1202–1210. [CrossRef] [PubMed]

180. Zaitsev, M.; MacLaren, J.; Herbst, M. Motion artifacts in MRI: A complex problem with many partial solutions. *J. Magn. Reson. Imaging* **2015**, *42*, 887–901. [CrossRef]

181. Havsteen, I.; Ohlhues, A.; Madsen, K.H.; Nybing, J.D.; Christensen, H.; Christensen, A. Are movement artifacts in magnetic resonance imaging a real problem? A narrative review. *Front. Neurol.* **2017**, *8*, 232. [CrossRef]

182. Noël, P.; Bammer, R.; Reinhold, C.; Haider, M.A. Parallel imaging artifacts in body magnetic resonance imaging. *Can. Assoc. Radiol. J.* **2009**, *60*, 91–98. [CrossRef]

183. Godenschweger, F.; Kägebein, U.; Stucht, D.; Yarach, U.; Sciarra, A.; Yakupov, R.; Lüsebrink, F.; Schulze, P.; Speck, O. Motion correction in MRI of the brain. *Phys. Med. Biol.* **2016**, *61*, R32–R56. [CrossRef] [PubMed]

184. Callaghan, M.F.; Ejosephs, O.; Eherbst, M.; Ezaitsev, M.; Etodd, N.; Eweiskopf, N. An evaluation of prospective motion correction (PMC) for high resolution quantitative MRI. *Front. Neuroscience* **2015**, *9*, 97. [CrossRef] [PubMed]

185. MacLaren, J.; Herbst, M.; Speck, O.; Zaitsev, M. Prospective motion correction in brain imaging: A review. *Magn. Reson. Med.* **2012**, *69*, 621–636. [CrossRef] [PubMed]

186. Wadghiri, Y.Z.; Johnson, G.; Turnbull, D.H. Sensitivity and performance time in MRI dephasing artifact reduction methods. *Magn. Reson. Med.* **2001**, *45*, 470–476. [CrossRef]

187. Duerk, J.L.; Simonetti, O.P. Theoretical aspects of motion sensitivity and compensation in echo-planar imaging. *J. Magn. Reson. Imaging* **1991**, *1*, 643–650. [CrossRef]

188. Felmlee, J.P.; Ehman, R.L.; Riederer, S.J.; Korin, H.W. Adaptive motion compensation in MRI: Accuracy of motion measurement. *Magn. Reson. Med.* **1991**, *18*, 207–213. [CrossRef]

189. Mirzadeh, Z.; Chapple, K.; Lambert, M.; Dhall, R.; Ponce, F.A. Validation of CT-MRI fusion for intraoperative assessment of stereotactic accuracy in DBS surgery. *Mov. Disord.* **2014**, *29*, 1788–1795. [CrossRef]

190. Geevarghese, R.; O'Gorman, R.; Lumsden, D.E.; Samuel, M.; Ashkan, K. Registration accuracy of CT/MRI fusion for localisation of deep brain stimulation electrode position: An imaging study and systematic review. *Ster. Funct. Neurosurg.* **2016**, *94*, 159–163. [CrossRef]

191. Nandish, S.; Prabhu, K.G.; Rajagopal, K.V. Multiresolution image registration for multimodal brain images and fusion for better neurosurgical planning. *Biomed. J.* **2017**, *40*, 329–338. [CrossRef]

192. Doltra, A.; Stawowy, P.; Dietrich, T.; Schneeweis, C.; Fleck, E.; Kelle, S. Magnetic resonance imaging of cardiovascular fibrosis and inflammation: From clinical practice to animal studies and back cardiovascular MRI view project magnetic resonance imaging of cardiovascular fibrosis and inflammation: From clinical practice to ani. *Biomed Res Int.* **2013**, *2013*, 676489. [CrossRef]

193. Charles Stud, A.; Ramamurthy, N. Interpolation of the histogramed MR brain images for resolution enhancement. *Int. J. Innov. Technol. Explor. Eng.* **2019**, *8*, 1253–1256. [CrossRef]

194. Woods, R.P.; Grafton, S.T.; Holmes, C.J.; Cherry, S.R.; Mazziotta, J.C. Automated image registration: I. general methods and intrasubject, intramodality validation. *J. Comput. Assist. Tomogr.* **1998**, *22*, 139–152. [CrossRef] [PubMed]

195. Glasser, M.F.; Sotiropoulos, S.; Wilson, J.A.; Coalson, T.S.; Fischl, B.; Andersson, J.L.; Xu, J.; Jbabdi, S.; Webster, M.; Polimeni, J.R.; et al. The minimal preprocessing pipelines for the human connectome project. *NeuroImage* **2013**, *80*, 105–124. [CrossRef]

196. Greve, D.N.; Fischl, B. Accurate and robust brain image alignment using boundary-based registration. *NeuroImage* **2009**, *48*, 63–72. [CrossRef] [PubMed]

197. Iglesias, J.E.; Sabuncu, M.R. Multi-atlas segmentation of biomedical images: A survey. *Med. Image Anal.* **2015**, *24*, 205–219. [CrossRef] [PubMed]

198. Ou, Y.; Sotiras, A.; Paragios, N.; Davatzikos, C. DRAMMS: Deformable registration via attribute matching and mutual-saliency weighting. *Med. Image Anal.* **2011**, *15*, 622–639. [CrossRef] [PubMed]

199. El-Gamal, F.E.Z.A.; Elmogy, M.; Atwan, A. Current trends in medical image registration and fusion. *Egypt. Inform. J.* **2016**, *17*, 99–124. [CrossRef]

200. De Hollander, G.; Keuken, M.C.; Forstmann, B.U. The subcortical cocktail problem; mixed signals from the subthalamic nucleus and substantia nigra. *PLoS ONE* **2015**, *10*, e0120572. [CrossRef]

201. Alkemade, A.; Mulder, M.J.; Groot, J.M.; Isaacs, B.R.; van Berendonk, N.; Lute, N.; Isherwood, S.J.S.; Bazin, P.-L.; Forstmann, B.U. The Amsterdam Ultra-high field adult lifespan database (AHEAD): A freely available multimodal 7 Tesla submillimeter magnetic resonance imaging database. *NeuroImage* **2002**, *221*, 117200. [CrossRef]

202. Lambert, C.; Lutti, A.; Helms, G.; Frackowiak, R.; Ashburner, J. Multiparametric brainstem segmentation using a modified multivariate mixture of Gaussians. *NeuroImage Clin.* **2013**, *2*, 684–694. [CrossRef]

203. Jara, H. *Theory of Quantitative Magnetic Resonance Imaging*; World Scientific Publishing Co.: New Jersey, NJ, USA, 2013.

204. Stüber, C.; Morawski, M.; Schäfer, A.; Labadie, C.; Wähnert, M.; Leuze, C.; Streicher, M.; Barapatre, N.; Reimann, K.; Geyer, S.; et al. Myelin and iron concentration in the human brain: A quantitative study of MRI contrast. *Neuroimage* **2014**, *93*, 95–106. [CrossRef] [PubMed]

205. Harkins, K.D.; Xu, J.; Dula, A.N.; Li, K.; Valentine, W.M.; Gochberg, D.F.; Gore, J.C.; Does, M.D. The microstructural correlates of T1 in white matter. *Magn Reson Med.* **2016**, *75*, 1341–1345. [CrossRef] [PubMed]

206. Polders, D. Quantitative MRI of the Human Brain at 7 tesla. Ph.D. Thesis, Utrecht University, Utrecht, The Netherlands, 2012.

207. Deoni, S.C.; Peters, T.M.; Rutt, B.K. High-resolutionT1 andT2 mapping of the brain in a clinically acceptable time with DESPOT1 and DESPOT2. *Magn. Reson. Med.* **2005**, *53*, 237–241. [CrossRef] [PubMed]

208. Deoni, S.C. High-resolution T1 mapping of the brain at 3T with driven equilibrium single pulse observation of T1 with high-speed incorporation of RF field inhomogeneities (DESPOT1-HIFI). *J. Magn. Reson. Imaging* **2007**, *26*, 1106–1111. [CrossRef] [PubMed]

209. Dekkers, I.A.; De Boer, A.; Sharma, K.; Cox, E.F.; Lamb, H.J.; Buckley, D.L.; Bane, O.; Morris, D.M.; Prasad, P.V.; Semple, S.I.K.; et al. Consensus-based technical recommendations for clinical translation of renal T1 and T2 mapping MRI. *Magn. Reson. Mater. Physics Biol. Med.* **2020**, *33*, 163–176. [CrossRef] [PubMed]

210. Keuken, M.C.; Bazin, P.-L.; Backhouse, K.; Beekhuizen, S.; Himmer, L.; Kandola, A.; Lafeber, J.J.; Prochazkova, L.; Trutti, A.C.; Schäfer, A.; et al. Effects of aging on T_1, T_2*, and QSM MRI values in the subcortex. *Brain Struct. Funct.* **2017**, *222*, 2487–2505. [CrossRef]

211. Milford, D.; Rosbach, N.; Bendszus, M.; Heiland, S. Mono-exponential fitting in T2-relaxometry: Relevance of offset and first echo. *PLoS ONE* **2015**, *10*, e0145255. [CrossRef]

212. Schweser, F.; Sommer, K.; Deistung, A.; Reichenbach, J.R. Quantitative susceptibility mapping for investigating subtle susceptibility variations in the human brain. *NeuroImage* **2012**, *62*, 2083–2100. [CrossRef]

213. Cronin, M.J.; Wharton, S.; Al-Radaideh, A.; Constantinescu, C.S.; Evangelou, N.; Bowtell, R.; Gowland, P. A comparison of phase imaging and quantitative susceptibility mapping in the imaging of multiple sclerosis lesions at ultrahigh field. *Magn. Reson. Mater. Physics Biol. Med.* **2016**, *29*, 543–557. [CrossRef]

214. Acosta-Cabronero, J.; Milovic, C.; Mattern, H.; Tejos, C.; Speck, O.; Callaghan, M.F. A robust multi-scale approach to quantitative susceptibility mapping. *NeuroImage* **2018**, *183*, 7–24. [CrossRef]

215. Liu, C.; Li, W.; Tong, K.A.; Yeom, K.W.; Kuzminski, S. Susceptibility-weighted imaging and quantitative susceptibility mapping in the brain. *J. Magn. Reson. Imaging* **2014**, *42*, 23–41. [CrossRef] [PubMed]

216. Langkammer, C.; Schweser, F.; Krebs, N.; Deistung, A.; Goessler, W.; Scheurer, E.; Sommer, K.; Reishofer, G.; Yen, K.; Fazekas, F.; et al. Quantitative susceptibility mapping (QSM) as a means to measure brain iron? A post mortem validation study. *NeuroImage* **2012**, *62*, 1593–1599. [CrossRef] [PubMed]

217. Fang, J.; Bao, L.; Li, X.; Van Zijl, P.C.; Chen, Z. Background field removal for susceptibility mapping of human brain with large susceptibility variations. *Magn. Reson. Med.* **2019**, *81*, 2025–2037. [CrossRef] [PubMed]

218. Fortier, V.; Levesque, I.R. Phase processing for quantitative susceptibility mapping of regions with large susceptibility and lack of signal. *Magn. Reson. Med.* **2017**, *79*, 3103–3113. [CrossRef]

219. Wang, Y.; Liu, T. Quantitative susceptibility mapping (QSM): Decoding MRI data for a tissue magnetic biomarker. *Magn. Reson. Med.* **2014**, *73*, 82–101. [CrossRef]

220. Zhou, N.; Liu, T.; Spincemaille, P.; Wang, Y. Background field removal by solving the Laplacian boundary value problem. *NMR Biomed.* **2014**, *27*, 312–319. [CrossRef]

221. Li, W.; Avram, A.V.; Wu, B.; Xiao, X.; Liu, C. Integrated Laplacian-based phase unwrapping and background phase removal for quantitative susceptibility mapping. *NMR Biomed.* **2013**, *27*, 219–227. [CrossRef]

222. Liu, T.; Spincemaille, P.; De Rochefort, L.; Kressler, B.; Wang, Y. Calculation of susceptibility through multiple orientation sampling (COSMOS): A method for conditioning the inverse problem from measured magnetic field map to susceptibility source image in MRI. *Magn. Reson. Med.* **2009**, *61*, 196–204. [CrossRef]

223. Schäfer, A.; Forstmann, B.U.; Neumann, J.; Wharton, S.; Mietke, A.; Bowtell, R.; Turner, R. Direct visualization of the subthalamic nucleus and its iron distribution using high-resolution susceptibility mapping. *Neuroimage* **2012**, *46*, 2831–2842. [CrossRef]

224. Schweser, F.; Zivadinov, R. Quantitative susceptibility mapping (QSM) with an extended physical model for MRI frequency contrast in the brain: A proof-of-concept of quantitative susceptibility and residual (QUASAR) mapping. *NMR Biomed.* **2018**, *31*, e3999. [CrossRef]

225. Chatnuntawech, I.; McDaniel, P.; Cauley, S.F.; Gagoski, B.A.; Langkammer, C.; Martin, A.; Grant, P.E.; Wald, L.L.; Setsompop, K.; Adalsteinsson, E.; et al. Single-step quantitative susceptibility mapping with variational penalties. *NMR Biomed.* **2017**, *30*, e3570. [CrossRef] [PubMed]

226. Langkammer, C.; Schweser, F.; Shmueli, K.; Kames, C.; Li, X.; Guo, L.; Milovic, C.; Kim, J.; Wei, H.; Bredies, K.; et al. Quantitative susceptibility mapping: Report from the 2016 reconstruction challenge. *Magn. Reson. Med.* **2017**, *79*, 1661–1673. [CrossRef] [PubMed]

227. Tabelow, K.; Balteau, E.; Ashburner, J.; Callaghan, M.F.; Draganski, B.; Helms, G.; Kherif, F.; Leutritz, T.; Lutti, A.; Phillips, C.; et al. hMRI—A toolbox for quantitative MRI in neuroscience and clinical research. *NeuroImage* **2019**, *194*, 191–210. [CrossRef]

228. Wang, Y.; Spincemaille, P.; Liu, Z.; Dimov, A.; Deh, K.; Li, J.; Zhang, Y.; Yao, Y.; Gillen, K.M.; Wilman, A.H.; et al. Clinical quantitative susceptibility mapping (QSM): Biometal imaging and its emerging roles in patient care. *J. Magn. Reson. Imaging* **2017**, *46*, 951–971. [CrossRef] [PubMed]

229. Fan, A.P.; Bilgic, B.; Gagnon, L.; Witzel, T.; Bhat, H.; Rosen, B.R.; Adalsteinsson, E. Quantitative oxygenation venography from MRI phase. *Magn. Reson. Med.* **2014**, *72*, 149–159. [CrossRef] [PubMed]

230. Wharton, S.; Bowtell, R. Effects of white matter microstructure on phase and susceptibility maps. *Magn. Reson. Med.* **2015**, *73*, 1258–1269. [CrossRef]

231. Alkemade, A.; De Hollander, G.; Keuken, M.C.; Schäfer, A.; Ott, D.V.M.; Schwarz, J.; Weise, D.; Kotz, S.A.; Forstmann, B.U. Comparison of T2*-weighted and QSM contrasts in Parkinson's disease to visualize the STN with MRI. *PLoS ONE* **2017**, *12*, e0176130. [CrossRef]

232. Schweser, F.; Deistung, A.; Lehr, B.W.; Reichenbach, J.R. Differentiation between diamagnetic and paramagnetic cerebral lesions based on magnetic susceptibility mapping. *Med. Phys.* **2010**, *37*, 5165–5178. [CrossRef]

233. Lönnfors-Weitzel, T.; Weitzel, T.; Slotboom, J.; Kiefer, C.; Pollo, C.; Schüpbach, M.; Oertel, M.; Kaelin, A.; Wiest, R. T2-relaxometry predicts outcome of DBS in idiopathic Parkinson's disease. *NeuroImage: Clin.* **2016**, *12*, 832–837. [CrossRef]

234. Xiao, Y.; Lau, J.C.; Hemachandra, D.; Gilmore, G.; Khan, A.; Peters, T.M. Image guidance in deep brain stimulation surgery to treat Parkinson's disease: A review. *arXiv preprint* **2020**, arXiv:2003.04822. [CrossRef]

235. Bernstein, J.E.; Kashyap, S.; Ray, K.; Ananda, A.K. Infections in Deep Brain Stimulator Surgery. *Cureus* **2019**, *11*, e5440. [CrossRef] [PubMed]

236. Vedam-Mai, V.; Rodgers, C.; Gureck, A.; Vincent, M.; Ippolito, G.; Elkouzi, A.; Yachnis, A.T.; Foote, K.D.; Okun, M. Deep Brain Stimulation associated gliosis: A post-mortem study. *Park. Relat. Disord.* **2018**, *54*, 51–55. [CrossRef] [PubMed]

237. Park, C.K.; Jung, N.Y.; Kim, M.; Chang, J.W. Analysis of delayed intracerebral hemorrhage associated with deep brain stimulation surgery. *World Neurosurg.* **2017**, *104*, 537–544. [CrossRef] [PubMed]

238. Albano, L.; Rohatgi, P.; Kashanian, A.; Bari, A.; Pouratian, N. Symptomatic pneumocephalus after deep brain stimulation surgery: Report of 2 cases. *Ster. Funct. Neurosurg.* **2020**, *98*, 30–36. [CrossRef] [PubMed]

239. Mao, Z.; Ling, Z.; Pan, L.; Xu, X.; Cui, Z.; Liang, S.; Yu, X. Comparison of efficacy of deep brain stimulation of different targets in Parkinson's disease: A network meta-analysis. *Front. Aging Neurosci.* **2019**, *11*, 23. [CrossRef] [PubMed]

240. Anderson, D.; Beecher, G.; Ba, F. Deep brain stimulation in Parkinson's disease: New and emerging targets for refractory motor and nonmotor symptoms. *Park. Dis.* **2017**, *2017*, 5124328. [CrossRef] [PubMed]

## 10

Deep Brain Stimulation is Effective for Treatment-Resistant Depression

Frederick L. Hitti [1,*], Andrew I. Yang [1], Mario A. Cristancho [2] and Gordon H. Baltuch [1]

[1] Department of Neurosurgery, Pennsylvania Hospital, University of Pennsylvania, 800 Spruce St, Philadelphia, PA 19107, USA; andrew.yang@pennmedicine.upenn.edu (A.I.Y.); gordon.baltuch@pennmedicine.upenn.edu (G.H.B.)

[2] Department of Psychiatry, University of Pennsylvania, 3535 Market Street, Philadelphia, PA 19104, USA; marioc@pennmedicine.upenn.edu

* Correspondence: Frederick.Hitti@uphs.upenn.edu

Abstract: Major depressive disorder (MDD) is a leading cause of disability and a significant cause of mortality worldwide. Approximately 30–40% of patients fail to achieve clinical remission with available pharmacological treatments, a clinical course termed treatment-resistant depression (TRD). Numerous studies have investigated deep brain stimulation (DBS) as a therapy for TRD. We performed a meta-analysis to determine efficacy and a meta-regression to compare stimulation targets. We identified and screened 1397 studies. We included 125 citations in the qualitative review and considered 26 for quantitative analysis. Only blinded studies that compared active DBS to sham stimulation (k = 12) were included in the meta-analysis. The random-effects model supported the efficacy of DBS for TRD (standardized mean difference = −0.75, <0 favors active stimulation; $p = 0.0001$). The meta-regression did not demonstrate a statistically significant difference between stimulation targets ($p = 0.45$). While enthusiasm for DBS treatment of TRD has been tempered by recent randomized trials, this meta-analysis reveals a significant effect of DBS for the treatment of TRD. Additionally, the majority of trials have demonstrated the safety and efficacy of DBS for this indication. Further trials are required to determine the optimal stimulation parameters and patient populations for which DBS would be effective. Particular attention to factors including electrode placement technique, patient selection, and long-term follow-up is essential for future trial design.

Keywords: deep brain stimulation; treatment-resistant depression; depression; meta-analysis; meta-regression; subcallosal cingulate gyrus; medial forebrain bundle; inferior thalamic peduncle; ventral capsule; ventral striatum

1. Introduction

Major depressive disorder (MDD) is one of the most common psychiatric diseases, and while a number of therapies are available, many patients remain symptomatic despite treatment [1,2]. Well-established treatment modalities for MDD include psychotherapy, medication, and electroconvulsive therapy (ECT) [3–9]. While ECT is efficacious for many patients resistant to medication and therapy, there are significant adverse effects associated with ECT, including cognitive and memory dysfunction [3]. Furthermore, there are patients who are refractory to multiple available therapies, including ECT. Patients who fail to improve following treatment with two or more therapies are considered to have treatment-resistant depression (TRD) [5,8,10–12]. Due to the considerable number of treatment non-remitters (30–40% of patients with MDD), developing novel therapies for TRD represents a major unmet need.

Deep brain stimulation (DBS) is a technique that uses implanted intracranial electrodes to modulate neural activity. It is currently a well-established, FDA-approved treatment for movement disorders such as Parkinson's disease (PD) and essential tremor (ET) [13,14]. In addition to movement disorders, DBS has been explored as a treatment modality for psychiatric conditions. Multiple human trials have explored the efficacy of DBS for TRD. Anatomic targets have included the ventral anterior limb of the internal capsule (vALIC) [15], ventral capsule/ventral striatum (VC/VS) [16], subcallosal cingulate (SCC) [17–22], inferior thalamic peduncle (ITP) [23], medial forebrain bundle (MFB) [24,25], and lateral habenula [26]. Reports regarding the efficacy of DBS for TRD have been mixed, with some studies demonstrating encouraging results, while others have shown a lack of efficacy relative to sham stimulation. To leverage all of the available data, we performed a meta-analysis to determine the efficacy of DBS for TRD. We then performed a meta-regression to compare stimulation targets. While prior meta-analyses have been undertaken [27–29], here we included only studies that compared active to sham stimulation in a blinded fashion. Furthermore, our analysis includes more recent studies.

2. Methods

2.1. Search Strategy

We used the PubMed database to identify studies investigating DBS for MDD and screened all studies for inclusion. We used the following search terms to identify relevant studies: ("deep brain stimulation"[MeSH Terms] OR ("deep"[All Fields] AND "brain"[All Fields] AND "stimulation"[All Fields]) OR "deep brain stimulation"[All Fields] OR "DBS"[All Fields]) AND ("depressive disorder"[MeSH Terms] OR ("depressive"[All Fields] AND "disorder"[All Fields]) OR "depressive disorder"[All Fields] OR "depression"[All Fields] OR "depression"[MeSH Terms]). All studies were considered, including studies written in other languages. The search was conducted on 10/16/2019, and the analysis followed the Preferred Reporting Items for Systematic reviews and Meta-Analyses (PRISMA) guidelines.

2.2. Study Inclusion and Exclusion Criteria

Only studies that investigated the efficacy of DBS for MDD were included. We excluded studies that utilized other therapies to treat MDD (e.g., ECT, epidural stimulation, vagal nerve stimulation, transcranial magnetic stimulation, or tDCS). We also excluded studies that investigated comorbid depression in the context of other disorders, such as epilepsy, dystonia, Tourette syndrome, anorexia nervosa, obsessive–compulsive disorder, schizophrenia, headache, ET, and PD. We excluded all non-human studies. Of the studies relevant to DBS as a treatment for MDD, we excluded case reports, non-systematic reviews, perspectives, commentaries, editorials, and opinions. We included the remainder of the studies for our qualitative review. For the quantitative meta-analysis, we only included studies in which sham stimulation was compared to active stimulation in a blinded fashion (either single- or double-blind). The clinical trial designs were varied and included both crossover and parallel studies.

2.3. Data Extraction and Outcome Measures

Our primary outcome was the efficacy of DBS as a treatment for depression as assessed by changes in the Hamilton Depression Rating Scale (HDRS) or Montgomery–Åsberg Depression Rating Scale (MADRS) scores. We compared sham stimulation scores to active stimulation scores. The data were extracted from tables when provided. If tables with the raw data were not provided, the WebPlotDigitizer tool was used to extract data from published graphs. We also extracted the number of patients, stimulation target, side effects of treatment, adverse events, study design, and depression rating scale used.

2.4. Statistical Methods

Statistical analysis was conducted in R using the meta, metaphor, and dmetar packages. We followed the guide published by Harrer et al. to conduct the analysis [30]. A random-effects model was employed for the meta-analysis to account for differences in study populations. We used the DerSimonian–Laird estimator for τ^2 (variance of true effect magnitude distributions), as it is the most widely used estimator. The studies included in the quantitative analysis used different depression rating scales. Therefore, we computed standardized mean differences so that the studies could be compared. We also calculated heterogeneity (I^2) of the studies in R. The differential efficacies of the various stimulation targets were compared with mixed-effects meta-regression. R was used to generate funnel plots and conduct Egger's test. Means are presented with their corresponding standard deviations. A p-value < 0.05 was considered statistically significant.

3. Results

We used fairly broad search terms (see Section 2) to ensure the inclusion of all studies relevant to the use of DBS as a therapy for depression. Our search identified 1397 studies, and all were screened for inclusion (Figure 1). We excluded 964 studies at the abstract/title level because these studies either did not use DBS as the therapeutic modality, examined depressive symptomatology in the context of other diseases, or were non-human animal studies. Of the remaining relevant studies, 308 were excluded because they were case reports, non-systematic reviews, perspectives, commentaries, editorials, or opinions. The remaining 125 studies were included in our qualitative review. We then screened these studies for inclusion in our quantitative meta-analysis. Twenty-six studies were candidates for inclusion at the abstract level. Thirteen studies were excluded because they did not compare active to sham stimulation [31–43], and one study was excluded as it included only three patients [44]. Therefore, 12 studies [15–25] (186 unique patients) were included in the meta-analysis and meta-regression (Table 1). The Raymaekers et al. study was analyzed as two separate studies, because this study included two anatomically distinct stimulation targets, and both targets were evaluated with blinded stimulation periods.

Figure 1. Flowchart of studies selected for inclusion in the qualitative review and quantitative meta-analysis.

Table 1. Studies included in meta-analysis and meta-regression.

Study	Location	N	Blinded Crossover
Bergfeld et al. 2016	vALIC	16	Yes
Coenen et al. 2019	MFB	16	No
Dougherty et al. 2015	VC/VS	29	No
Fenoy et al. 2018	MFB	6	Yes
Holtzheimer et al. 2012	SCC	10	Yes
Holtzheimer et al. 2017	SCC	85	No
Merkl et al. 2013	SCC	6	Yes
Merkl et al. 2018	SCC	4	Yes *
Puigdemont et al. 2015	SCC	5	Yes
Ramasubbu et al. 2013	SCC	4	Yes
Raymaekers et al. 2017	IC/BST	5	Yes
Raymaekers et al. 2017	ITP	5	Yes

* Only half of the patients crossed over. IC/BST: internal capsule/bed nucleus of the stria terminalis; ITP: inferior thalamic peduncle; MFB: medial forebrain bundle; SCC: subcallosal cingulate; vALIC: ventral anterior limb of the internal capsule; VC/VS: ventral capsule/ventral striatum.

The studies included in the meta-analysis had varied trial designs (Table 1). Due to our inclusion criteria, all studies contained a period of blinded sham stimulation and blinded active stimulation. The duration of the active and sham stimulation periods, however, was heterogeneous. The average blinded stimulation duration was 7.5 ± 6.6 weeks. All studies contained an open-label period of long-term active stimulation following the blinded phases. These long-term data were not included in the meta-analysis, since the goal of the present study was to compare blinded active stimulation to blinded sham stimulation. The majority of the trials (75%) were done in a crossover fashion (Table 1). Thus, all of the patients in these studies received both active and sham stimulation in a blinded fashion. Importantly, these study designs allow for within-subject comparisons and may enhance statistical power.

Using a random-effects model, our meta-analysis revealed that active stimulation results in a greater decline in HDRS/MADRS scores relative to sham stimulation (standardized mean difference (SMD) = −0.75; −1.13 to −0.36, 95% confidence interval (CI); *p*-value = 0.0001; Figure 2). There was moderate heterogeneity across studies (I^2 = 59%).

Figure 2. Meta-analysis forest plot depicting changes in HDRS/MADRS scores with active stimulation compared to sham stimulation. CI: confidence interval; IC: internal capsule; ITP: inferior thalamic peduncle; SMD: standardized mean difference; PI: prediction interval.

In addition to differences in study design, the studies also investigated the efficacy of DBS for TRD using different stimulation targets (Table 1). The most common target was the SCC (50% of studies), followed by the internal capsule (IC, 25%), MFB (17%), and ITP (8%). While there were a limited number of studies, we utilized meta-regression to determine if the available data would reveal an optimal stimulation target. The meta-regression, however, did not demonstrate a statistically significant difference ($p = 0.45$) between stimulation targets (Figure 3).

Figure 3. Meta-regression forest plot comparing various stimulation targets. CI: confidence interval; IC: internal capsule; ITP: inferior thalamic peduncle; MFB: medial forebrain bundle; SCC: subcallosal cingulate; SMD: standardized mean difference; TE: treatment effect; seTE: standard error of treatment effect.

Since the duration of stimulation during the blinded phase varied between studies, we performed another meta-regression to determine if there was an association between the duration of active stimulation and SMD. Our analysis did not reveal a significant effect of stimulation duration on SMD outcomes ($p = 0.20$).

Publication bias is an important concern when conducting a meta-analysis. We investigated for possible publication bias by first generating a funnel plot (Figure 4). We then tested for asymmetry of the funnel plot with Egger's test. The test revealed that there was no statistically significant asymmetry in the plot (intercept -1.9; 95% CI -3.864–0.056; $p = 0.07$), thus arguing against publication bias. Given the strong trend of Egger's test and the fact that one study (Fenoy et al. 2018) was a clear outlier, as depicted in the funnel plot, we re-analyzed the data with this outlier study excluded. Using a random-effects model, a meta-analysis of the pared data confirmed that active stimulation results in a greater decline in HDRS/MADRS scores relative to sham stimulation (SMD = −0.62; 95% CI −0.95 to −0.30; p = 0.0002). Removing the outlier study decreased study heterogeneity (I^2 = 45%) and decreased the likelihood of publication bias as estimated by Egger's test (intercept −1.3; 95% CI −3.26–0.66; p = 0.21).

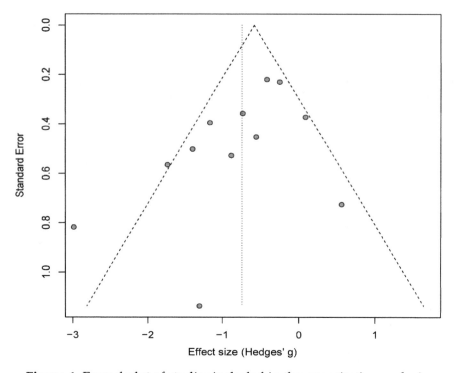

Figure 4. Funnel plot of studies included in the quantitative analysis.

We examined and compiled the adverse events reported in the studies included in the quantitative meta-analysis. The adverse events occurring in greater than 1% of patients are listed in Table 2, and the full list of adverse events in each study is detailed in Supplementary Table S1. The most common complaint was headache (26% of patients), followed by visual disturbances (21%), worsening depression (16%), sleep disturbances (16%), and anxiety (14%). All other adverse events were only seen in less than 10% of patients (Table 2). The authors of the original studies reported that the vast majority of adverse events were transient and were often resolved by stimulation parameter adjustment. The headaches were often postoperative and resolved a few days after surgery. A significant number of patients (n = 16, 8%) expressed suicidal ideation, and a similar number of patients (n = 15, 8%) attempted suicide. Completed suicides were rare. In two studies, one patient from each study who had no response to DBS committed suicide [15,16]. In one large study, there were two deaths by suicide in the control group during the open-label phase [17]. Finally, in another study, two patients committed suicide [23]. These suicides were deemed to be unrelated to DBS, because both patients had a history of suicide attempts and DBS did not appear to increase impulsivity [23].

Table 2. Adverse events.

Adverse Event	Patients (N)	Patients (%)
Headache	50	26
Blurred Vision/Diplopia	41	21
Worsening depression	31	16
Sleep Disturbances	30	16
Anxiety	26	14
Pain Around Neurostimulator	17	9
Nausea	16	8
Suicidal Ideation	16	8
Pain Around Incisions	16	8
Post-operative discomfort	16	8
Suicide Attempt	15	8
Device Infection	15	8
Balance/Gait Problems	13	7
Non-Specific Somatic Complaints	12	6
Pain/pulling sensation around Extension Wires	11	6
Other infections	10	5
Agitation	9	5
Paresthesias	9	5
Restlessness	8	4
Disinhibition/Impulsivity	8	4
Hypomania	8	4
Confusion/Cognitive impairment	8	4
Swollen Eyes	6	3
Excessive Sweating	6	3
Memory Disturbance	6	3
Weight Gain/hyperphagia	6	3
Lethargy	6	3
Abnormal Body Temperature	5	3
Hypertension	5	3
Postoperative Delirium	4	2
Constipation	4	2
Speech difficulties	4	2
Panic attack	4	2
Diarrhea	4	2
Irritability	4	2
Libido decrease/increase	4	2
Increase in drug side effects	4	2
Skin Disorder	4	2
Neuralgia	4	2
Drowsiness	4	2
Palpations Around Neurostimulator	3	2
Neck Pain	3	2
Mania	3	2
Hallucinations	3	2
Palpitations	3	2
Weakness	3	2
Mood swings	3	2
Difficulty voiding/urinary retention	3	2
Back pain	3	2
Electrode revision	3	2
Elective hospitalization	3	2

4. Discussion

MDD is a very prevalent neuropsychiatric condition. Although there are a number of existing treatment modalities, many patients remain symptomatic despite adequate treatment protocols. There is an urgent need for additional treatment options for TRD, since it is a significant source of morbidity and mortality.

Pathological neural activity (either hyperactivity or hypoactivity) may lead to neurological or psychiatric disease, and non-pharmacological neuromodulatory techniques may be used to ameliorate these conditions. DBS is a neuromodulatory approach that is an FDA-approved treatment for movement disorders, so multiple investigators have trialed DBS as a therapy for TRD. Initial open-label reports regarding the efficacy of DBS for TRD were encouraging [36,45], and subsequently, multiple randomized trials were initiated and completed [16,17]. The large-scale trials, however, did not reveal a significant difference between the control and treatment groups. A number of reasons have been posited to explain these negative results, including choice of stimulation target, electrode placement technique, patient selection, and short-term follow-up of patients [43,46–52].

Due to the discrepancy between earlier reports and larger trials, we undertook a meta-analysis to investigate the efficacy of DBS for TRD. In agreement with prior analyses [27–29], we found a significant effect of DBS on TRD. Specifically, active stimulation was associated with an improvement in depression scores relative to sham stimulation. The effect size of this treatment is medium to large, as indicated by the SMD of −0.75 [53]. This effect size is much larger than the small effect sizes (~0.3) seen with pharmacologic antidepressant treatment of patients with MDD [54]. Our findings extend those of prior analyses by including all currently available studies and by only including blinded studies that utilized a trial design in which active stimulation was compared to sham stimulation. Importantly, analyzing the data in this manner allows for the control of placebo effects. While some patients are able to detect active stimulation due to side effects such as visual disturbances, these effects are largely absent with a stimulation parameter adjustment [24,25]. With most studies including an optimization phase prior to the blinded assessments, it is reasonable to propose that comparing active stimulation to sham stimulation controls for placebo effects.

We conducted a meta-regression to determine if the data would reveal an optimal stimulation target. Due to the limited number of available studies, our analysis did not demonstrate an optimal target. With further research, the answer to this question may be elucidated in the future; however, a significant limitation is the heterogeneous nature of MDD neurobiology (i.e., symptoms of depression as a common manifestation of multiple brain functional abnormalities). It may be that instead of one optimal stimulation target for all patients, the optimal stimulation target varies across individuals [46,55–58].

As with any therapy, there is a risk of publication bias since studies with positive results and large effect sizes are more likely to be published than studies with small effect sizes or negative results [59]. To investigate publication bias in DBS for depression, we plotted the studies in a funnel plot and used Egger's test to assess for asymmetry. We did not find evidence of publication bias in this series of studies.

DBS is a well-tolerated treatment for movement disorders, but it is important to critically evaluate potential side effects of DBS for depression. The thoroughness of adverse event reporting varied between the studies. Nonetheless, the majority of adverse events were transient. Furthermore, many side effects were relieved by a stimulation parameter adjustment, as is seen with DBS for movement disorders. Patients with MDD are at significant risk for suicide, and patients with TRD have an even higher risk of suicide [60,61]. Currently available data do not demonstrate an increased risk of suicide with DBS, since suicide was rare in these studies and occurred at a lower rate than in patients with severe MDD not receiving DBS [62]. Moreover, the completed suicides occurred in non-responders or were deemed unrelated to DBS. As an invasive therapy, DBS may be perceived by patients as a "last resort" for recovery. Therefore, non-responders may represent a particularly high-risk group for suicide. Psychoeducation and adequate discussion of post DBS treatment options to reframe those perceptions may decrease the risk of suicide. In summary, published trials have demonstrated the safety of DBS for TRD.

While the results of this meta-analysis are encouraging, additional large-scale clinical trials demonstrating the efficacy of DBS for TRD are essential. Crucial to these efforts will be careful consideration of future trial design [24,63]. The large-scale clinical trials of DBS for TRD conducted to date have utilized a parallel trial design, whereas many of the smaller trials employed a crossover design (Table 1). Given the negative outcomes of the large-scale trials, a crossover design may be optimal to investigate the efficacy of DBS for TRD. As a therapy, DBS is unique in that sham stimulation and active stimulation may be compared within individuals, thereby facilitating crossover trial design. Crossover studies require fewer patients to achieve significance, so this design optimizes statistical power [64]. Some studies have used customized trial designs with a variable optimization period [15,65]. Ensuring proper optimization prior to randomization may be necessary to determine the efficacy of DBS for TRD. Another important factor in trial design is the length of time that the patient undergoes therapy. Long-term open-label studies have demonstrated that the efficacy of DBS for TRD improves over time, so longer trials may be necessary [17,18,38,66,67]. Finally, depression severity waxes and wanes throughout a patient's disease course. Therefore, trial designs that compare groups at specific time points may not be optimal. Integrating scores over predefined time periods may enhance outcome assessment.

In addition to trial design, proper electrode targeting is important for the efficacy of DBS for the treatment of depression. Instead of targeting brain nuclei, as is routinely done, targeting fiber tracts using patient-specific tractography may be important for therapeutic efficacy [49–52,58,68]. Furthermore, stereotactic accuracy of electrode placement is essential. For example, intraoperative phenomena, such as brain shift, should be accounted for [48]. Patient selection is also a critical consideration for future studies. The available data have demonstrated that there is a subgroup of patients that respond to this therapy and a subgroup that does not. Determining patient-specific factors (e.g., anatomical or symptom-based) that predict response to DBS for TRD may enable targeted selection of patients for whom DBS would be therapeutic [43,69–75]. These patient-specific factors could then be used as study inclusion criteria to enhance the probability of study success.

5. Conclusions

While enthusiasm for DBS as a therapy for TRD has been tempered by recent randomized trials, this meta-analysis reveals that active stimulation significantly ameliorates depression in patients with TRD. The meta-regression did not reveal an optimal stimulation target to treat depression due to the small size and number of available studies, and also likely due to the heterogeneous nature of this condition's neurobiology. Additional trials are needed to determine optimal stimulation targets. Further studies are also required to establish the patient populations for whom DBS would be effective. Particular attention to factors that include electrode placement technique, patient selection, and long-term observation is essential for future trial design.

Author Contributions: Conceptualization, F.L.H. and G.H.B.; methodology, F.L.H.; validation, F.L.H., A.I.Y., M.A.C., G.H.B.; formal analysis, F.L.H and A.I.Y; investigation, F.L.H.; data curation, F.L.H.; writing—Original draft preparation, F.L.H. and A.I.Y.; writing—Review and editing, F.L.H., A.I.Y., M.A.C., G.H.B.; visualization, F.L.H.; supervision, G.H.B.; project administration, G.H.B. All authors have read and agreed to the published version of the manuscript.

References

1. Ferrari, A.J.; Charlson, F.J.; Norman, R.E.; Patten, S.B.; Freedman, G.; Murray, C.J.L.; Vos, T.; Whiteford, H.A. Burden of Depressive Disorders by Country, Sex, Age, and Year: Findings from the Global Burden of Disease Study 2010. *PLoS Med.* **2013**, *10*, e1001547. [CrossRef] [PubMed]

2. Steel, Z.; Marnane, C.; Iranpour, C.; Chey, T.; Jackson, J.W.; Patel, V.; Silove, D. The global prevalence of common mental disorders: A systematic review and meta-analysis 1980–2013. *Int. J. Epidemiol.* **2014**, *43*, 476–493. [CrossRef] [PubMed]

3. Bailine, S.H.; Rifkin, A.; Kayne, E.; Selzer, J.A.; Vital-Herne, J.; Blieka, M.; Pollack, S. Comparison of Bifrontal and Bitemporal ECT for Major Depression. *Am. J. Psychiatry* **2000**, *157*, 121–123. [CrossRef] [PubMed]

4. Fava, M.; Rush, A.J.; Wisniewski, S.R.; Nierenberg, A.A.; Alpert, J.E.; McGrath, P.J.; Thase, M.E.; Warden, D.; Biggs, M.; Luther, J.F.; et al. A comparison of mirtazapine and nortriptyline following two consecutive failed medication treatments for depressed outpatients: A STAR*D report. *Am. J. Psychiatry* **2006**, *163*, 1161–1172. [CrossRef]

5. Hollon, S.D.; Jarrett, R.B.; Nierenberg, A.A.; Thase, M.E.; Trivedi, M.; Rush, A.J. Psychotherapy and Medication in the Treatment of Adult and Geriatric Depression: Which Monotherapy or Combined Treatment? *J. Clin. Psychiatry* **2005**, *66*, 455–468. [CrossRef]

6. Nierenberg, A.A.; Fava, M.; Trivedi, M.H.; Wisniewski, S.R.; Thase, M.E.; McGrath, P.J.; Alpert, J.E.; Warden, D.; Luther, J.F.; Niederehe, G.; et al. A Comparison of Lithium and T 3 Augmentation Following Two Failed Medication Treatments for Depression: A STAR*D Report. *Am. J. Psychiatry* **2006**, *163*, 1519–1530. [CrossRef]

7. Rush, A.J.; Trivedi, M.H.; Wisniewski, S.R.; Stewart, J.W.; Nierenberg, A.A.; Thase, M.E.; Ritz, L.; Biggs, M.M.; Warden, D.; Luther, J.F.; et al. Bupropion-SR, sertraline, or venlafaxine-XR after failure of SSRIs for depression. *N. Engl. J. Med.* **2006**, *354*, 1231–1242. [CrossRef]

8. Thase, M.E.; Friedman, E.S.; Biggs, M.M.; Wisniewski, S.R.; Trivedi, M.H.; Luther, J.F.; Fava, M.; Nierenberg, A.A.; McGrath, P.J.; Warden, D.; et al. Cognitive Therapy Versus Medication in Augmentation and Switch Strategies as Second-Step Treatments: A STAR*D Report. *Am. J. Psychiatry* **2007**, *164*, 739–752. [CrossRef]

9. Trivedi, M.H.; Rush, A.J.; Wisniewski, S.R.; Nierenberg, A.A.; Warden, D.; Ritz, L.; Norquist, G.; Howland, R.H.; Lebowitz, B.; McGrath, P.J.; et al. Evaluation of Outcomes With Citalopram for Depression Using Measurement-Based Care in STAR*D: Implications for Clinical Practice. *Am. J. Psychiatry* **2006**, *163*, 28–40. [CrossRef]

10. Souery, D.; Papakostas, G.I.; Trivedi, M.H. Treatment-resistant depression. *J. Clin. Psychiatry* **2006**, *67* (Suppl. 6), 16–22.

11. Greden, J.F. The burden of disease for treatment-resistant depression. *J. Clin. Psychiatry* **2001**, *62* (Suppl. 16), 26–31.

12. Taipale, H.; Reutfors, J.; Tanskanen, A.; Brandt, L.; Tiihonen, J.; DiBernardo, A.; Mittendorfer-Rutz, E.; Brenner, P. Risk and risk factors for disability pension among patients with treatment resistant depression- a matched cohort study. *BMC Psychiatry* **2020**, *20*, 232. [CrossRef] [PubMed]

13. Hitti, F.L.; Ramayya, A.G.; McShane, B.J.; Yang, A.I.; Vaughan, K.A.; Baltuch, G.H. Long-term outcomes following deep brain stimulation for Parkinson's disease. *J. Neurosurg.* **2019**. [CrossRef] [PubMed]

14. Miocinovic, S.; Somayajula, S.; Chitnis, S.; Vitek, J.L. History, Applications, and Mechanisms of Deep Brain Stimulation. *JAMA Neurol.* **2013**, *70*, 163–171. [CrossRef] [PubMed]

15. Bergfeld, I.O.; Mantione, M.; Hoogendoorn, M.L.C.; Ruhe, H.G.; Notten, P.; van Laarhoven, J.; Visser, I.; Figee, M.; de Kwaasteniet, B.P.; Horst, F.; et al. Deep Brain Stimulation of the Ventral Anterior Limb of the Internal Capsule for Treatment-Resistant Depression: A Randomized Clinical Trial. *JAMA Psychiatry* **2016**, *73*, 456–464. [CrossRef] [PubMed]

16. Dougherty, D.D.; Rezai, A.R.; Carpenter, L.L.; Howland, R.H.; Bhati, M.T.; O'Reardon, J.P.; Eskandar, E.N.; Baltuch, G.H.; Machado, A.D.; Kondziolka, D.; et al. A Randomized Sham-Controlled Trial of Deep Brain Stimulation of the Ventral Capsule/Ventral Striatum for Chronic Treatment-Resistant Depression. *Biol. Psychiatry* **2015**, *78*, 240–248. [CrossRef]

17. Holtzheimer, P.E.; Husain, M.M.; Lisanby, S.H.; Taylor, S.F.; Whitworth, L.A.; McClintock, S.; Slavin, K.V.; Berman, J.; McKhann, G.M.; Patil, P.G.; et al. Subcallosal cingulate deep brain stimulation for treatment-resistant depression: A multisite, randomised, sham-controlled trial. *Lancet Psychiatry* **2017**, *4*, 839–849. [CrossRef]

18. Holtzheimer, P.E.; Kelley, M.E.; Gross, R.E.; Filkowski, M.M.; Garlow, S.J.; Barrocas, A.; Wint, D.; Craighead, M.C.; Kozarsky, J.; Chismar, R.; et al. Subcallosal cingulate deep brain stimulation for treatment-resistant unipolar and bipolar depression. *Arch. Gen. Psychiatry* **2012**, *69*, 150–158. [CrossRef]

19. Merkl, A.; Schneider, G.-H.; Schonecker, T.; Aust, S.; Kuhl, K.-P.; Kupsch, A.; Kuhn, A.A.; Bajbouj, M. Antidepressant effects after short-term and chronic stimulation of the subgenual cingulate gyrus in treatment-resistant depression. *Exp. Neurol.* **2013**, *249*, 160–168. [CrossRef]

20. Merkl, A.; Aust, S.; Schneider, G.-H.; Visser-Vandewalle, V.; Horn, A.; Kuhn, A.A.; Kuhn, J.; Bajbouj, M. Deep brain stimulation of the subcallosal cingulate gyrus in patients with treatment-resistant depression: A double-blinded randomized controlled study and long-term follow-up in eight patients. *J. Affect. Disord.* **2018**, *227*, 521–529. [CrossRef]

21. Puigdemont, D.; Portella, M.; Perez-Egea, R.; Molet, J.; Gironell, A.; de Diego-Adelino, J.; Martin, A.; Rodriguez, R.; Alvarez, E.; Artigas, F.; et al. A randomized double-blind crossover trial of deep brain stimulation of the subcallosal cingulate gyrus in patients with treatment-resistant depression: A pilot study of relapse prevention. *J. Psychiatry Neurosci. JPN* **2015**, *40*, 224–231. [CrossRef] [PubMed]

22. Ramasubbu, R.; Anderson, S.; Haffenden, A.; Chavda, S.; Kiss, Z.H.T. Double-blind optimization of subcallosal cingulate deep brain stimulation for treatment-resistant depression: A pilot study. *J. Psychiatry Neurosci. JPN* **2013**, *38*, 325–332. [CrossRef] [PubMed]

23. Raymaekers, S.; Luyten, L.; Bervoets, C.; Gabriels, L.; Nuttin, B. Deep brain stimulation for treatment-resistant major depressive disorder: A comparison of two targets and long-term follow-up. *Transl. Psychiatry* **2017**, *7*, e1251. [CrossRef] [PubMed]

24. Coenen, V.A.; Bewernick, B.H.; Kayser, S.; Kilian, H.; Bostrom, J.; Greschus, S.; Hurlemann, R.; Klein, M.E.; Spanier, S.; Sajonz, B.; et al. Superolateral medial forebrain bundle deep brain stimulation in major depression: A gateway trial. *Neuropsychopharmacol. Off. Publ. Am. Coll. Neuropsychopharmacol.* **2019**, *44*, 1224–1232. [CrossRef]

25. Fenoy, A.J.; Schulz, P.E.; Selvaraj, S.; Burrows, C.L.; Zunta-Soares, G.; Durkin, K.; Zanotti-Fregonara, P.; Quevedo, J.; Soares, J.C. A longitudinal study on deep brain stimulation of the medial forebrain bundle for treatment-resistant depression. *Transl. Psychiatry* **2018**, *8*, 111. [CrossRef] [PubMed]

26. Sartorius, A.; Kiening, K.L.; Kirsch, P.; von Gall, C.C.; Haberkorn, U.; Unterberg, A.W.; Henn, F.A.; Meyer-Lindenberg, A. Remission of Major Depression Under Deep Brain Stimulation of the Lateral Habenula in a Therapy-Refractory Patient. *Biol. Psychiatry* **2010**, *67*, e9–e11. [CrossRef]

27. Zhou, C.; Zhang, H.; Qin, Y.; Tian, T.; Xu, B.; Chen, J.; Zhou, X.; Zeng, L.; Fang, L.; Qi, X.; et al. A systematic review and meta-analysis of deep brain stimulation in treatment-resistant depression. *Prog. Neuropsychopharmacol. Biol. Psychiatry* **2018**, *82*, 224–232. [CrossRef]

28. Kisely, S.; Li, A.; Warren, N.; Siskind, D. A systematic review and meta-analysis of deep brain stimulation for depression. *Depress. Anxiety* **2018**, *35*, 468–480. [CrossRef]

29. Berlim, M.T.; McGirr, A.; Van den Eynde, F.; Fleck, M.P.A.; Giacobbe, P. Effectiveness and acceptability of deep brain stimulation (DBS) of the subgenual cingulate cortex for treatment-resistant depression: A systematic review and exploratory meta-analysis. *J. Affect. Disord.* **2014**, *159*, 31–38. [CrossRef]

30. Harrer, M.; Cuijpers, P.; Furukawa, T.; Ebert, D. Doing Meta-Analysis in R: A Hands-on Guide. Available online: https://bookdown.org/MathiasHarrer/Doing_Meta_Analysis_in_R/ (accessed on 26 June 2020).

31. Lozano, A.M.; Mayberg, H.S.; Giacobbe, P.; Hamani, C.; Craddock, R.C.; Kennedy, S.H. Subcallosal cingulate gyrus deep brain stimulation for treatment-resistant depression. *Biol. Psychiatry* **2008**, *64*, 461–467. [CrossRef]

32. Lozano, A.M.; Giacobbe, P.; Hamani, C.; Rizvi, S.J.; Kennedy, S.H.; Kolivakis, T.T.; Debonnel, G.; Sadikot, A.F.; Lam, R.W.; Howard, A.K.; et al. A multicenter pilot study of subcallosal cingulate area deep brain stimulation for treatment-resistant depression. *J. Neurosurg.* **2012**, *116*, 315–322. [CrossRef] [PubMed]

33. Puigdemont, D.; Perez-Egea, R.; Portella, M.J.; Molet, J.; de Diego-Adelino, J.; Gironell, A.; Radua, J.; Gomez-Anson, B.; Rodriguez, R.; Serra, M.; et al. Deep brain stimulation of the subcallosal cingulate gyrus: Further evidence in treatment-resistant major depression. *Int. J. Neuropsychopharmacol.* **2012**, *15*, 121–133. [CrossRef] [PubMed]

34. Bewernick, B.H.; Hurlemann, R.; Matusch, A.; Kayser, S.; Grubert, C.; Hadrysiewicz, B.; Axmacher, N.; Lemke, M.; Cooper-Mahkorn, D.; Cohen, M.X.; et al. Nucleus accumbens deep brain stimulation decreases ratings of depression and anxiety in treatment-resistant depression. *Biol. Psychiatry* **2010**, *67*, 110–116. [CrossRef] [PubMed]

35. Millet, B.; Jaafari, N.; Polosan, M.; Baup, N.; Giordana, B.; Haegelen, C.; Chabardes, S.; Fontaine, D.; Devaux, B.; Yelnik, J.; et al. Limbic versus cognitive target for deep brain stimulation in treatment-resistant depression: Accumbens more promising than caudate. *Eur. Neuropsychopharmacol. J. Eur. Coll. Neuropsychopharmacol.* **2014**, *24*, 1229–1239. [CrossRef]

36. Malone, D.A.J.; Dougherty, D.D.; Rezai, A.R.; Carpenter, L.L.; Friehs, G.M.; Eskandar, E.N.; Rauch, S.L.; Rasmussen, S.A.; Machado, A.G.; Kubu, C.S.; et al. Deep brain stimulation of the ventral capsule/ventral striatum for treatment-resistant depression. *Biol. Psychiatry* **2009**, *65*, 267–275. [CrossRef]

37. Bewernick, B.H.; Kayser, S.; Gippert, S.M.; Switala, C.; Coenen, V.A.; Schlaepfer, T.E. Deep brain stimulation to the medial forebrain bundle for depression- long-term outcomes and a novel data analysis strategy. *Brain Stimulat.* **2017**, *10*, 664–671. [CrossRef]

38. Crowell, A.L.; Riva-Posse, P.; Holtzheimer, P.E.; Garlow, S.J.; Kelley, M.E.; Gross, R.E.; Denison, L.; Quinn, S.; Mayberg, H.S. Long-Term Outcomes of Subcallosal Cingulate Deep Brain Stimulation for Treatment-Resistant Depression. *Am. J. Psychiatry* **2019**. [CrossRef]

39. Schlaepfer, T.E.; Bewernick, B.H.; Kayser, S.; Madler, B.; Coenen, V.A. Rapid effects of deep brain stimulation for treatment-resistant major depression. *Biol. Psychiatry* **2013**, *73*, 1204–1212. [CrossRef]

40. Bewernick, B.H.; Kayser, S.; Sturm, V.; Schlaepfer, T.E. Long-term effects of nucleus accumbens deep brain stimulation in treatment-resistant depression: Evidence for sustained efficacy. *Neuropsychopharmacol. Off. Publ. Am. Coll. Neuropsychopharmacol.* **2012**, *37*, 1975–1985. [CrossRef]

41. Eitan, R.; Fontaine, D.; Benoit, M.; Giordana, C.; Darmon, N.; Israel, Z.; Linesky, E.; Arkadir, D.; Ben-Naim, S.; Iserlles, M.; et al. One year double blind study of high vs low frequency subcallosal cingulate stimulation for depression. *J. Psychiatr. Res.* **2018**, *96*, 124–134. [CrossRef]

42. Accolla, E.A.; Aust, S.; Merkl, A.; Schneider, G.-H.; Kuhn, A.A.; Bajbouj, M.; Draganski, B. Deep brain stimulation of the posterior gyrus rectus region for treatment resistant depression. *J. Affect. Disord.* **2016**, *194*, 33–37. [CrossRef] [PubMed]

43. Sankar, T.; Chakravarty, M.M.; Jawa, N.; Li, S.X.; Giacobbe, P.; Kennedy, S.H.; Rizvi, S.J.; Mayberg, H.S.; Hamani, C.; Lozano, A.M. Neuroanatomical predictors of response to subcallosal cingulate deep brain stimulation for treatment-resistant depression. *J. Psychiatry Neurosci. JPN* **2019**, *44*, 1–10. [CrossRef] [PubMed]

44. Schlaepfer, T.E.; Cohen, M.X.; Frick, C.; Kosel, M.; Brodesser, D.; Axmacher, N.; Joe, A.Y.; Kreft, M.; Lenartz, D.; Sturm, V. Deep Brain Stimulation to Reward Circuitry Alleviates Anhedonia in Refractory Major Depression. *Neuropsychopharmacology* **2008**, *33*, 368–377. [CrossRef] [PubMed]

45. Mayberg, H.S.; Lozano, A.M.; Voon, V.; McNeely, H.E.; Seminowicz, D.; Hamani, C.; Schwalb, J.M.; Kennedy, S.H. Deep brain stimulation for treatment-resistant depression. *Neuron* **2005**, *45*, 651–660. [CrossRef]

46. Dandekar, M.P.; Fenoy, A.J.; Carvalho, A.F.; Soares, J.C.; Quevedo, J. Deep brain stimulation for treatment-resistant depression: An integrative review of preclinical and clinical findings and translational implications. *Mol. Psychiatry* **2018**, *23*, 1094–1112. [CrossRef]

47. Fins, J.J.; Kubu, C.S.; Mayberg, H.S.; Merkel, R.; Nuttin, B.; Schlaepfer, T.E. Being open minded about neuromodulation trials: Finding success in our "failures". *Brain Stimulat.* **2017**, *10*, 181–186. [CrossRef]

48. Choi, K.S.; Noecker, A.M.; Riva-Posse, P.; Rajendra, J.K.; Gross, R.E.; Mayberg, H.S.; McIntyre, C.C. Impact of brain shift on subcallosal cingulate deep brain stimulation. *Brain Stimulat.* **2018**, *11*, 445–453. [CrossRef]

49. Noecker, A.M.; Choi, K.S.; Riva-Posse, P.; Gross, R.E.; Mayberg, H.S.; McIntyre, C.C. StimVision Software: Examples and Applications in Subcallosal Cingulate Deep Brain Stimulation for Depression. *Neuromodulation J. Int. Neuromodulation Soc.* **2018**, *21*, 191–196. [CrossRef]

50. Riva-Posse, P.; Choi, K.S.; Holtzheimer, P.E.; Crowell, A.L.; Garlow, S.J.; Rajendra, J.K.; McIntyre, C.C.; Gross, R.E.; Mayberg, H.S. A connectomic approach for subcallosal cingulate deep brain stimulation surgery: Prospective targeting in treatment-resistant depression. *Mol. Psychiatry* **2018**, *23*, 843–849. [CrossRef]

51. Tsolaki, E.; Espinoza, R.; Pouratian, N. Using probabilistic tractography to target the subcallosal cingulate cortex in patients with treatment resistant depression. *Psychiatry Res. Neuroimaging* **2017**, *261*, 72–74. [CrossRef]

52. Coenen, V.A.; Sajonz, B.; Reisert, M.; Bostroem, J.; Bewernick, B.; Urbach, H.; Jenkner, C.; Reinacher, P.C.; Schlaepfer, T.E.; Madler, B. Tractography-assisted deep brain stimulation of the superolateral branch of the medial forebrain bundle (slMFB DBS) in major depression. *NeuroImage Clin.* **2018**, *20*, 580–593. [CrossRef] [PubMed]

53. Faraone, S.V. Interpreting Estimates of Treatment Effects. *Pharm. Ther.* **2008**, *33*, 700–711.

54. Locher, C.; Koechlin, H.; Zion, S.R.; Werner, C.; Pine, D.S.; Kirsch, I.; Kessler, R.C.; Kossowsky, J. Efficacy and Safety of Selective Serotonin Reuptake Inhibitors, Serotonin-Norepinephrine Reuptake Inhibitors, and Placebo for Common Psychiatric Disorders Among Children and Adolescents. *JAMA Psychiatry* **2017**, *74*, 1011–1020. [CrossRef] [PubMed]

55. Drobisz, D.; Damborska, A. Deep brain stimulation targets for treating depression. *Behav. Brain Res.* **2019**, *359*, 266–273. [CrossRef]

56. Guo, C.C.; Hyett, M.P.; Nguyen, V.T.; Parker, G.B.; Breakspear, M.J. Distinct neurobiological signatures of brain connectivity in depression subtypes during natural viewing of emotionally salient films. *Psychol. Med.* **2016**, *46*, 1535–1545. [CrossRef]

57. Williams, N.R.; Okun, M.S. Deep brain stimulation (DBS) at the interface of neurology and psychiatry. *J. Clin. Investig.* **2013**, *123*, 4546–4556. [CrossRef]

58. Coenen, V.A.; Schlaepfer, T.E.; Reinacher, P.C.; Mast, H.; Urbach, H.; Reisert, M. Machine learning-aided personalized DTI tractographic planning for deep brain stimulation of the superolateral medial forebrain bundle using HAMLET. *Acta Neurochir. (Wien)* **2019**, *161*, 1559–1569. [CrossRef]

59. van Aert, R.C.M.; Wicherts, J.M.; van Assen, M.A.L.M. Publication bias examined in meta-analyses from psychology and medicine: A meta-meta-analysis. *PLoS ONE* **2019**, *14*, e0215052. [CrossRef]

60. Bergfeld, I.O.; Mantione, M.; Figee, M.; Schuurman, P.R.; Lok, A.; Denys, D. Treatment-resistant depression and suicidality. *J. Affect. Disord.* **2018**, *235*, 362–367. [CrossRef]

61. Seo, H.-J.; Jung, Y.-E.; Jeong, S.; Kim, J.-B.; Lee, M.-S.; Kim, J.-M.; Yim, H.W.; Jun, T.-Y. Persistence and resolution of suicidal ideation during treatment of depression in patients with significant suicidality at the beginning of treatment: The CRESCEND study. *J. Affect. Disord.* **2014**, *155*, 208–215. [CrossRef]

62. Wulsin, L.R.; Vaillant, G.E.; Wells, V.E. A systematic review of the mortality of depression. *Psychosom. Med.* **1999**, *61*, 6–17. [CrossRef] [PubMed]

63. Bari, A.A.; Mikell, C.B.; Abosch, A.; Ben-Haim, S.; Buchanan, R.J.; Burton, A.W.; Carcieri, S.; Cosgrove, G.R.; D'Haese, P.-F.; Daskalakis, Z.J.; et al. Charting the road forward in psychiatric neurosurgery: Proceedings of the 2016 American Society for Stereotactic and Functional Neurosurgery workshop on neuromodulation for psychiatric disorders. *J. Neurol. Neurosurg. Psychiatry* **2018**, *89*, 886–896. [CrossRef] [PubMed]

64. Jones, B.; Lewis, J.A. The case for cross-over trials in phase III. *Stat. Med.* **1995**, *14*, 1025–1038. [CrossRef] [PubMed]

65. Mayberg, H.S.; Riva-Posse, P.; Crowell, A.L. Deep Brain Stimulation for Depression: Keeping an Eye on a Moving Target. *JAMA Psychiatry* **2016**, *73*, 439–440. [CrossRef]

66. Kennedy, S.H.; Giacobbe, P.; Rizvi, S.J.; Placenza, F.M.; Nishikawa, Y.; Mayberg, H.S.; Lozano, A.M. Deep brain stimulation for treatment-resistant depression: Follow-up after 3 to 6 years. *Am. J. Psychiatry* **2011**, *168*, 502–510. [CrossRef]

67. van der Wal, J.M.; Bergfeld, I.O.; Lok, A.; Mantione, M.; Figee, M.; Notten, P.; Beute, G.; Horst, F.; van den Munckhof, P.; Schuurman, P.R.; et al. Long-term deep brain stimulation of the ventral anterior limb of the internal capsule for treatment-resistant depression. *J. Neurol. Neurosurg. Psychiatry* **2020**, *91*, 189–195. [CrossRef]

68. Bhatia, K.D.; Henderson, L.; Ramsey-Stewart, G.; May, J. Diffusion tensor imaging to aid subgenual cingulum target selection for deep brain stimulation in depression. *Stereotact. Funct. Neurosurg.* **2012**, *90*, 225–232. [CrossRef]

69. Coenen, V.A.; Schlaepfer, T.E.; Bewernick, B.; Kilian, H.; Kaller, C.P.; Urbach, H.; Li, M.; Reisert, M. Frontal white matter architecture predicts efficacy of deep brain stimulation in major depression. *Transl. Psychiatry* **2019**, *9*, 197. [CrossRef]

70. Riva-Posse, P.; Choi, K.S.; Holtzheimer, P.E.; McIntyre, C.C.; Gross, R.E.; Chaturvedi, A.; Crowell, A.L.; Garlow, S.J.; Rajendra, J.K.; Mayberg, H.S. Defining critical white matter pathways mediating successful subcallosal cingulate deep brain stimulation for treatment-resistant depression. *Biol. Psychiatry* **2014**, *76*, 963–969. [CrossRef]

71. Howell, B.; Choi, K.S.; Gunalan, K.; Rajendra, J.; Mayberg, H.S.; McIntyre, C.C. Quantifying the axonal pathways directly stimulated in therapeutic subcallosal cingulate deep brain stimulation. *Hum. Brain Mapp.* **2019**, *40*, 889–903. [CrossRef]

72. McInerney, S.J.; McNeely, H.E.; Geraci, J.; Giacobbe, P.; Rizvi, S.J.; Ceniti, A.K.; Cyriac, A.; Mayberg, H.S.; Lozano, A.M.; Kennedy, S.H. Neurocognitive Predictors of Response in Treatment Resistant Depression to Subcallosal Cingulate Gyrus Deep Brain Stimulation. *Front. Hum. Neurosci.* **2017**, *11*, 74. [CrossRef] [PubMed]

73. Quraan, M.A.; Protzner, A.B.; Daskalakis, Z.J.; Giacobbe, P.; Tang, C.W.; Kennedy, S.H.; Lozano, A.M.; McAndrews, M.P. EEG power asymmetry and functional connectivity as a marker of treatment effectiveness in DBS surgery for depression. *Neuropsychopharmacol. Off. Publ. Am. Coll. Neuropsychopharmacol.* **2014**, *39*, 1270–1281. [CrossRef] [PubMed]

74. Broadway, J.M.; Holtzheimer, P.E.; Hilimire, M.R.; Parks, N.A.; Devylder, J.E.; Mayberg, H.S.; Corballis, P.M. Frontal theta cordance predicts 6-month antidepressant response to subcallosal cingulate deep brain stimulation for treatment-resistant depression: A pilot study. *Neuropsychopharmacol. Off. Publ. Am. Coll. Neuropsychopharmacol.* **2012**, *37*, 1764–1772. [CrossRef]

75. Lujan, J.L.; Chaturvedi, A.; Malone, D.A.; Rezai, A.R.; Machado, A.G.; McIntyre, C.C. Axonal pathways linked to therapeutic and nontherapeutic outcomes during psychiatric deep brain stimulation. *Hum. Brain Mapp.* **2012**, *33*, 958–968. [CrossRef] [PubMed]

## 11

Deep Brain Stimulation Selection Criteria for Parkinson's Disease: Time to go beyond CAPSIT-PD

Carlo Alberto Artusi [1],*, Leonardo Lopiano [1] and Francesca Morgante [2,3]

[1] Department of Neuroscience 'Rita Levi Montalcini', University of Torino, 10126 Torino, Italy; Leonardo.lopiano@unito.it

[2] Neurosciences Research Centre, Molecular and Clinical Sciences Research Institute, St George's University of London, London SW17 0RE, UK; fmorgante@gmail.com

[3] Department of Clinical and Experimental Medicine, University of Messina, 98125 Messina, Italy

* Correspondence: caartusi@gmail.com

Abstract: Despite being introduced in clinical practice more than 20 years ago, selection criteria for deep brain stimulation (DBS) in Parkinson's disease (PD) rely on a document published in 1999 called 'Core Assessment Program for Surgical Interventional Therapies in Parkinson's Disease'. These criteria are useful in supporting the selection of candidates. However, they are both restrictive and out-of-date, because the knowledge on PD progression and phenotyping has massively evolved. Advances in understanding the heterogeneity of PD presentation, courses, phenotypes, and genotypes, render a better identification of good DBS outcome predictors a research priority. Additionally, DBS invasiveness, cost, and the possibility of serious adverse events make it mandatory to predict as accurately as possible the clinical outcome when informing the patients about their suitability for surgery. In this viewpoint, we analyzed the pre-surgical assessment according to the following topics: early versus delayed DBS; the evolution of the levodopa challenge test; and the relevance of axial symptoms; patient-centered outcome measures; non-motor symptoms; and genetics. Based on the literature, we encourage rethinking of the selection process for DBS in PD, which should move toward a broad clinical and instrumental assessment of non-motor symptoms, quantitative measurement of gait, posture, and balance, and in-depth genotypic and phenotypic characterization.

Keywords: Parkinson's disease; deep brain stimulation; selection; levodopa; axial symptoms; non motor symptoms; genetics

1. Introduction

Despite having being introduced in clinical practice more than 20 years ago, selection criteria for deep brain stimulation (DBS) as an effective treatment for advanced Parkinson's disease (PD) still rely on the 'Core Assessment Program for Surgical Interventional Therapies in Parkinson's Disease' (CAPSIT-PD) published in 1999 [1]. These criteria were primarily designed to facilitate clinical research, harmonizing the cohorts of clinical trials. However, most of the indications provided in the CAPSIT-PD document were introduced as guidance into the clinical practice of DBS centers worldwide, being extremely useful in supporting the selection of candidates [2]. Twenty years later, these indications could be considered both restrictive and out-of-date, because the knowledge on PD progression, phenotyping, and genotyping has strongly evolved over the last 20 years. Indeed, according to CAPSIT-PD, only 1.6% of PD subjects would be eligible for DBS, rising to 4.5% when applying more flexible criteria [3].

Moreover, a growing number of studies have reported novel data on the outcome of DBS in the short- and long-term follow-up and proposed predictors of DBS response [4,5]. However, evidence on how to improve and refine the selection process based on these insights for candidates to DBS is still lacking. Finally, despite the consolidated efficacy of DBS in improving PD cardinal symptoms and motor complications, the factors predicting a successful outcome on activities of daily living (ADL) and quality of life (QoL) have been addressed only by a few studies so far [6].

Advances in understanding the heterogeneity of PD presentation, courses, phenotypes, and genotypes impose a better identification of DBS candidates as a research priority. Additionally, DBS invasiveness, cost, and the possibility of serious adverse events make it mandatory to predict as accurately as possible the clinical outcome when informing the patients about their suitability for surgery.

Here, we appraised the DBS pre-surgical assessment for PD starting from the original CAPSIT-PD document and addressed the following topics which may impact on the selection process: early versus delayed DBS; the evolution of the levodopa challenge test; the relevance of axial symptoms; new focus on patient-centered outcome measures; the relevance of non-motor symptoms; and a new role for genetics. Our main aim was to highlight current pitfalls and potentialities in the DBS selection process, stimulating future randomized control trials (RCT) to address specific needs.

2. Early Versus Delayed DBS: How Early?

2.1. The Standard Rule

The CAPSIT-PD document recommended that a patient considered for interventional surgery should have a diagnosis of idiopathic PD and a minimum disease duration of five years [1]. These requirements were developed to exclude people with atypical parkinsonism, given the absence of benefits and the risk to harm patients with no idiopathic PD [7].

2.2. Pros and Cons

The concept of a five-year disease duration has been challenged upon the results of a large RCT published in 2013 (the EARLY-STIM trial) [8]. In this trial demonstrating the superiority of subthalamic (STN) DBS compared to medical therapy alone, patients were included when having a PD diagnosis of ≥4 years, and fluctuations or dyskinesia present for four years or less [8].

The EARLY-STIM trial endorsed a conceptual change about the use of DBS for PD favoring a paradigm shift from DBS as the last therapeutic option for advanced disease stages toward an earlier approach for patients experiencing motor complications. This paradigm change is based on three relevant points: (1) the confirmation of DBS safety over the years, even in the long term; (2) the great efficacy of DBS in improving the QoL of patients, even superior to levodopa alone [9]; (3) an earlier intervention could preserve functional capacity. The evidence of efficacy provided by the EARLY-STIM trial led the U.S. Food and Drug Administration (FDA) to extend the DBS indication to patients with a four year PD diagnosis in the presence of at least four months of uncontrolled motor complications [10].

The EARLY-STIM trial has triggered discussion as to whether its findings should be translated into clinical practice [11]. Firstly, the shorter disease duration at the time of surgery might pose the risks of including subjects with atypical parkinsonism for which the five-year rule has been developed for CAPSIT-PD. However, in the EARLY-STIM cohort, the mean disease duration of the surgically-treated group was 7.3 ± 3.1 years and only three cases (0.8% of the cohort) were re-diagnosed as non-idiopathic PD eight years after the first randomization and approximately 15 years after diagnosis [12]. However, it should be noted that the issue of a shorter disease duration at the time of surgery might mirror a greater and faster burden of disability which is also associated with specific genotypes associated to PD, such as severe and complex glucocerobrosidase (*GBA*) gene variants [13], which have been associated to poor DBS functional outcome [14].

A related matter is the difficulty in predicting the trajectory of disease progression at such an early stage, either for more benign or rapidly progressing phenotypes [15], with the consequent risk of referring to surgery patients whose motor fluctuations could remain mild for a long time, or vice-versa, those who may develop symptoms non-responsive to DBS and severely impacting ADL and QoL.

However, when looking carefully into the EARLY-STIM cohort, all patients had experienced either motor or psychiatric disability due to PD. Accordingly, further analyses on this population have demonstrated that STN-DBS was successful in improving freezing of gait (FoG) in OFF medication condition [16], which affected 52% of the patients at baseline. Remarkably, behavioral complications linked to dopaminergic overmedication had a better outcome in the neurostimulation group [17].

How early should DBS be considered in PD? A pilot open label study on 28 patients suggested to consider DBS even earlier, before motor complications arose [18]. However, despite long term follow-up data on the same cohort [19], the impact of early surgical intervention in such earlier stages is still unknown and should be carefully interpreted including the risks we mentioned above but also a presumptive neuroprotective effect [20]. Finally, it should be taken into account that DBS (STN-DBS in particular) allows a reduction in dose of dopaminergic therapies in most patients [21]. Although favoring the improvement of dyskinesia, the reduction in antiparkinsonian drugs could have role in improving impulsive-compulsive behaviors and obsessive-compulsive and paranoid traits [22,23].

2.3. Recommendations

There is evidence for an earlier use of DBS as a treatment option to improve patients' QoL and early levodopa-responsive axial symptoms, while minimizing the psychiatric consequences of overtreatment. Long-term results from the EARLY-STIM trial would allow the better defining of which PD features are associated to a long-term successful outcome. However, there is not enough knowledge on how early into the disease history DBS should be considered, given the paucity of published data and the current lack of knowledge on how to predict disease progression and DBS response in such early stages. We recommend considering each case singularly, according to the patient's phenotype, age, needs, and expectations in patients whose symptoms significantly impact ADL and QoL despite a reasonable number of attempts to provide the best medical therapy.

3. The Evolution of the Levodopa Challenge Test

3.1. The Standard Rule

The second recommendation of CAPSIT-PD is dopaminergic responsiveness confirmed by a levodopa/apomorphine challenge test (LCT). Accordingly, the test has to demonstrate at least a 33% decrease in the Unified Parkinson's Disease Rating Scale (UPDRS) part III score in the "defined-on condition" (best therapeutic effect after medication agreed by patient and physician) compared to the "defined-off condition" (at least 12 h after receiving the last medication dose).

3.2. Pros and Cons

The threshold of 33% for UPDRS improvement is considered relevant to rule out possible misdiagnoses (i.e., identifying atypical parkinsonism for which DBS is not recommended). The LCT is also important to inform the possible outcome of surgery, showing the likely extent of symptom improvement after surgery, and to establish realistic expectations from DBS [24]. Indeed, it is generally accepted that symptoms improving with levodopa are likely to respond to DBS [25]. However, there are some exceptions and caveats to these widely accepted concepts. Firstly, levodopa-resistant tremor represents one of the indications of DBS, even in the absence of disabling motor fluctuations [26,27], given its excellent effect in controlling or even suppressing tremors, regardless of the deep nuclei targeted [28].

Another relevant challenge related to the LCT is the cut-off of 33%. This value has been validated by a study based on its ability to predict chronic levodopa responsiveness, with a positive predictive value for the PD diagnosis of 88.6% [29]. Notably, the Movement Disorders Society (MDS)-sponsored UPDRS scale introduced in 2008 has some differences in the scoring of the part-III (motor part), and a study analyzing the MDS-UPDRS scores with the old UPDRS [30] ones after an acute LCT found an excellent correlation between the two scales, with the 30% UPDRS score variation used for predicting sustained long-term levodopa response equivalent to 24% in MDS-UPDRS [31]. However, data from STN-DBS clinical trials seems to indicate that an excellent response to levodopa (i.e., >50% UPDRS part-III improvement) could be associated with a better DBS motor outcome [32]. A meta-analysis published in 2006 on the STN-DBS outcomes supports this hypothesis, demonstrating that the magnitude of decrease in both UPDRS part-II and part-III scores exhibits a dose–response relationship with the presurgical response to the levodopa challenge test [33]. However, it is unknown whether the magnitude of response at the LCT may predict better ADL and QoL after DBS. Moreover, the relevance of axial symptoms as a source of disability, their heterogenous response to dopaminergic therapies, and their influence on the trajectory of the PD course put in light further considerations on the usefulness of the presurgical LCT simplistically considered as a >30% motor response.

3.3. Recommendations

We recommend using LCT as a key tool to obtain relevant presurgical information on the patient's status and the possibility of improvement after DBS. However, the rule of UPDRS part-III improvement >30% should not be strictly applied. Although patients affected by disabling dopa-resistant tremor could represent an exception to this rule, improvement >50% can be associated with greater overall benefit in most patients. The LCT response of disabling axial symptoms, such as FoG, is important and should be weighted independently from the percentage UPDRS part-III total score improvement.

4. The Relevance of Axial Symptoms: How Sensitive Is Current Clinical Assessment?

4.1. The Standard Rule

The term 'axial symptoms' is commonly referred to as a group of PD motor features encompassing gait impairment, postural instability, postural abnormalities, and speech disorders, especially dysarthria and stuttering. These are a major source of disability because they are associated with reduced mobility, communication difficulties, recurrent falls, and subsequent injuries [34]. Moreover, they are markers of advanced disease and are often resistant to dopaminergic therapies or exhibit an heterogenous pattern of response to levodopa [35]. There are no precise indications on how to consider these symptoms and their pre-surgical response to levodopa in the clinical practice.

4.2. Pros and Cons

The evidence on the effect of DBS on axial symptoms is controversial. A meta-analysis published in 2004 showed that one year after surgery, STN-DBS or globus pallidus pars interna (GPi) DBS can improve gait and balance symptoms, with an effect size similar to the preoperative effects of dopaminergic medication [36]. However, the improvement provided by DBS seems not sustained over the years. Evidence for axial symptom progression, despite a good control of PD appendicular motor symptoms, has been shown in open-label, long-term follow-up studies, although some extent of axial improvement related to stimulation is reported in the first years after surgery [37–40].

The relevance of axial symptoms as a marker of disease progression was disclosed in a cohort of 143 PD patients treated with STN-DBS [5], in whom axial disability during the follow-up period was strongly associated with an increased risk of death (hazard ratio of 4.3), proving to be the most accurate mortality predictor, even superior to the cognitive status.

Axial symptoms track disease progression and disability, therefore an accurate presurgical evaluation of levodopa-responsiveness would be necessary for estimating the extent of response after DBS. Indeed, worsening or amelioration after DBS of speech, posture and gait disorders is multifactorial and depends upon clinical variables such as disease duration [16,41], the type of axial symptom (gait often improves after DBS, speech may worsen as a stimulus-related side effect), their interplay with dopaminergic medications [42,43], the brain target employed for DBS, the frequency [44,45] and distribution of stimulation [46], and placement of active electrode contact [41].

Levodopa-resistant axial symptoms are considered a relative contraindication for surgery [47]; however, the current pre-surgical clinical examination is unable to detect early axial signs which may foster worse DBS outcomes. In particular, FoG evaluation poses great challenges, given the episodic nature of this phenomenon and the complex relationship with dopaminergic medications. Trunk postural abnormalities also represent a source of difficulty at the time of DBS selection (including on which target to choose), because camptocormia and Pisa syndrome might be responsive to STN-DBS, even with poor or no amelioration after LCT [48,49].

These difficulties which impact on the selection process might be overcome by integrating objective evaluation involving kinematic analysis and wearable sensors to the pre-operative clinical examination. Specifically, novel technological developments on wearable sensors for home-monitoring have the potential to provide a measure of axial symptoms and their relation to levodopa intake in a naturalistic way [50,51]. These technologies should be employed to detect early axial signs which might predict worsening after DBS and assist the identification of the best candidates. Indeed, a study employing kinematic assessment of gait demonstrated a correlation between presurgical levodopa response of stride length and range of motion and FoG outcome after DBS [52].

4.3. Recommendations

The global burden of axial symptoms can be considered a proxy for disease stage because of their correlation with disability and death. A fine-grained assessment of each axial symptom, the accurate evaluation of their relationship with dopaminergic therapy, and the integration of technology outcome measures into the clinical practice should favor a better understanding of candidates to DBS, with the potential to predict their disease course and the probability to improve after DBS. Pending clinical trials aiming at the evaluation of the effect of DBS on PD-related axial symptoms, we recommend to accurately evaluate in clinical practice the presence, severity, and impact on patient's daily life and independence of axial symptoms before surgery, and discuss the weight of each symptom with the patient, clarifying its poor, good, or indeterminate probability of improvement after DBS. Severe FoG and speech issues, in particular, represent a potential challenge in the management of patients undergoing DBS, while camptocormia and Pisa syndrome could have good chances of improvement and should not be considered contraindications for DBS.

5. The Need for Patient-Centered Outcome Measures

5.1. The Standard Rule

From a regulatory point of view, the FDA and European Medicine Agency (EMA) request the presence of motor fluctuations as a mandatory criterion for DBS indication in PD [10]. Reduction in severity and frequency of motor fluctuations represents one of the most relevant achievements obtained by DBS, which translates into the improvement of QoL revealed by randomized controlled trials [8,53].

5.2. Pros and Cons

In CAPSIT-PD, it is recommended that the patients perform the self-reporting diary one week per month during the three preoperative months, indicating the presence of four conditions: complete OFF, partial OFF, complete ON, and ON with dyskinesias [1]. However, these measures are highly subjective, and wrong or missed entries may occur in about one third of cases—also when using electronic motor diaries [54]. That is, objective home-based quantification by wearable sensors of PD motor symptoms [55], including FoG [56], should be explored carefully in patients considered for DBS, also with respect to the predictive value of these measures. Indeed, when it comes to predicting the outcome of DBS in PD and patient-centered outcome measures are employed, some discrepancies arise. Patient-centered outcome measures are represented by QoL, evaluated by the validated Parkinson's Disease Questionnaire 39 (PDQ-39) [57] or by its short form (PDQ-8) [58], and ADL functioning or independence, typically measured by UPDRS part-II and the Schwab and England (S&E) scale [59]. The importance of measuring patient-centered outcomes relates to the discrepancy between the judgment made in-clinic by the neurologist and the degree of satisfaction [60] and independence obtained by the patient during daily life [54]. Two key factors may account for this discrepancy: (1) motor symptoms observed by clinicians explain only a small part of the complex picture of PD, which encompasses several non-motor symptoms; (2) the standardized tasks assessed during in-clinic visits and the non-quantitative, non-continuous, non-ecologic in-clinic examinations may not represent a comprehensive measure of the patient situation and condition during daily life. This last aspect is true even when limiting the evaluation to motor symptoms, in particular episodic motor symptoms such as FoG [61], which are not adequately captured during in-clinic standard assessments [54].

When it comes to analyzing determinants of improvement in QoL after STN DBS, a post-hoc analysis of the EARLY-STIM trial found smaller QoL improvement at 24-months follow-up in patients with better pre-surgical PDQ-39 scores [6]. Interestingly, patients with pre-surgical PDQ-39 scores ≤ 15 had no significant change in QoL following surgery. This finding is not meant to be caused by a ceiling effect of STN-DBS to improve motor symptoms in the EARLY-STIM cohort, because the change in QoL over the two years was independent of the severity of parkinsonian motor signs assessed by UPDRS-III [8]. Accordingly, in another study analyzing a cohort of 85 PD patients treated with DBS, the magnitude of motor symptom improvement with a pre-surgical LCT was only borderline associated with improvement of QoL after DBS ($p = 0.053$) [62].

A systematic review [63] demonstrated that higher baseline QoL predicted larger QoL changes after surgery in three out of four studies. The analysis of the 18 studies included in this review yielded mixed results with respect to the predictive value of other clinical and demographical features. There are two main explanations for such discrepant findings: (1) most of these studies were not primarily designed to detect predictors of QoL change after DBS and results are influenced by the main a priori hypothesis tested in each study; (2) factors contributing to QoL in PD include not only motor disability but also non-motor symptoms [64], and the interplay between these domains might be individualized and have a different weight in each subject. Moreover, among motor symptoms, axial disability (and its response to therapies) might have a high impact, which has not been yet explored carefully in regard to QoL or ADL outcome after DBS.

5.3. Recommendations

Future studies should be designed to capture predictors of QoL and ADL improvements after DBS, taking into account the heterogeneity of the disease, the contribution of non-motor symptoms, and the impact of axial symptoms. We recommend evaluating both the ADL and QoL of candidates for DBS by means of validated scales (e.g., UPDRS part-II and PDQ-39 or PDQ-8) and carefully discuss with patients the disease burden and their determinants. After surgery, these scales can inform more than the in-clinic motor assessment about the clinical status of the patient and the impact of stimulation on their functioning in daily life, guiding possible changes in stimulation parameters, medical therapy or non-medical interventions, such as psychological support, physiotherapy, and emotional and social stimulation.

6. The Complexity of PD Spectrum Integrated into the Selection Process: Relevance of Non-Motor Symptoms

6.1. The Standard Rule

Despite the fact that DBS was developed to treat motor symptoms, the growing relevance given to non-motor symptoms (NMS) in the last 15 years fostered investigations into the effect of DBS for these features as well [65,66]. There are no indications nor clues so far on how to consider the presence and burden of non-motor symptoms in PD candidates for DBS.

6.2. Pros and Cons

A few studies have demonstrated the improvement of different NMS (cardiovascular, sleep/fatigue, perceptual problems/hallucinations, gastrointestinal, urinary, and miscellaneous domains) six months after surgery [65], which were maintained at 24 months for the sleep/fatigue, urinary and miscellaneous domains [66], and at 36 months for the sleep domain [67]. These findings were confirmed in a small cohort of young onset PD patients, for whom STN-DBS provided sustained improvement of the sleep domain of the Non-Motor Symptoms Scale and Parkinson's disease sleep scale-2 up to 24 months and correlated to the decrease in dopamine-agonist medication [68].

Remarkably, change in NMS frequency and severity after STN-DBS is strongly correlated to the improvement in QoL both in uncontrolled [66] and controlled studies [67,69] performed in the same STN-treated cohort at different follow-up.

In the attempt to define profiles for the best DBS candidates which may encompass the complexity of PD clinical spectrum and its heterogeneity, a new data-driven approach to PD, supported by biomarkers and neuropathology, disclosed three different PD subtypes: mild-motor predominant, intermediate, and diffuse malignant [70,71]. These three groups, defined based on the progression of disability and mortality, differ in the presentation of motor and non-motor symptoms at onset, in particular for the contribution of three types of NMS: cognitive impairment, rapid eye movement sleep behavior disorder, and dysautonomia. When the same subtyping criteria were applied to a cohort of STN-DBS patients at the time of the surgical selection, the mild phenotype seem to perform better on ADL independence at the short and long-term follow-up compared to the malignant phenotype, despite similar efficacy of stimulation on motor symptoms, fluctuations, and ambulatory capacity [72].

6.3. Recommendations

More efforts are needed to understand which NMS are predictors of good or poor outcome, how different targets of DBS (STN or GPi) should be indicated to treat different NMS based on the ability to decrease total LEDD and dopamine-agonists LEDD [17], or directly treat particular symptoms by means of the stimulation of specific networks involved in pain or mood, apathy and attention [73]. We recommend to carefully assess the presence and severity of non-motor symptoms before surgery and explain to the patients that when the disease burden is mainly driven by non-motor symptoms, DBS might not be the best therapeutic option to consider.

7. A New Role for Genetics

7.1. The Standard Rule

One of the most remarkable advances in our understanding of PD pathogenesis in the last 20 years is represented by genetics. The increasing power of genetic analyses led to the identification of several chromosomal loci that cause or modulate the risk for PD [74]. Moreover, specific genetic mutations have been associated to specific clinical features and different disease courses, which could have an impact on the selection for DBS.

That is, only some evidence on the differential DBS response in different forms of monogenic PD has been put forward, suggesting some differences in the magnitude of response [14,75–77]. However, in this case there are no specific recommendations on the use of genetics in the clinical practice of DBS centers.

7.2. Pros and Cons

The main advantage of knowing the genotype of a PD patient appraised for DBS is related to the knowledge of disease evolution associated to a particular gene variant. However, despite the effort of systematic reviews [76,77] and one meta-analysis [14], the small size of the cohorts reported and the paucity of data on different gene variants and brain targets other than STN, do not allow researchers to reach firm conclusions. For example, *LRRK2*-G2019S variant carriers, described in 44 out of 50 *LRRK2* subjects with DBS reported in the literature, show an excellent response to STN DBS, which is also the most reported target [76]. G2019S is the most frequent *LRRK2* variant and produces a phenotype overlapping to late-onset, non-mutated PD with frequent presence of tremor and good response to dopaminergic medications [78]. However, in three out of four reported cases with *LRRK2*-R1441G variant, a mutation variant rarely found outside northern Spain, poor response to STN-DBS was reported [76]. The paucity of data characterizing the phenotype of *LRRK2*-R1441G variant makes it impossible to assume that the poor DBS outcome was due to more severe disease progression and development of DBS resistant features. A similar issue applies to carriers of glucocerebrosidase (*GBA*) gene variants which have a high prevalence of neuropsychiatric symptoms, especially impulsive compulsive behavior and hallucinations, and a higher risk to develop early over disease course cognitive disturbances [13]. Indeed, *GBA*-associated PD showed worse cognitive and functional performances and lower reductions in dopaminergic medication after surgery [14]. However, it is unknown which variants mostly contribute to this result. Remarkably, the risk of hallucinations and cognitive impairment, as well as survival, differs across *GBA* subjects, being higher in subjects carrying complex and severe variants [13,79].

7.3. Recommendations

Genetic testing is becoming accessible and affordable in clinical practice in many countries and may be used to inform PD candidates for their suitability for DBS. Evidence is still weak to opt for either endorsing DBS or not for a certain patient only relying on the genetic background, but in the future it is probable that certain genotypes will be considered not suitable for DBS on the basis of their improbability to benefit from the effects. To date, genetic testing of patients undergoing DBS might be proposed in those manifesting specific phenotype features (e.g., rapid development of disability, susceptibility to behavioral complications and hallucinations) consistent with particular gene variants, such as severe *GBA* mutations, which may determine possible issues presented in the post-operative follow-up (Figure 1).

Figure 1. Core Assessment Program for Surgical Interventional Therapies in Parkinson's Disease (CAPSIT-PD) and recommendations on challenging areas related to the deep brain stimulation (DBS) selection.

8. Conclusions

Advances in understanding both the complexity of PD and the effect of DBS in PD patients have provided new evidence for a better stratification of patients and a more conscious use of this therapeutic option.

It is critical to take into account that the multifaceted symptomatology of PD, encompassing motor, non-motor, and behavioral issues, makes a candidate's selection for advanced therapies a process difficult to fit in fixed and precise borders. Additionally, the probability of improving or worsening certain symptoms according to clinical trials (or to post-hoc analysis of trials) cannot capture the full clinical complexity and heterogeneity of the PD clinical spectrum and should be used cautiously for making a decision at a single level. To date, in addition to studies supporting a better comprehension of pre-surgical predictors of DBS outcomes, we also need a shift in the statistical approach to improve the decision-making from a group to an individual level.

In conclusion, the improvement in the stratification of PD patients according to their clinical features and genetic background can inform the disease course, and more-in-depth knowledge on patients most probable to benefit from DBS. A redefinition of CAPSIT-PD criteria for DBS should be pursued based on the new knowledge gained on PD clinical spectrum and DBS long term follow-up studies. This would allow surgical centers to be more accurate in predicting the outcome after functional neurosurgery and choosing the best target for stimulation. We can now estimate the probability to improve specific disabling symptoms and choose integrated approaches, combining stimulation of specific targets according to patients' issues (e.g., ventral STN for high non-motor burden [73]) with other therapeutic options (e.g., rehabilitation), with the ultimate goal of improving ADL, mental wellbeing, and eventually the QoL of PD patients. This viewpoint provided updated recommendations for a more accurate and fine-grained assessment of PD patients considered as potential candidates for DBS and highlighted the need for further studies to strengthen the evidence on predictors of DBS outcomes at an individual level, encompassing the complex and multifaceted syndromic picture of the disease and the new possibilities offered by validated clinical scales, technological devices, and genetic analysis.

Author Contributions: C.A.A.: conception, design and organization of the study, literature search, writing of the first draft; L.L.: data interpretation, review and critique; F.M.: conception, design and organization of the study, literature search, review and critique. All authors have read and agreed to the published version of the manuscript.

References

1.   Defer, G.L.; Widner, H.; Marie, R.M.; Remy, P.; Levivier, M. Core assessment program for surgical interventional therapies in Parkinson's disease (CAPSIT-PD). *Mov. Disord.* **1999**, *14*, 572–584. [CrossRef]

2.   Munhoz, R.P.; Picillo, M.; Fox, S.H.; Bruno, V.; Panisset, M.; Honey, C.R.; Fasano, A. Eligibility Criteria for Deep Brain Stimulation in Parkinson's Disease, Tremor, and Dystonia. *Can. J. Neurol. Sci.* **2016**, *43*, 462–471. [CrossRef]

3.   Morgante, L.; Morgante, F.; Moro, E.; Epifanio, A.; Girlanda, P.; Ragonese, P.; Antonini, A.; Barone, P.; Bonuccelli, U.; Contarino, M.F.; et al. How many parkinsonian patients are suitable candidates for deep brain stimulation of subthalamic nucleus? Results of a questionnaire. *Parkinsonism Relat. Disord.* **2007**, *13*, 528–531. [CrossRef] [PubMed]

4.   Abboud, H.; Genc, G.; Thompson, N.R.; Oravivattanakul, S.; Alsallom, F.; Reyes, D.; Wilson, K.; Cerejo, R.; Yu, X.X.; Floden, D.; et al. Predictors of Functional and Quality of Life Outcomes following Deep Brain Stimulation Surgery in Parkinson's Disease Patients: Disease, Patient, and Surgical Factors. *Parkinsons Dis.* **2017**, *2017*, 5609163. [CrossRef] [PubMed]

5.   Lau, B.; Meier, N.; Serra, G.; Czernecki, V.; Schuepbach, M.; Navarro, S.; Cornu, P.; Grabli, D.; Agid, Y.;
      Vidailhet, M.; et al. Axial symptoms predict mortality in patients with Parkinson disease and subthalamic
      stimulation. *Neurology* **2019**, *92*, e2559–e2570. [CrossRef] [PubMed]

6.   Schuepbach, W.M.M.; Tonder, L.; Schnitzler, A.; Krack, P.; Rau, J.; Hartmann, A.; Halbig, T.D.; Pineau, F.;
      Falk, A.; Paschen, L.; et al. Quality of life predicts outcome of deep brain stimulation in early Parkinson
      disease. *Neurology* **2019**, *92*, e1109–e1120. [CrossRef] [PubMed]

7.   Lopez-Cuina, M.; Fernagut, P.O.; Canron, M.H.; Vital, A.; Lannes, B.; De Paula, A.M.; Streichenberger, N.;
      Guehl, D.; Damier, P.; Eusebio, A.; et al. Deep brain stimulation does not enhance neuroinflammation in
      multiple system atrophy. *Neurobiol. Dis.* **2018**, *118*, 155–160. [CrossRef]

8.   Schuepbach, W.M.; Rau, J.; Knudsen, K.; Volkmann, J.; Krack, P.; Timmermann, L.; Halbig, T.D.; Hesekamp, H.;
      Navarro, S.M.; Meier, N.; et al. Neurostimulation for Parkinson's disease with early motor complications.
      N. Engl. J. Med. **2013**, *368*, 610–622. [CrossRef]

9.   Vizcarra, J.A.; Situ-Kcomt, M.; Artusi, C.A.; Duker, A.P.; Lopiano, L.; Okun, M.S.; Espay, A.J.; Merola, A.
      Subthalamic deep brain stimulation and levodopa in Parkinson's disease: A meta-analysis of combined
      effects. *J. Neurol.* **2019**, *266*, 289–297. [CrossRef]

10.   Cabrera, L.Y.; Goudreau, J.; Sidiropoulos, C. Critical appraisal of the recent US FDA approval for earlier DBS
      intervention. *Neurology* **2018**, *91*, 133–136. [CrossRef]

11.   Mestre, T.A.; Espay, A.J.; Marras, C.; Eckman, M.H.; Pollak, P.; Lang, A.E. Subthalamic nucleus-deep brain
      stimulation for early motor complications in Parkinson's disease-the EARLYSTIM trial: Early is not always
      better. *Mov. Disord.* **2014**, *29*, 1751–1756. [CrossRef] [PubMed]

12.   Schupbach, W.M.; Rau, J.; Houeto, J.L.; Krack, P.; Schnitzler, A.; Schade-Brittinger, C.; Timmermann, L.;
      Deuschl, G. Myths and facts about the EARLYSTIM study. *Mov. Disord.* **2014**, *29*, 1742–1750. [CrossRef]
      [PubMed]

13.   Petrucci, S.; Ginevrino, M.; Trezzi, I.; Monfrini, E.; Ricciardi, L.; Albanese, A.; Avenali, M.; Barone, P.;
      Bentivoglio, A.R.; Bonifati, V.; et al. GBA-Related Parkinson's Disease: Dissection of Genotype-Phenotype
      Correlates in a Large Italian Cohort. *Mov. Disord.* **2020**. [CrossRef] [PubMed]

14.   Artusi, C.A.; Dwivedi, A.K.; Romagnolo, A.; Pal, G.; Kauffman, M.; Mata, I.; Patel, D.; Vizcarra, J.A.;
      Duker, A.; Marsili, L.; et al. Association of Subthalamic Deep Brain Stimulation With Motor, Functional,
      and Pharmacologic Outcomes in Patients With Monogenic Parkinson Disease: A Systematic Review and
      Meta-analysis. *JAMA Netw. Open* **2019**, *2*, e187800. [CrossRef] [PubMed]

15.   Merola, A.; Romagnolo, A.; Dwivedi, A.K.; Padovani, A.; Berg, D.; Garcia-Ruiz, P.J.; Fabbri, M.; Artusi, C.A.;
      Zibetti, M.; Lopiano, L.; et al. Benign versus malignant Parkinson disease: The unexpected silver lining of
      motor complications. *J. Neurol.* **2020**. [CrossRef]

16.   Barbe, M.T.; Tonder, L.; Krack, P.; Debu, B.; Schupbach, M.; Paschen, S.; Dembek, T.A.; Kuhn, A.A.; Fraix, V.;
      Brefel-Courbon, C.; et al. Deep Brain Stimulation for Freezing of Gait in Parkinson's Disease With Early
      Motor Complications. *Mov. Disord.* **2020**, *35*, 82–90. [CrossRef]

17.   Lhommee, E.; Wojtecki, L.; Czernecki, V.; Witt, K.; Maier, F.; Tonder, L.; Timmermann, L.; Halbig, T.D.;
      Pineau, F.; Durif, F.; et al. Behavioural outcomes of subthalamic stimulation and medical therapy versus
      medical therapy alone for Parkinson's disease with early motor complications (EARLYSTIM trial): Secondary
      analysis of an open-label randomised trial. *Lancet Neurol.* **2018**, *17*, 223–231. [CrossRef]

18.   Charles, D.; Konrad, P.E.; Neimat, J.S.; Molinari, A.L.; Tramontana, M.G.; Finder, S.G.; Gill, C.E.; Bliton, M.J.;
      Kao, C.; Phibbs, F.T.; et al. Subthalamic nucleus deep brain stimulation in early stage Parkinson's disease.
      Parkinsonism Relat. Disord. **2014**, *20*, 731–737. [CrossRef]

19.   Hacker, M.L.; Turchan, M.; Heusinkveld, L.E.; Currie, A.D.; Millan, S.H.; Molinari, A.L.; Konrad, P.E.;
      Davis, T.L.; Phibbs, F.T.; Hedera, P.; et al. Deep brain stimulation in early-stage Parkinson disease: Five-year
      outcomes. *Neurology* **2020**, *95*, e393–e401. [CrossRef]

20.   Fasano, A.; Merello, M. Fading of Deep Brain Stimulation Efficacy Versus Disease Progression: Untangling a
      Gordian Knot. *Mov. Disord. Clin. Pract.* **2020**, *7*, 747–749. [CrossRef]

21.   Zibetti, M.; Pesare, M.; Cinquepalmi, A.; Rosso, M.; Bergamasco, B.; Ducati, A.; Lanotte, M.; Lopiano, L. Antiparkinsonian therapy modifications in PD patients after STN DBS: A retrospective observational analysis. *Parkinsonism Relat. Disord.* **2008**, *14*, 608–612. [CrossRef] [PubMed]

22.   Castelli, L.; Perozzo, P.; Zibetti, M.; Crivelli, B.; Morabito, U.; Lanotte, M.; Cossa, F.; Bergamasco, B.; Lopiano, L. Chronic deep brain stimulation of the subthalamic nucleus for Parkinson's disease: Effects on cognition, mood, anxiety and personality traits. *Eur. Neurol.* **2006**, *55*, 136–144. [CrossRef] [PubMed]

23.   Merola, A.; Romagnolo, A.; Rizzi, L.; Rizzone, M.G.; Zibetti, M.; Lanotte, M.; Mandybur, G.; Duker, A.P.; Espay, A.J.; Lopiano, L. Impulse control behaviors and subthalamic deep brain stimulation in Parkinson disease. *J. Neurol.* **2017**, *264*, 40–48. [CrossRef] [PubMed]

24.   Saranza, G.; Lang, A.E. Levodopa challenge test: Indications, protocol, and guide. *J. Neurol.* **2020**. [CrossRef]

25.   Machado, A.G.; Deogaonkar, M.; Cooper, S. Deep brain stimulation for movement disorders: Patient selection and technical options. *Clevel. Clin. J. Med.* **2012**, *79* (Suppl. S2), S19–S24. [CrossRef]

26.   Bronstein, J.M.; Tagliati, M.; Alterman, R.L.; Lozano, A.M.; Volkmann, J.; Stefani, A.; Horak, F.B.; Okun, M.S.; Foote, K.D.; Krack, P.; et al. Deep brain stimulation for Parkinson disease: An expert consensus and review of key issues. *Arch. Neurol.* **2011**, *68*, 165. [CrossRef]

27.   Armstrong, M.J.; Okun, M.S. Choosing a Parkinson Disease Treatment. *JAMA* **2020**, *323*, 1420. [CrossRef]

28.   Benabid, A.L.; Benazzouz, A.; Hoffmann, D.; Limousin, P.; Krack, P.; Pollak, P. Long-term electrical inhibition of deep brain targets in movement disorders. *Mov. Disord.* **1998**, *13* (Suppl. S3), 119–125. [CrossRef]

29.   Merello, M.; Nouzeilles, M.I.; Arce, G.P.; Leiguarda, R. Accuracy of acute levodopa challenge for clinical prediction of sustained long-term levodopa response as a major criterion for idiopathic Parkinson's disease diagnosis. *Mov. Disord.* **2002**, *17*, 795–798. [CrossRef]

30.   Fahn, S.; Elton, R.; Members of the UPDRS Development Committee. The Unified Parkison's Disease Rating Scale. In *Recent Developments in Parkinson's Disease*; Fahn, S., Marsden, C.D., Calne, D.B., Goldstein, M., Eds.; Macmillan Health Care Information: Florham Park, NJ, USA, 1987; Volume 2, pp. 153–163, 293–304.

31.   Merello, M.; Gerschcovich, E.R.; Ballesteros, D.; Cerquetti, D. Correlation between the Movement Disorders Society Unified Parkinson's Disease rating scale (MDS-UPDRS) and the Unified Parkinson's Disease rating scale (UPDRS) during L-dopa acute challenge. *Parkinsonism Relat. Disord.* **2011**, *17*, 705–707. [CrossRef]

32.   Deuschl, G.; Follett, K.A.; Luo, P.; Rau, J.; Weaver, F.M.; Paschen, S.; Steigerwald, F.; Tonder, L.; Stoker, V.; Reda, D.J. Comparing two randomized deep brain stimulation trials for Parkinson's disease. *J. Neurosurg.* **2019**, 1–9. [CrossRef] [PubMed]

33.   Kleiner-Fisman, G.; Herzog, J.; Fisman, D.N.; Tamma, F.; Lyons, K.E.; Pahwa, R.; Lang, A.E.; Deuschl, G. Subthalamic nucleus deep brain stimulation: Summary and meta-analysis of outcomes. *Mov. Disord.* **2006**, *21* (Suppl. S14), S290–S304. [CrossRef]

34.   Fasano, A.; Aquino, C.C.; Krauss, J.K.; Honey, C.R.; Bloem, B.R. Axial disability and deep brain stimulation in patients with Parkinson disease. *Nat. Rev. Neurol.* **2015**, *11*, 98–110. [CrossRef] [PubMed]

35.   Fasano, A.; Bloem, B.R. Gait disorders. *Contin. Lifelong Learn. Neurol.* **2013**, *19*, 1344–1382. [CrossRef] [PubMed]

36.   Bakker, M.; Esselink, R.A.; Munneke, M.; Limousin-Dowsey, P.; Speelman, H.D.; Bloem, B.R. Effects of stereotactic neurosurgery on postural instability and gait in Parkinson's disease. *Mov. Disord.* **2004**, *19*, 1092–1099. [CrossRef] [PubMed]

37.   Zibetti, M.; Merola, A.; Rizzi, L.; Ricchi, V.; Angrisano, S.; Azzaro, C.; Artusi, C.A.; Arduino, N.; Marchisio, A.; Lanotte, M.; et al. Beyond nine years of continuous subthalamic nucleus deep brain stimulation in Parkinson's disease. *Mov. Disord.* **2011**, *26*, 2327–2334. [CrossRef] [PubMed]

38.   Rizzone, M.G.; Fasano, A.; Daniele, A.; Zibetti, M.; Merola, A.; Rizzi, L.; Piano, C.; Piccininni, C.; Romito, L.M.; Lopiano, L.; et al. Long-term outcome of subthalamic nucleus DBS in Parkinson's disease: From the advanced phase towards the late stage of the disease? *Parkinsonism Relat. Disord.* **2014**, *20*, 376–381. [CrossRef]

39.   Castrioto, A.; Lozano, A.M.; Poon, Y.Y.; Lang, A.E.; Fallis, M.; Moro, E. Ten-year outcome of subthalamic stimulation in Parkinson disease: A blinded evaluation. *Arch. Neurol.* **2011**, *68*, 1550–1556. [CrossRef] [PubMed]

40.   Fasano, A.; Romito, L.M.; Daniele, A.; Piano, C.; Zinno, M.; Bentivoglio, A.R.; Albanese, A. Motor and cognitive outcome in patients with Parkinson's disease 8 years after subthalamic implants. *Brain* **2010**, *133*, 2664–2676. [CrossRef]

41. Tripoliti, E.; Limousin, P.; Foltynie, T.; Candelario, J.; Aviles-Olmos, I.; Hariz, M.I.; Zrinzo, L. Predictive factors of speech intelligibility following subthalamic nucleus stimulation in consecutive patients with Parkinson's disease. *Mov. Disord.* **2014**, *29*, 532–538. [CrossRef]

42. Mei, S.; Li, J.; Middlebrooks, E.H.; Almeida, L.; Hu, W.; Zhang, Y.; Ramirez-Zamora, A.; Chan, P. New Onset On-Medication Freezing of Gait After STN-DBS in Parkinson's Disease. *Front. Neurol.* **2019**, *10*, 659. [CrossRef] [PubMed]

43. Vercruysse, S.; Vandenberghe, W.; Munks, L.; Nuttin, B.; Devos, H.; Nieuwboer, A. Effects of deep brain stimulation of the subthalamic nucleus on freezing of gait in Parkinson's disease: A prospective controlled study. *J. Neurol. Neurosurg. Psychiatry* **2014**, *85*, 871–877. [CrossRef] [PubMed]

44. Moreau, C.; Pennel-Ployart, O.; Pinto, S.; Plachez, A.; Annic, A.; Viallet, F.; Destee, A.; Defebvre, L. Modulation of dysarthropneumophonia by low-frequency STN DBS in advanced Parkinson's disease. *Mov. Disord.* **2011**, *26*, 659–663. [CrossRef] [PubMed]

45. Zibetti, M.; Moro, E.; Krishna, V.; Sammartino, F.; Picillo, M.; Munhoz, R.P.; Lozano, A.M.; Fasano, A. Low-frequency Subthalamic Stimulation in Parkinson's Disease: Long-term Outcome and Predictors. *Brain Stimul.* **2016**, *9*, 774–779. [CrossRef] [PubMed]

46. Golfre Andreasi, N.; Rispoli, V.; Contaldi, E.; Colucci, F.; Mongardi, L.; Cavallo, M.A.; Sensi, M. Deep brain stimulation and refractory freezing of gait in Parkinson's disease: Improvement with high-frequency current steering co-stimulation of subthalamic nucleus and substantia Nigra. *Brain Stimul.* **2020**, *13*, 280–283. [CrossRef]

47. Antonini, A.; Stoessl, A.J.; Kleinman, L.S.; Skalicky, A.M.; Marshall, T.S.; Sail, K.R.; Onuk, K.; Odin, P.L.A. Developing consensus among movement disorder specialists on clinical indicators for identification and management of advanced Parkinson's disease: A multi-country Delphi-panel approach. *Curr. Med. Res. Opin.* **2018**, *34*, 2063–2073. [CrossRef]

48. Artusi, C.A.; Zibetti, M.; Romagnolo, A.; Rizzone, M.G.; Merola, A.; Lopiano, L. Subthalamic deep brain stimulation and trunk posture in Parkinson's disease. *Acta Neurol. Scand.* **2018**, *137*, 481–487. [CrossRef]

49. Roediger, J.; Artusi, C.A.; Romagnolo, A.; Boyne, P.; Zibetti, M.; Lopiano, L.; Espay, A.J.; Fasano, A.; Merola, A. Effect of subthalamic deep brain stimulation on posture in Parkinson's disease: A blind computerized analysis. *Parkinsonism Relat. Disord.* **2019**, *62*, 122–127. [CrossRef]

50. Silva de Lima, A.L.; Evers, L.J.W.; Hahn, T.; Bataille, L.; Hamilton, J.L.; Little, M.A.; Okuma, Y.; Bloem, B.R.; Faber, M.J. Freezing of gait and fall detection in Parkinson's disease using wearable sensors: A systematic review. *J. Neurol.* **2017**, *264*, 1642–1654. [CrossRef]

51. Silva de Lima, A.L.; Smits, T.; Darweesh, S.K.L.; Valenti, G.; Milosevic, M.; Pijl, M.; Baldus, H.; de Vries, N.M.; Meinders, M.J.; Bloem, B.R. Home-based monitoring of falls using wearable sensors in Parkinson's disease. *Mov. Disord.* **2020**, *35*, 109–115. [CrossRef]

52. Cebi, I.; Scholten, M.; Gharabaghi, A.; Weiss, D. Clinical and Kinematic Correlates of Favorable Gait Outcomes From Subthalamic Stimulation. *Front. Neurol.* **2020**, *11*, 212. [CrossRef] [PubMed]

53. Deuschl, G.; Schade-Brittinger, C.; Krack, P.; Volkmann, J.; Schafer, H.; Botzel, K.; Daniels, C.; Deutschlander, A.; Dillmann, U.; Eisner, W.; et al. A randomized trial of deep-brain stimulation for Parkinson's disease. *N. Engl. J. Med.* **2006**, *355*, 896–908. [CrossRef] [PubMed]

54. Erb, M.K.; Karlin, D.R.; Ho, B.K.; Thomas, K.C.; Parisi, F.; Vergara-Diaz, G.P.; Daneault, J.F.; Wacnik, P.W.; Zhang, H.; Kangarloo, T.; et al. mHealth and wearable technology should replace motor diaries to track motor fluctuations in Parkinson's disease. *NPJ Digit. Med.* **2020**, *3*, 6. [CrossRef] [PubMed]

55. Espay, A.J.; Hausdorff, J.M.; Sanchez-Ferro, A.; Klucken, J.; Merola, A.; Bonato, P.; Paul, S.S.; Horak, F.B.; Vizcarra, J.A.; Mestre, T.A.; et al. A roadmap for implementation of patient-centered digital outcome measures in Parkinson's disease obtained using mobile health technologies. *Mov. Disord.* **2019**, *34*, 657–663. [CrossRef]

56. Capecci, M.; Pepa, L.; Verdini, F.; Ceravolo, M.G. A smartphone-based architecture to detect and quantify freezing of gait in Parkinson's disease. *Gait Posture* **2016**, *50*, 28–33. [CrossRef]

57. Jenkinson, C.; Fitzpatrick, R.; Peto, V.; Greenhall, R.; Hyman, N. The Parkinson's Disease Questionnaire (PDQ-39): Development and validation of a Parkinson's disease summary index score. *Age Ageing* **1997**, *26*, 353–357. [CrossRef]

58. Jenkinson, C.; Fitzpatrick, R. Cross-cultural evaluation of the short form 8-item Parkinson's Disease Questionnaire (PDQ-8): Results from America, Canada, Japan, Italy and Spain. *Parkinsonism Relat. Disord.* **2007**, *13*, 22–28. [CrossRef]

59. Schwab, R.S.; England, A.C. Projection techniques for evaluating surgery in Parkinson's Disease. In Proceedings of the Third Symposium on Parkinson's Disease, Royal College of Surgeons in Edinburgh, Edinburgh, UK, 20–22 May 1968.

60. Karl, J.A.; Ouyang, B.; Colletta, K.; Verhagen Metman, L. Long-Term Satisfaction and Patient-Centered Outcomes of Deep Brain Stimulation in Parkinson's Disease. *Brain Sci.* **2018**, *8*, 60. [CrossRef]

61. Barthel, C.; Mallia, E.; Debu, B.; Bloem, B.R.; Ferraye, M.U. The Practicalities of Assessing Freezing of Gait. *J. Parkinsons Dis.* **2016**, *6*, 667–674. [CrossRef]

62. Floden, D.; Cooper, S.E.; Griffith, S.D.; Machado, A.G. Predicting quality of life outcomes after subthalamic nucleus deep brain stimulation. *Neurology* **2014**, *83*, 1627–1633. [CrossRef]

63. Geraedts, V.J.; Feleus, S.; Marinus, J.; van Hilten, J.J.; Contarino, M.F. What predicts quality of life after subthalamic deep brain stimulation in Parkinson's disease? A systematic review. *Eur. J. Neurol.* **2020**, *27*, 419–428. [CrossRef]

64. Barone, P.; Antonini, A.; Colosimo, C.; Marconi, R.; Morgante, L.; Avarello, T.P.; Bottacchi, E.; Cannas, A.; Ceravolo, G.; Ceravolo, R.; et al. The PRIAMO study: A multicenter assessment of nonmotor symptoms and their impact on quality of life in Parkinson's disease. *Mov. Disord.* **2009**, *24*, 1641–1649. [CrossRef] [PubMed]

65. Dafsari, H.S.; Reddy, P.; Herchenbach, C.; Wawro, S.; Petry-Schmelzer, J.N.; Visser-Vandewalle, V.; Rizos, A.; Silverdale, M.; Ashkan, K.; Samuel, M.; et al. Beneficial Effects of Bilateral Subthalamic Stimulation on Non-Motor Symptoms in Parkinson's Disease. *Brain Stimul.* **2016**, *9*, 78–85. [CrossRef] [PubMed]

66. Dafsari, H.S.; Silverdale, M.; Strack, M.; Rizos, A.; Ashkan, K.; Mahlstedt, P.; Sachse, L.; Steffen, J.; Dembek, T.A.; Visser-Vandewalle, V.; et al. Nonmotor symptoms evolution during 24 months of bilateral subthalamic stimulation in Parkinson's disease. *Mov. Disord.* **2018**, *33*, 421–430. [CrossRef] [PubMed]

67. Jost, S.T.; Ray Chaudhuri, K.; Ashkan, K.; Loehrer, P.A.; Silverdale, M.; Rizos, A.; Evans, J.; Petry-Schmelzer, J.N.; Barbe, M.T.; Sauerbier, A.; et al. Subthalamic Stimulation Improves Quality of Sleep in Parkinson Disease: A 36-Month Controlled Study. *J. Parkinsons Dis.* **2020**, 1–13. [CrossRef]

68. Ricciardi, L.; Sorbera, C.; Barbuto, M.; Morgante, F. Sleep disturbances are mainly improved by deep brain stimulation of the subthalamic nucleus. *Mov. Disord.* **2019**, *34*, 154–155. [CrossRef]

69. Jost, S.T.; Sauerbier, A.; Visser-Vandewalle, V.; Ashkan, K.; Silverdale, M.; Evans, J.; Loehrer, P.A.; Rizos, A.; Petry-Schmelzer, J.N.; Reker, P.; et al. A prospective, controlled study of non-motor effects of subthalamic stimulation in Parkinson's disease: Results at the 36-month follow-up. *J. Neurol. Neurosurg. Psychiatry* **2020**, *91*, 687–694. [CrossRef]

70. Fereshtehnejad, S.M.; Zeighami, Y.; Dagher, A.; Postuma, R.B. Clinical criteria for subtyping Parkinson's disease: Biomarkers and longitudinal progression. *Brain* **2017**, *140*, 1959–1976. [CrossRef]

71. De Pablo-Fernandez, E.; Lees, A.J.; Holton, J.L.; Warner, T.T. Prognosis and Neuropathologic Correlation of Clinical Subtypes of Parkinson Disease. *JAMA Neurol.* **2019**, *76*, 470–479. [CrossRef]

72. Parkinson Disease Phenotype Classification Predicts the Outcome of Deep Brain Stimulation. Available online: https://www.mdsabstracts.org/abstract/parkinson-disease-phenotype-classification-predicts-the-outcome-of-deep-brain-stimulation/ (accessed on 3 December 2020).

73. Petry-Schmelzer, J.N.; Krause, M.; Dembek, T.A.; Horn, A.; Evans, J.; Ashkan, K.; Rizos, A.; Silverdale, M.; Schumacher, W.; Sack, C.; et al. Non-motor outcomes depend on location of neurostimulation in Parkinson's disease. *Brain* **2019**, *142*, 3592–3604. [CrossRef]

74. Bandres-Ciga, S.; Diez-Fairen, M.; Kim, J.J.; Singleton, A.B. Genetics of Parkinson's disease: An introspection of its journey towards precision medicine. *Neurobiol. Dis.* **2020**, *137*, 104782. [CrossRef] [PubMed]

75. Rizzone, M.G.; Martone, T.; Balestrino, R.; Lopiano, L. Genetic background and outcome of Deep Brain Stimulation in Parkinson's disease. *Parkinsonism Relat. Disord.* **2019**, *64*, 8–19. [CrossRef] [PubMed]

76. De Oliveira, L.M.; Barbosa, E.R.; Aquino, C.C.; Munhoz, R.P.; Fasano, A.; Cury, R.G. Deep Brain Stimulation in Patients With Mutations in Parkinson's Disease-Related Genes: A Systematic Review. *Mov. Disord. Clin. Pract.* **2019**, *6*, 359–368. [CrossRef] [PubMed]

77. Kuusimaki, T.; Korpela, J.; Pekkonen, E.; Martikainen, M.H.; Antonini, A.; Kaasinen, V. Deep brain stimulation for monogenic Parkinson's disease: A systematic review. *J. Neurol.* **2020**, *267*, 883–897. [CrossRef] [PubMed]

78.   Marras, C.; Schule, B.; Munhoz, R.P.; Rogaeva, E.; Langston, J.W.; Kasten, M.; Meaney, C.; Klein, C.; Wadia, P.M.; Lim, S.Y.; et al. Phenotype in parkinsonian and nonparkinsonian LRRK2 G2019S mutation carriers. *Neurology* **2011**, *77*, 325–333. [CrossRef]

79.   Cilia, R.; Tunesi, S.; Marotta, G.; Cereda, E.; Siri, C.; Tesei, S.; Zecchinelli, A.L.; Canesi, M.; Mariani, C.B.; Meucci, N.; et al. Survival and dementia in GBA-associated Parkinson's disease: The mutation matters. *Ann. Neurol.* **2016**, *80*, 662–673. [CrossRef]

Deep Brain Stimulation for Treatment-Resistant Depression: Towards a More Personalized Treatment Approach

Milaine Roet [1,2], **Jackson Boonstra** [1,2], **Erdi Sahin** [3], **Anne E.P. Mulders** [1,2,4],
Albert F.G. Leentjens [2,4] **and Ali Jahanshahi** [1,2,*]

1   Department of Neurosurgery, Maastricht University Medical Center, P. Debyelaan 25,
    6202 AZ Maastricht, The Netherlands; m.roet@maastrichtuniversity.nl (M.R.);
    j.boonstra@maastrichtuniversity.nl (J.B.); a.mulders@maastrichtuniversity.nl (A.E.P.M.)
2   European Graduate School of Neuroscience (EURON); 6229 ER Maastricht, The Netherlands;
    a.leentjens@maastrichtuniversity.nl
3   Department of Neurology, Istanbul Faculty of Medicine, Istanbul University Capa, Istanbul 34093, Turkey;
    erdisahin@gmail.com
4   Department of Psychiatry and Psychology, Maastricht University Medical Center, P. Debyelaan 25,
    6202 AZ Maastricht, The Netherlands
*   Correspondence: a.jahanshahi@maastrichtuniversity.nl

Abstract: Major depressive disorder (MDD) affects approximately 4.4% of the world's population. One third of MDD patients do not respond to routine psychotherapeutic and pharmacotherapeutic treatment and are said to suffer from treatment-resistant depression (TRD). Deep brain stimulation (DBS) is increasingly being investigated as a treatment modality for TRD. Although early case studies showed promising results of DBS, open-label trials and placebo-controlled studies have reported inconsistent outcomes. This has raised discussion about the correct interpretation of trial results as well as the criteria for patient selection, the choice of stimulation target, and the optimal stimulation parameters. In this narrative review, we summarize recent studies of the effectiveness of DBS in TRD and address the relation between the targeted brain structures and clinical outcomes. Elaborating upon that, we hypothesize that the effectiveness of DBS in TRD can be increased by a more personalized and symptom-based approach. This may be achieved by using resting-state connectivity mapping for neurophysiological subtyping of TRD, by using individualized tractography to help decisions about stimulation target and electrode placement, and by using a more detailed registration of symptomatic improvements during DBS, for instance by using 'experience sampling' methods.

Keywords: major depressive disorder; treatment resistant depression; deep brain stimulation; neuropsychological subtypes; personalized treatment approach

1. Introduction

Major depressive disorder (MDD) is a common mood disorder that affects one's feelings, thoughts, and behavior. According to the DSM-5, for a diagnosis of MDD, five of the following symptoms need to be present for at least two weeks: depressed mood, reduced interest or pleasure, weight loss or reduced appetite, insomnia or hypersomnia, psychomotor agitation or retardation, fatigue or loss of energy, worthlessness or excessive guilt, impaired concentration or indecisiveness, and recurrent thoughts of death or suicidal ideation or attempts. Either 'depressed mood' or 'loss of interest or pleasure' is essential for a diagnosis [1]. The total number of people suffering from MDD worldwide was estimated to be 322 million in 2015 and its prevalence increased by 18.4% between 2005 and 2015 [2]. Therefore, effective treatment of MDD merits intense consideration.

Whereas psychotherapy and antidepressant medication are effective in the majority of patients, approximately one third of patients do not respond to these therapies. In the Sequenced Treatment Alternatives to Relieve Depression (STAR*D) trial, the cumulative remission rate of MDD patients after four successive treatments was 67% [3]. In line with this, a meta-analysis of 92 studies of the effectiveness of psychotherapy showed that 62% of patients no longer met the criteria of depression after treatment [4]. Failure to respond to a treatment algorithm of several steps is commonly referred to as treatment resistance, although there is still discussion about the exact definition of treatment refractoriness [5]. Treatment-resistant depression (TRD) is associated with more (comorbid) mental health disorders, a higher number of hospitalizations, and more suicide attempts, leading to higher treatment costs compared to non-TRD [6]. In addition, patients with TRD show a higher demand of healthcare resources and costs of health care compared to non-TRD patients [7]. Various alternative treatment options for TRD are currently being investigated, including vagal nerve stimulation [8], repetitive transcranial magnetic stimulation (rTMS) [9], and deep brain stimulation (DBS) [10].

The aim of this narrative review is to provide an overview of recent studies of the effectiveness of DBS in TRD with a special focus on the relationship between the targeted brain structures and clinical outcomes. Based on these findings, we discuss the importance of distinguishing between different clinical phenotypes of depression that would allow for more personalized symptom-based treatment approaches, which may be a key factor in improving treatment outcomes.

2. Recent Insights on the Pathophysiology of Depression

It is hypothesized that in depression, there is an imbalance in the limbic cortico-striatal-thalamo-cortical (CSTC) mood circuits [11,12], yet many aspects of circuitopathy in MDD remain largely unknown. Based on different models [11,12], three main components of the CSTC mood circuits have been proposed (Figure 1). First, the ventral component is essential for recognizing emotions and initiating an adequate emotional and behavioral response. In this circuit, the amygdala, ventral striatum, ventral part of the anterior cingulate cortex, orbitofrontal cortex, ventrolateral prefrontal cortex, and downstream structures such as the hypothalamus and locus coeruleus are involved. Second, the dorsal component that regulates the emotional responses and requires cognitive processing. Here, the dorsolateral and dorsomedial prefrontal cortex, the dorsal part of the anterior cingulate cortex, and the hippocampus are involved. Third, a modulating region is present, although no consensus has been made about its precise anatomical organization and function. Some have suggested that this component consists of the thalamus and the rostral part of the anterior cingulate cortex [11–13]. As implied by Mayberg et al., the model of depression indicates that depression is associated with a decreased activity in dorsal limbic and neocortical regions and a relative increase in ventral paralimbic regions. Treatment of depression therefore requires the inhibition of the overactive ventral regions, resulting in the disinhibition of the underactive dorsal regions. To mediate this process, proper functioning of the rostral cingulate cortex is required [12]. These mood circuits overlap with the circuitry involved in compulsive traits; DBS of the ventral capsule/ventral striatum (VC/VS) in treatment resistant obsessive-compulsive disorder (OCD) patients has led to improvements in mood which prompted studying the application of DBS in TRD patients [14,15].

Figure 1. Schematic representation of emotional processing and its neurobiological base. Figure from Moonen et al. (2017) [16] with permission.

Expanding the Cortico-Striatal-Thalamo-Cortical Mood Circuits

One region that is not included in the CSTC mood circuits and yet has been a region of interest for DBS targeting in depression for over a decade is the subgenual cingulate gyrus/cortex (SCG/SCC) [10]. This region has shown hyperactivity in untreated depressed patients [17], is part of the ventral component, and has projections to the amygdala, hippocampus, superior and medial temporal gyri, ventral striatum, mid- and posterior cingulate cortex, thalamus, hypothalamus, periaqueductal gray, and lateral habenula [18,19]. Furthermore, in recent years, it has become known that several other brain areas all belonging to the ventral component play a role in the pathophysiology of depression. Among these are the thalamic peduncles (THp) that interconnects with the prefrontal cortex including the orbitofrontal cortex (OFC) [20], the medial forebrain bundle (MFB) that projects to the frontal cortex, the NAcc and ventral striatum [21], and the ventral part of the anterior limb of the internal capsule (vALIC) which forms a homeostatic system with the MFB and the bed nucleus of the stria terminalis (BNST) [22] (Figure 2).

Figure 2. Cortico-striatal-thalamic-cortico mood circuits divided in a dorsal, ventral, and modulating compartment based on Alexander et al. [11], Mayberg et al. [12], and Moonen et al. [16] expanded with regions researched with deep brain stimulation (DBS) for treatment-resistant depression (TRD). DLPFC; dorsolateral prefrontal cortex, DMPFC; dorsomedial prefrontal cortex, ACC; anterior cingulate cortex, THp; thalamic peduncles, OFC; orbitofrontal cortex, VLPFC; ventrolateral prefrontal cortex, MFB; medial forebrain bundle, vALIC, ventral part of the anterior limb of the internal capsule, BNST; bed nucleus of the stria terminalis, SCG; subgenual cingulate gyrus, HPA axis; hypothalamic pituitary adrenal axis.

3. Deep Brain Stimulation for Treatment-Resistant Depression

DBS is an invasive neuromodulation technique that is effective in managing clinical symptoms of neurological and psychiatric disorders, such as Parkinson's disease (PD) [23,24] and OCD [25]. At stimulation settings commonly used in clinical practice, DBS decreases the spontaneous firing of neuronal populations and activates axonal projections near the electrode [26]. This modulates pathological activity and replaces it with regular patterns of discharge with intervals of burst activity [27, 28]. More recent theories suggest that DBS destabilizes abnormal synchronous oscillatory activity within the basal ganglia circuitry improving hyperkinetic symptomology [24]. However, the exact mechanism(s) by which DBS normalizes electrical activity in the basal ganglia and exerts beneficial effects on PD symptoms remain unknown. In DBS for TRD, target selection has mostly been based on either neuroimaging studies or clinical observations of mood improvement following DBS in OCD [10,15,29]. For these reasons, the underlying mechanisms of action are poorly studied. DBS studies for TRD (Table 1) and the outcomes for selected brain targets (Table 2) are described below.

Table 1. DBS in treatment-resistant depression (TRD); published open-label and randomized clinical trials.

Region (DBS)	Study	Open-Labeled, RCT or Case-Report	N	Follow-Up	Age (Mean)	Length of Current Depressive Episode, Years (Mean)	Response Rate (%) in HDRS or MADRS Scores	Remission Rate (%)	Serious Adverse Events (N)
SCG	Mayberg et al., 2005	Open-label	6	6 months	46	5.58	33.3 (1 month), # 83 (2 months), # 66.6 (6 months), #	0 (1 month) 33.3 (3 months) 33.3 (6 months)	Suicidal ideation: 2 Syncope: 1 Lead problem: 1
	Lozano et al., 2008	Open-label	20	12 months	47.4	6.9	60 (6 months), # 55 (12 months), #	35 (6 months) 35 (12 months)	Seizure: 1 Lead problem: 3
	Kennedy et al., 2011	Open-label	20	1, 2 and 3 years, last follow-up (3–6 years)	47.4	6.9	62.5 (1 year), # 46.2 (2 year), # 75 (3 years), # 64.3 (last follow-up), #	18.8 (1 year) 15.4 (2 years) 50 (3 years)	Worsening depression:3 Suicidal ideation:3
	Puigdemont et al., 2012	Open-label	8	12 months	47.4	6.3	87.5 (1 week), # 37.5 (1 month), # 87.5 (6 months), # 62.5 (12 months), #	50 (1 week) 37.5 (6 months) 50 (12 months)	Suicide attempt: 1
	Lozano et al., 2012	Open-label	21	12 months	47.3	5.0	57 (1 month), # 48 (6 months), # 29 (12 months), #	-	Suicide: 1 Suicide attempt: 1
	Holtzheimer et al., 2012	Open-label	17	24 months	42	5.34	41 (6 months), # 36 (12 months), # 92 (24 months), #	18 (6 months) 36 (12 months) 58 (24 months)	Suicidal ideation: 1 Suicide attempt: 2
	Merkl et al., 2013	Open-label	6	24 h Last follow up (24–36 weeks)	50.66	2.13	33.33 (36 weeks), #	33.33 (36 weeks)	Headaches: 6 Tenseness in neck region: 1
	Holtzheimer et al., 2017	RCT	60 (52)	6 months (24 months)	50.53	12.62	22 (6 months), ‡ 54 (12 months), ‡ 48 (24 months), ‡	10 (6 months) 17 (12 months) 25 (24 months)	Suicide attempt: 2 Suicidal ideation: 2 Seizure: 2
	Eitan et al., 2018	RCT HF vs. LF DBS	9	13 months	46	-	44.44 (13 months), ‡	-	-

Table 1. *Cont.*

Region (DBS)	Study	Open-Labeled, RCT or Case-Report	N	Follow-Up	Age (Mean)	Length of Current Depressive Episode, Years (Mean)	Response Rate (%) in HDRS or MADRS Scores	Remission Rate (%)	Serious Adverse Events (N)
	Merkl et al., 2018	RCT	8	28 months ($n = 6$) 4 years ($n = 2$)	48.25	2	37.5 (6 months), # 43.0 (12 months), # 23.0 (28 months), #	12.5 (6 months) 14.2 (12 months) 33.0 (24 months) 33.3 (28 months)	Manic episode: 1
	Crowell et al., 2019	Open-label	28	4 ($n = 14$) 8 ($n = 11$) years	44.9 (45.9)	45.1 (46.6)	18 #	21	Suicide attempt: 6 Suicidal ideation: 8 Anxiety: 6 Worsening depression: 2
PGR	Accolla et al., 2016	Open-label	5 (1)	6 months (24 months)	45.20	-	-	-	-
NAcc	Schlaepfer et al., 2008	Open-label	3	6–24 weeks	46.7	7.2	-	-	None
	Bewernick et al., 2010	Open-label	10	10 months	48.6	10.8	50 (1 month), # 50 (6 months), # 50 (12 months), #	30 (1 month)	Suicide: 1 Suicide attempt: 1
	Bewernick et al., 2012	Open-label	11	12 months 24 months Last follow up (max 4 years)	48.36	9.26	45 (12 months), #	9.1 (24 months)	Pain: 4 Seizure: 1 Agitation: 3 Suicide:1 Suicide attempt: 1
VC/VS	Malone et al., 2009	Open-label	15	6 months ($n = 15$) 12 months ($n = 11$)	46.3	21	20 (1 month), # 40 (6 months), # 53.3 (last follow-up) #	20 (6 months) 40 (last follow-up)	Suicidal ideation: 2 Syncope: 1 Lead problem: 1
	Dougherty et al., 2015	RCT	30	24 months	47.7	11.4	20 (16 weeks), ¥ 20 (12 months), ¥ 23.3 (24 months), ¥	13 (12 months) 20 (24 months)	Suicide: 1 (stimulation off) Suicide attempt: 4 Suicidal ideation: 5 Lead revision: 3

Table 1. *Cont.*

Region (DBS)	Study	Open-Labeled, RCT or Case-Report	N	Follow-Up	Age (Mean)	Length of Current Depressive Episode, Years (Mean)	Response Rate (%) in HDRS or MADRS Scores	Remission Rate (%)	Serious Adverse Events (N)
vALIC	Van der Wal et al., 2020 (follow-up of the RCT Bergfeld et al. 2016)	Open-label	25	2 years	52.5	7.42	32.0 (2 years, ITT) #	20.0 (2 years, ITT)	Pain: 1 Agitation: 3 Suicidal ideation: 6 Fatigue: 4
	Bergfeld et al., 2016	RCT	25	52 weeks	53.2	6.98	40 (after optimization of DBS settings (T_2)) #	20 (T_2)	Suicide attempt: 4 Suicidal ideation: 3 Automutilation: 1
LHb	Sartorius et al., 2009	Case-report	1	60 weeks	64.0	9.0	-	-	-
MFB	Schlaepfer et al., 2013	Open-label	7	12–33 weeks	42.6	7.6	86, ¥	57	Cranial bleeding: 1
	Fenoy et al., 2016 (interim analysis)	Open-label	4	52 weeks	-	-	75 (7 days) ¥66 (26 weeks, OC) ¥	-	-

"-": has not been mentioned in this article, RCT; response criteria; #; 50% or greater reduction in Hamilton Depression Rating Scale (HDRS) (17 or 28) scores, ¥; 50% or greater reduction in MADRS scores, ‡; 40% or greater reduction in MADRS scores, RCT; randomized controlled trial, ITT; intention to treat, OC; observed case.

Table 2. Targets for DBS in treatment resistant depression (TRD), functions, pathophysiology and the effect of DBS.

Brain Region	Function	Pathological Activity in MDD	HF-DBS Effect
SCG	Contains three white matter bundles; forceps minor + uncinate fasciculus connecting to the medial frontal cortex, cingulum connecting to the rostral and dorsal ACC and fronto-striatal fibers connecting to the NAcc, CN, Pt and anterior Th. Connects higher 'top-down' cortical regions with subcortical modulatory regions. Involvement in brain DMN [30]	Increased activity [31] Reduced volume in familial depression [32] Projections to: (1) NAcc may play a role in lack of interest, disruption in reward and underlie anhedonia (2) Hth and brainstem may play a role in circadian and sleep disturbances, problems with appetite and an abnormal stress responds and cortisol metabolism [31].	Disruption of pathological activity Modulation of multiple regions connected to the SCG [31]
NAcc	Receives projections from VTA, AG, OFC, mPFC, dCN, GP and Hip and projects to Cg25, mPFC, VP, Th, AG and Hth. Transmits information from emotion centers to motor control regions, causing motivational behavior to obtain rewards [33] Processes reward and pleasure information	In severe anhedonia; smaller size and less activation to reward [34]	Acute: Increase in exploratory motivation Chronic: reduction in anhedonia PET Imaging: ↑ activity in VS, bilateral dlPFC and dmPFC, cingulate cortex and bilateral AG. ↓ activity in vmPFC and vlPFC, dCN and Th [33]
VC/VS	Contains fibers connecting the dPFC, dACC, OFC and vmPFC with THAL, AG, Hth and brainstem (SN, VTA, RN and PTN) [35]	Increased activity [36] Activation of the connection from left vs. to left caudate has been associated with anhedonia Increased connectivity of vs. to DMN is positively correlated to higher depression scores in the CES-D score [37]	-
vALIC	Contains two fiber bundles: the anterior thalamic radiation and the supero-lateral branch of the MFB connecting the PFC to different subcortical structures such as the Th, NAcc, VTA and VS. Decreased integrity of the right vALIC in depressed patients [38]	-	Decreased metabolism in OFC, subgenual ACC and right DLPFC in patients with OCD [39]
LHb	Activity corresponds negatively to anticipation and reception of a reward [40]	Increased activity [41] Possible down regulation of serotonergic, noradrenergic and dopaminergic systems [42], volume reduction [43]	Localized metabolic increase in one patient with FDG-PET, presumably due to functional inhibition [44]
ITP	Interconnects the intralaminar nucleus and TRN with the OFC [30,45]	Hyperactivation in both TRN and OFC [46]	Cortical desynchronization Disruption of adrenergic and serotonergic malfunction [46]

Table 2. *Cont.*

Brain Region	Function	Pathological Activity in MDD	HF-DBS Effect
MFB	Interconnects the Nacc, VTA, vmHth, lHth and AG ventromedial and lateral nuclei of the Hth and AG with convergence onto the PFC [47,48] Plays a crucial role in the reward pathway;	Dysfunctional reward system. Responders showed a strong connectivity between the active electrode contact and the mPFC pre-operatively using individual DTI [49]	Insignificant changes in metabolism in 3 patients with PET measurements pre-operatively, 6 and 12 months post-operatively [49]
BNST	Mayor output pathway of the AG Regulates stress response Integrates information from multiple brain areas to perform 'valence surveillance' [22,30]	Oscillatory activity with high α-power [50]	-

"-": not investigated; (d) ACC; (dorsal) anterior cingulate cortex, AG; amygdala, CES-D score; center for epidemiologic studies depression score, (d) CN; (dorsal) caudate nucleus, DMN; default mode network, DTI; deterministic diffusion tensor imaging, GP; globus pallidus, Hip; hippocampus, Hth; hypothalamus, MFB; medial forebrain bundle, OFC; Orbitofrontal cortex, (m/dl/dm/vm/vl) PFC (medial/dorsolateral/dorsomedial/ventromedial/ventrolateral) Prefrontal cortex, PGR; posterior gyrus rectus, PTN; pedunculopontine tegmental nucleus, Pt: putamen, RN; raphe nuclei, SN; substantia nigra, Th; thalamus, TRN; thalamic reticular nucleus, VP; ventral pallidum, VS; ventral striatum, VTA; ventral tegmental area.

3.1. Subgenual Cingulate Gyrus/Cortex

The first clinical trial of DBS of the SCG for TRD was performed in 2005 and included six patients with MDD [10]. The severity of depression was measured using the Hamilton Depression Rating Scale (HDRS) and the Montgomory Asberg Depression Rating Scale (MADRS). The HDRS has been the gold standard for the assessment of depression for years [51]. A clinical response is commonly defined as a decrease in the HDRS score of more than 50% compared to baseline, and clinical remission is defined as a decrease in the HDRS score to eight or less. After one month, two out of six patients met the criteria for response. At the end of the sixth month, a response was seen in four out of six patients, with three of the patients reaching remission or near remission. Preliminary observations with positron emission tomography (PET) showed a metabolic hyperactive SCG (Brodmann area 25, Cg 25) during depressive states. It was speculated that DBS would reduce this hyperactivity [17] (Table 2). The improvement in depression scores after DBS was thought to be due to effectively disrupting focal pathological activity in limbic-cortical circuits. After 3 months of stimulation of the subgenual cingulate region (CG25) in patients suffering from TRD, local cerebral blood flow (CBF) was decreased in CG25 and the adjacent orbitofrontal cortex (Brodmann area 11). Moreover, after three and six months of stimulation, CBF was decreased in the hypothalamus, anterior insula, and medial frontal cortex of long-term responders, while CBF increased in the dorsolateral prefrontal cortex (dlPFC), dorsal anterior, posterior cingulate, and premotor and parietal regions (Table 2) [10]. In the different open-label trials, response rates varied from 20 to 57% after 1 month, 33.3 to 87.5% after 6 months, and 29 to 62.5% after 12 months (Table 1) [10,33,49,52–61]. In a long term follow-up, Kennedy et al. (2011) reported response rates at 1, 2, and 3 years after DBS implantation in the SCC of TRD patients of 62.5%, 46,2%, and 75%, respectively [52] (Table 1). In a case series of DBS of the SCG in five TRD patients, a decrease in the score of the depression rating scale was only found in one of the five TRD patients. This patient turned out to be stimulated in the posterior gyrus rectus (PGR) based on single subject tractography results rather than the initially targeted CG25 [62]. A recent exploratory meta-analysis of four observational studies investigating DBS for TRD (Holtzheimer et al. 2012, Lozano et al. 2012, Puigdemont et al. 2012, and Kennedy et al. 2011) reported relatively large response and remission rates following DBS treatment: the twelve-month response and remission rates were 39.9% (95% CI = 28.4% to 52.8%) and 26.3% (95% CI = 13% to 45.9%). The included studies reported a significant decrease in depression scores between 3 and 6 months (Hedges' g = −0.27, p = 0.003), while no additional decrease was found between 6 and 12 months, suggesting that maximal antidepressant effects occur mostly within the first 6 months of treatment [63]. However, adverse events can occur, including worsening of depression, suicidal ideation, and seizures (Table 1). A study consisting of a double-blind active vs. sham stimulation phase of four weeks, followed by an open-label stimulation for up to 24 months, reported no significant differences between the active and sham stimulation of the SCG and no reduction in HDRS scores in the first four weeks. In the open-label phase, response rates were 37.5%, 43% and 23% after 6, 12 and 28 months, respectively. Remission rates were 12.5% and 14.2% at 6 and 12 months, respectively, and 33.3% at 24 and 28 months [64].

A randomized controlled trial (RCT) investigating DBS of the subcallosal cingulate, known as the BROADEN trial, was aborted prematurely. The study lasted six months, during which all patients should have received SCC implantation surgery. After six months, blinding would have been uncovered and both groups would have been offered open-label DBS for another six months. At the end of the first six months, responses of the treatment group and control group were predicted to be 40% and 18.5%, respectively. In this trial, the response rate was defined as more than or equal to a 40% decrease in MADRS scores from baseline. However, after six months, only 20% of patients (n = 12) in the treatment group showed a response versus 17% of patients (n = 5) in the control group. At that time, a futility analysis predicted the probability of a successful study outcome to be 17% or less leading to the funding for DBS electrodes for this study to be discontinued. The actual study was never published, but results were published and mentioned in Morishita et al. (2014) [65,66]. It has been postulated that the patients enrolled in the BROADEN trial had extreme and chronic depression with a mean duration of the current depressive episode of 12 years, nearly twice that of previous open-label studies. Therefore, these patients could have required a longer treatment period before significant results emerge. Long-term outcomes of SCG DBS in TRD patients for up to 8 years show that most patients have a sustained antidepressant response [60]. However, these results need to be interpreted carefully as the patient group consisted of both MDD and bipolar type-II disorder patients. Further comparison between high- and low frequency DBS in the SCG in TRD showed no significant difference in effectiveness between the two groups and a 44.44% response rate at 13 months of stimulation [67].

3.2. Nucleus Accumbens

Another brain region involved in MDD is the nucleus accumbens (NAcc), part of the mesolimbic dopaminergic circuit involved in different cognitive functions such as motivation and reward [33] (Table 2). DBS of the NAcc exerts immediate and long-term positive clinical effects in TRD and has been shown to significantly improve depression scores within one week [33]. Visualized with PET–computed tomography (PET-CT or PET/CT), NAcc-DBS increased metabolic activity in the ventral striatum, dlPFC, dorsomedial PFC (dmPFC), cingulate cortex, and the amygdala. Furthermore, metabolic activity in the vmPFC, ventrolateral prefrontal cortex (vlPFC), dorsal caudate nucleus, and part of the thalamus were decreased. Targeting the NAcc was essential for the effect of DBS on anhedonia (i.e., the inability to feel pleasure) in patients suffering from TRD. However, when Schlaepfer et al. (2008) looked at single items of depression rating scales, capturing aspects of anhedonia such as 'work and activities', 'apparent sadness', and the 'inability to feel', no significant improvements were found following NAcc-DBS. A follow-up study showed a 50% response rate in 10 patients suffering from TRD undergoing NAcc-DBS after 10 months [53]. In a more recent study reporting the long term effects of NAcc-DBS, 45% of TRD patients ($n = 11$) were classified as responders with a 50% reduction in HDRS scores after 12 months of stimulation, which remained until the last follow-up of 4 years [54] (Table 1). Several side effects were reported, such as seizure, agitation, and a transient increase in anxiety. In addition, one attempted suicide and one completed suicide were reported, for which the relation with the DBS treatment is uncertain.

3.3. Ventral Capsule/Ventral Striatum

The ventral capsule/ventral striatum (VC/VS) is thought to be hyperactive in MDD [36] (Table 2). Capsulotomy (i.e., lesioning) of the VC/VS improved not only OCD symptoms but also depressive symptoms, inspiring stimulation of the VC/VS for TRD [15]. In an open-label trial that stimulated the VC/VS in 15 TRD patients, responder rates at three months, six months, and 12 months were 53.3%, 46.7%, and 53.3%, respectively, using the MADRS as an outcome measure, and were 46.7%, 40%, and 53.3%, respectively, using the HDRS as an outcome measure [55]. Adverse events ranged from pain or discomfort at the incision site, to hypomania, mixed bipolar state, and increased depression due to battery depletion.

The first RCT of DBS of the VC/VS for TRD was performed by Dougherty et al. (2015) who stimulated 30 patients for 16 weeks. There were no significant differences in response rates between the intervention and sham group in the double-blind phase [68,69]. Another RCT of VC/VS DBS in eight TRD patients was discontinued after an interim futility analysis of active vs. sham stimulation showed no difference in effects between the two groups after 16 weeks. These results were never published but were discussed by Rezai et al. [70].

3.4. The Ventral Part of the Anterior Limb of the Internal Capsule

The anterior limb of the internal capsule (ALIC) is another brain region that was initially studied for DBS in OCD. One study aimed at stimulating the NAcc discovered that most treated OCD patients (9 out of 16) actually received DBS in the ventral part of the ALIC (vALIC), which improved obsessive compulsive scale scores, showed anti-depressive effects, and led to the clinical implementation of vALIC-DBS in TRD [29]. DBS of the vALIC has also been associated with a decreased metabolism in the OFC, subgenual anterior cingulate cortex, and right dlPFC [71–73] (Table 2).

The first RCT of DBS of the vALIC for TRD was conducted by Bergfeld et al. (2016), investigating 25 TRD patients during a 52 week open-label trial, which resulted in a significant decrease in HDRS scores in the whole group during the optimization phase, although overall HDRS scores were still in the depression range (22.2 at baseline vs. 15.9 after optimization phase). Ten of the 25 patients could be classified as responders, with a more than 50% decrease on the HDRS. After the optimization phase, a RCT with a cross-over design including nine responders and seven non-responders ensued and showed a significantly lower score in the active DBS phase compared with the sham DBS phase (mean HDRS score of 13.6 (95% CI; 9.8–17.4 vs. 23.1 (95% CI; 20.6–25.6)) (HDRS < 0.001). However, the scores on the HDRS in the active treatment group were still within the mild to moderate depression range [74]. Both crossover phases lasted approximately 21 and 18 days, respectively.

3.5. Lateral Habenula

The activity of the lateral habenula (LHb) is negatively associated with reward, meaning its neurons increase their firing rate in a non-reward situation or in the omission of a reward. LHb hyperactivity could therefore explain the lower reward-seeking behavior in TRD [75] (Table 2). Speculation that DBS of the LHb could lead to the inhibition of hyperactivity prompted the first case study of LHb-DBS in TRD, which notably led to full remission of the patients' depressive symptoms [44]. A clinical non-randomized study in six patients suffering from TRD is currently being held, investigating the safety, tolerability, and benefit of LHb DBS in TRD. Patients that respond at 12 months of stimulation will enter a randomized, staggered withdrawal phase. During this phase, a double-blind discontinuation will be attempted at month 12 or 13, decreasing the stimulation by 50% and then completely discontinuing it during the following two weeks. Evaluation will take place at 15 months, where, in the meantime, escape criteria are included, and if met, will stop the blinded phase in continuing with an open treatment [76].

3.6. Thalamic Peduncles

The inferior thalamic peduncle (ITP) is a bundle of fibers connecting the OFC to the thalamus. The OFC is thought to play a role in the non-reward tractor theory of depression, where the orbitofrontal non-reward system is more easily triggered in depression, causing negative emotional states [77] (Table 2). Stimulating the ITP could disrupt this enhanced triggering and lead to less depressive symptoms. ITP stimulation for OCD has already shown improvements of the score on the Yale-Brown Obsessive-Compulsive scale in five OCD patients [45]. A case study in one TRD patient reported that DBS of the ITP decreased depressive symptoms [78]. However, within this study, two brain regions were investigated, the second being the BNST.

3.7. Bed Nucleus of the Stria Terminalis

The BNST is involved in a range of behaviors, such as stress response, social behavior, and extended duration of fear states. This nucleus assesses sensory information from the environment, coupled together with the subjects current mood and arousal, integrating a proper response to environmental and social setting changes [22] (Table 2). Raymaekers et al. (2017) indicated that both BNST and ITP stimulation could alleviate depressive symptoms; however, due to a small sample size, no statistical analyses were conducted [78].

3.8. Medial Forebrain Bundle

The medial forebrain bundle (MFB) is a fiber tract connected to various parts of the limbic system thought to play a role in reward-seeking systems [21] (Table 2). In one trial, DBS of the superolateral branch of the MFB resulted in more than a 50% decrease in depressive symptoms in six out of seven TRD patients within seven days [47]. An additional interim analysis of MFB-DBS in TRD confirmed these findings, showing more than a 50% decrease in depressive symptoms in three out of four patients within seven days of stimulation. At 26 weeks follow-up, two patients showed more than an 80% decrease in depression rating scales [49] (Table 1).

Taken together, the results of the aforementioned studies of DBS for TRD imply that stimulation at a number of different brain areas can alleviate depressive symptoms, which is in line with the view that MDD is a circuitopathy involving various brain regions and networks mainly within the limbic CSTC mood circuits [12,79]. However, how DBS of those targets improves the depressive symptoms is not completely clear. Moreover, stimulation parameters vary between studies due to a need to adjust and balance therapeutic effects to side effects.

MDD is a circuitopathy that involves a wide range of brain structures and exhibits diverse clinical manifestations. Therefore, a one-size-fits-all approach to the DBS targeting may not be beneficial in all patients, whereas a patient-centric selection based on individually disrupted neurocircuits could improve therapeutic outcomes. In evaluating the effects of DBS, one needs to focus on overall improvement on depression rating scales as well as individual scores and symptom-specific improvements. This will enhance the understanding of the effects of DBS and eventually contribute to the development of more personalized treatment approaches. Seemingly, this also applies in other psychiatric disorders such as OCD, where personalized approaches with content-specific DBS targets have already proven to be beneficial [80].

4. Towards a More Personalized DBS Treatment Approach for Treatment-Resistant Depression

Since open-label trials and RCT data on DBS in TRD show inconsistent results, this gives rise to discussion about the chosen study designs, the correct interpretation of results, and the best target(s) for neuromodulation. Depression entails different clinical subtypes and looking at homogenous subgroups of depressed patients may lead to a personalized DBS approach. This would be superior to looking at primary outcomes across all participants. Importantly, a prerequisite to this approach is the ability to determine pathoanatomical substrates of specific subtypes. How to implement such a more personalized approach to DBS treatment for TRD is discussed below.

4.1. Clinical and Neurophysiological Subtypes of Depression

Most response rates in depression treatments to date have been measured with changes in average levels among all patients treated. However, depressive symptomatology varies highly among individuals, making the standardization of positive outcomes challenging. Mood, sleep rhythm, concentration, psychomotor, and cognitive domains can all be disturbed in depression, while treating one selected brain structure within the mood circuit may not have an effect on all aforementioned symptoms nor have an effect on the main symptomatology of all depressed patients.

Subdividing TRD into different subtypes, involving distinct clinical symptoms as well as distinct patterns of dysfunctional connectivity in limbic and frontal striatal networks, may reveal different subtype-related outcomes for each investigated brain region, and if so, patient selection for a given brain target could enhance treatment effectiveness [81]. Analysis of resting-state connectivity biomarkers previously revealed four connectivity-based biotypes of depression characterized by either anxiety, increased anhedonia, psychomotor retardation, and/or increased anergia and fatigue. Moreover, patients could not be differentiated into a particular subtype based on clinical features alone and clustering them based on functional connectivity was needed [82]. Therefore, imaging procedures as well as featured symptoms should be taken into account when treating TRD with DBS. It is conceivable that subdividing TRD patients according to connectivity-based biotypes will shed new light on the interpretation of previous DBS study results, and that the integration of functional connectivity in future DBS studies will reveal clinically relevant subgroups that might respond to DBS of a specific target within the mood circuit. Altogether, it can be suggested that better assessment of therapeutic outcomes at symptom level might be accomplished when TRD patients with dominant anergia/fatigue symptoms (biotype 2) are stimulated within the CG 25; and patients characterized by more anxiety (biotype 4) are stimulated within the thalamic region, as suggested by Drysdale and coworkers [82]. Likewise, SCG stimulation could alleviate sleep disturbances and NAcc stimulation could improve anhedonia (Table 2).

4.2. Individual Tractography

Another way in which DBS efficiency can be improved is to ameliorate the implantation of electrodes with the usage of individualized, patient-specific, deterministic tractography targeting. Riva-Posse et al. (2018) used individualized patient-specific tractography targeting for SCC-DBS surgeries in TRD patients, aiming at the convergence of the four white matter bundles: the forceps minor, uncinate fasciculus, cingulum, and fronto-striatal fibers. This resulted in a response rate of 81.8% and a remission rate of 54% after a one year trial period, which proved greater than the previous open-label trials [83]. In a recent study, diffusion tensor imaging (DTI) tractography was used to target SCC-DBS more optimally, and the authors examined the impact of tract activation on clinical response at 6 and 12 months. Stimulation of vmPFC pathways by SCC-DBS was associated with a positive response and stimulation of the cingulum was associated with a 6 month, but not a 12 months DBS response. Monopolar stimulation of 130 Hz was applied with either pulse width (90–450 μs) or amplitude (4–8 V) progressively increased every month, based on response status. Patients were changed to bipolar settings if monopolar stimulation caused adverse effects. It was speculated that targeting more ventral, rather than the dorsal mPFC projections, might improve the response [84].

4.3. Combining Deep Brain Stimulation with Cognitive-Behavioral Therapy

It is plausible that better therapeutic outcomes could be achieved if DBS is applied in combination with concurrent treatments, such as pharmacotherapy with antidepressants or cognitive-behavioral therapy (CBT) in TRD. Studies focusing on the added effect of concurrent treatments to DBS have not been conducted in patients with TRD. The results from studies in OCD patients treated with DBS show that adding CBT to DBS has added beneficial effects [85]. Studies targeted at revealing the added effects of concomitant treatments after DBS for TRD would also provide information that may facilitate establishing a treatment algorithm to determine the place of these treatments in DBS patients.

4.4. Biomarkers

Biomarkers are quantifiable characteristics of biological processes, which could prove helpful in improving diagnostic objectivity of MDD and TRD as well as help in personalizing its treatment. For MDD, no specific biomarkers have yet been found, though several markers have been shown to be potential candidates, such as brain-derived neurotrophic factor (BDNF), interleukins (IL) 1 and 6, tumor necrosis factor (TNF), malondialdehyde (MDA), hypothalamic-pituitary-adrenal (HPA) activity, and cortisol responses [86,87]. Every biomarker as a standalone shows a low sensitivity and specificity, partly explained by the heterogeneity of MDD. To overcome this shortcoming, either examining a biological panel of several markers [88] or phenotyping MDD and TRD into distinct subtypes could be considered. However, a recent meta-analysis showed that only cortisol has a predictive effect on onset/relapse and recurrence of MDD making the integration of biomarkers for personalizing TRD treatment a futuristic milestone yet to be discovered [89].

4.5. Insights into Symptomatic Improvement after Deep Brain Stimulation

For TRD, different regions in the mood circuit can be stimulated with DBS (Table 2), although it is still unclear which depressive-symptoms respond to the stimulation of a specific target. More research into the mood circuit is needed to untangle which emotions arise from specific brain regions. This may vary from basic animal research, disentangling neuronal function per brain region, and ultra-high field MR studies in humans, all of which could shed light on the dysfunctional brain circuits in TRD. In contrast to the motor system that is studied thoroughly [90,91], emotional circuitry is far less understood. One reason for this is that animal research into mood circuitry remains complicated as there is considerable heterogeneity between species [92]. Modeling depression in animals is complex as there are several depressive-like behavior models, such as the chronic unpredictable stress paradigm (CUS), which give insight into depression pathology [93]. DBS is investigated within these models to unravel behavioral and cellular changes following DBS [94].

Alongside the standard clinical rating scales, the use of momentary assessment techniques, such as the experience sampling method (ESM), could enhance the documentation of the momentary mood states [95]. The ESM includes short repeated assessments of experiences and behaviors, as well as moment-to-moment changes in mental states in the context of daily life. Research has shown that depressed patients can improve their depressive symptomology while using weekly ESM for six weeks, and add-on ESM derived feedback resulted in a significant decrease in HDRS scores compared to controls ($p < 0.01$; −5.5 point reduction in HDRS at 6 months) [96]. In add-on-derived feedback, a psychologist or psychiatrist gives feedback on the association between the participants momentary affective states and specific daily life contexts [97]. ESM-derived feedback could further improve treatment by showing within-subject changes in a heterogeneous TRD population and contribute to clinical decision-making [97]. In the case of DBS, the use of ESM may reveal specific response patterns depending on the brain region that is stimulated, which can provide valuable information about emotional circuitry. This can be done using well-evaluated day-to-day scores, including questionnaires that go into detail on current mood and adaptive functioning.

5. Conclusions

More personalized treatment approaches hold the potential to increase the overall efficacy of DBS for TRD. Precise evaluations of symptoms, biomarkers, and resting-state connectivity patterns are essential when distinguishing clinical subtypes of TRD. Moreover, subtyping may provide more insight into the working mechanisms of DBS and help in selecting optimal targets in patients. Monitoring of biomarkers at multiple time points during treatment along with evaluation of ESM data, in parallel with clinical assessments of mood using standardized depression-rating scales, will lead to a better understanding of symptom changes when stimulating specific brain regions. Such considerations could further lead to optimal adjustments of stimulation parameters as long-term effects of DBS on mood occur.

Author Contributions: M.R. and E.S. prepared the first draft. J.B., A.E.P.M., A.F.G.L. and A.J. provided inputs and revised the manuscript. A.J. supervised the process. All authors have read and agreed to the published version of the manuscript.

References

1. Uher, R.; Payne, J.L.; Pavlova, B.; Perlis, R.H. Major depressive disorder in DSM-5: Implications for clinical practice and research of changes from DSM-IV. *Depress. Anxiety* **2014**, *31*, 459–471. [CrossRef] [PubMed]

2. WHO. *Depression and Other Common Mental Disorders Global Health Estimates*; World Health Organization: Geneva, Switzerland, 2017.

3. Rush, A. Acute and Longer-Term Outcomes in Depressed Outpatients Requiring One or Several Treatment Steps: A STAR*D Report. *Am. J. Psychiatry* **2006**, *163*, 1905. [CrossRef] [PubMed]

4. Cuijpers, P.; Karyotaki, E.; Weitz, E.; Andersson, G.; Hollon, S.D.; van Straten, A. The effects of psychotherapies for major depression in adults on remission, recovery and improvement: A meta-analysis. *J. Affect. Disord.* **2014**, *159*, 118–126. [CrossRef] [PubMed]

5. Gaynes, B.N.; Asher, G.; Gartlehner, G.; Hoffman, V.; Green, J.; Boland, E.; Lux, L.; Weber, R.P.; Randolph, C.; Bann, C.; et al. *Definition of Treatment-Resistant Depression in the Medicare Population*; Agency for Healthcare Research and Quality: Rockville, MD, USA, 2018.

6. Amital, D.; Fostick, L.; Silberman, A.; Beckman, M.; Spivak, B. Serious life events among resistant and non-resistant MDD patients. *J. Affect. Disord.* **2008**, *110*, 260–264. [CrossRef]

7.   Ivanova, J.I.; Birnbaum, H.G.; Kidolezi, Y.; Subramanian, G.; Khan, S.A.; Stensland, M.D. Direct and indirect costs of employees with treatment-resistant and non-treatment-resistant major depressive disorder. *Curr. Med. Res. Opin.* **2010**, *26*, 2475–2484. [CrossRef]

8.   Johnson, R.L.; Wilson, C.G. A review of vagus nerve stimulation as a therapeutic intervention. *J. Inflamm. Res.* **2018**, *11*, 203–213. [CrossRef]

9.   George, M.S.; Taylor, J.J.; Short, E.B. The expanding evidence base for rTMS treatment of depression. *Curr. Opin. Psychiatry* **2013**, *26*, 13–18. [CrossRef]

10. Mayberg, H.S.; Lozano, A.M.; Voon, V.; McNeely, H.E.; Seminowicz, D.; Hamani, C.; Schwalb, J.M.; Kennedy, S.H. Deep brain stimulation for treatment-resistant depression. *Neuron* **2005**, *45*, 651–660. [CrossRef]

11. Alexander, G.E.; DeLong, M.R.; Strick, P.L. Parallel organization of functionally segregated circuits linking basal ganglia and cortex. *Annu. Rev. Neurosci.* **1986**, *9*, 357–381. [CrossRef]

12. Mayberg, H.S. Limbic-cortical dysregulation: A proposed model of depression. *J. Neuropsychiatry Clin. Neurosci.* **1997**, *9*, 471–481.

13. Temel, Y.; Leentjens, A.F.G.; de Bie, R.M.A. *Handboek Diepe Hersenstimulatie Bij Neurologische En Psychiatrische Aandoeningen*; Bohn Stafleu van Loghum: Houten, The Netherlands, 2016; pp. 137–142.

14. Gabriels, L.; Cosyns, P.; Nuttin, B.; Demeulemeester, H.; Gybels, J. Deep brain stimulation for treatment-refractory obsessive-compulsive disorder: Psychopathological and neuropsychological outcome in three cases. *Acta Psychiatry Scand.* **2003**, *107*, 275–282. [CrossRef]

15. Greenberg, B.D.; Malone, D.A.; Friehs, G.M.; Rezai, A.R.; Kubu, C.S.; Malloy, P.F.; Salloway, S.P.; Okun, M.S.; Goodman, W.K.; Rasmussen, S.A. Three-year outcomes in deep brain stimulation for highly resistant obsessive-compulsive disorder. *Neuropsychopharmacology* **2006**, *31*, 2384–2393. [CrossRef] [PubMed]

16. Moonen, A.J.H.; Wijers, A.; Dujardin, K.; Leentjens, A.F.G. Neurobiological correlates of emotional processing in Parkinson's disease: A systematic review of experimental studies. *J. Psychosom. Res.* **2017**, *100*, 65–76. [CrossRef]

17. Mayberg, H.S.; Liotti, M.; Brannan, S.K.; McGinnis, S.; Mahurin, R.K.; Jerabek, P.A.; Silva, J.A.; Tekell, J.L.; Martin, C.C.; Lancaster, J.L.; et al. Reciprocal limbic-cortical function and negative mood: Converging PET findings in depression and normal sadness. *Am. J. Psychiatry* **1999**, *156*, 675–682. [PubMed]

18. Drevets, W.C.; Savitz, J.; Trimble, M. The subgenual anterior cingulate cortex in mood disorders. *CNS Spectr.* **2008**, *13*, 663–681. [CrossRef]

19. Ongur, D.; Ferry, A.T.; Price, J.L. Architectonic subdivision of the human orbital and medial prefrontal cortex. *J. Comp. Neurol.* **2003**, *460*, 425–449. [CrossRef]

20. Sun, C.; Wang, Y.; Cui, R.; Wu, C.; Li, X.; Bao, Y.; Wang, Y. Human Thalamic-Prefrontal Peduncle Connectivity Revealed by Diffusion Spectrum Imaging Fiber Tracking. *Front. Neuroanat.* **2018**, *12*, 24. [CrossRef]

21. Coenen, V.A.; Panksepp, J.; Hurwitz, T.A.; Urbach, H.; Madler, B. Human medial forebrain bundle (MFB) and anterior thalamic radiation (ATR): Imaging of two major subcortical pathways and the dynamic balance of opposite affects in understanding depression. *J. Neuropsychiatry Clin. Neurosci.* **2012**, *24*, 223–236. [CrossRef]

22. Lebow, M.A.; Chen, A. Overshadowed by the amygdala: The bed nucleus of the stria terminalis emerges as key to psychiatric disorders. *Mol. Psychiatry* **2016**, *21*, 450–463. [CrossRef]

23. Lozano, A.M.; Lipsman, N.; Bergman, H.; Brown, P.; Chabardes, S.; Chang, J.W.; Matthews, K.; McIntyre, C.C.; Schlaepfer, T.E.; Schulder, M.; et al. Deep brain stimulation: Current challenges and future directions. *Nat. Rev. Neurol.* **2019**, *15*, 148–160. [CrossRef]

24. Daneshzand, M.; Faezipour, M.; Barkana, B.D. Robust desynchronization of Parkinson's disease pathological oscillations by frequency modulation of delayed feedback deep brain stimulation. *PLoS ONE* **2018**, *13*, e0207761. [CrossRef] [PubMed]

25. Vicheva, P.; Butler, M.; Shotbolt, P. Deep brain stimulation for obsessive-compulsive disorder: A systematic review of randomised controlled trials. *Neurosci. Biobehav. Rev.* **2020**, *109*, 129–138. [CrossRef] [PubMed]

26. Agnesi, F.; Johnson, M.D.; Vitek, J.L. Deep brain stimulation: How does it work? *Handb. Clin. Neurol.* **2013**, *116*, 39–54. [PubMed]

27. Cheney, P.D.; Griffin, D.M.; Van Acker, G.M., III. Neural hijacking: Action of high-frequency electrical stimulation on cortical circuits. *Neuroscientist* **2013**, *19*, 434–441. [CrossRef]

28. Ashkan, K.; Rogers, P.; Bergman, H.; Ughratdar, I. Insights into the mechanisms of deep brain stimulation. *Nat. Rev. Neurol.* **2017**, *13*, 548–554. [CrossRef]

29. Van den Munckhof, P.; Bosch, D.A.; Mantione, M.H.; Figee, M.; Denys, D.A.; Schuurman, P.R. Active stimulation site of nucleus accumbens deep brain stimulation in obsessive-compulsive disorder is localized in the ventral internal capsule. *Acta Neurochir. Suppl.* **2013**, *117*, 53–59.

30. Drobisz, D.; Damborska, A. Deep brain stimulation targets for treating depression. *Behav. Brain Res.* **2019**, *359*, 266–273. [CrossRef]

31. Hamani, C.; Mayberg, H.; Stone, S.; Laxton, A.; Haber, S.; Lozano, A.M. The subcallosal cingulate gyrus in the context of major depression. *Biol. Psychiatry* **2011**, *69*, 301–308. [CrossRef]

32. Coryell, W.; Nopoulos, P.; Drevets, W.; Wilson, T.; Andreasen, N.C. Subgenual prefrontal cortex volumes in major depressive disorder and schizophrenia: Diagnostic specificity and prognostic implications. *Am. J. Psychiatry* **2005**, *162*, 1706–1712. [CrossRef]

33. Schlaepfer, T.E.; Cohen, M.X.; Frick, C.; Kosel, M.; Brodesser, D.; Axmacher, N.; Joe, A.Y.; Kreft, M.; Lenartz, D.; Sturm, V. Deep brain stimulation to reward circuitry alleviates anhedonia in refractory major depression. *Neuropsychopharmacology* **2008**, *33*, 368–377. [CrossRef]

34. Wacker, J.; Dillon, D.G.; Pizzagalli, D.A. The role of the nucleus accumbens and rostral anterior cingulate cortex in anhedonia: Integration of resting EEG, fMRI, and volumetric techniques. *Neuroimage* **2009**, *46*, 327–337. [CrossRef] [PubMed]

35. Makris, N.; Rathi, Y.; Mouradian, P.; Bonmassar, G.; Papadimitriou, G.; Ing, W.I.; Yeterian, E.H.; Kubicki, M.; Eskandar, E.N.; Wald, L.L.; et al. Variability and anatomical specificity of the orbitofrontothalamic fibers of passage in the ventral capsule/ventral striatum (VC/VS): Precision care for patient-specific tractography-guided targeting of deep brain stimulation (DBS) in obsessive compulsive disorder (OCD). *Brain Imaging Behav.* **2016**, *10*, 1054–1067.

36. Quevedo, K.; Ng, R.; Scott, H.; Kodavaganti, S.; Smyda, G.; Diwadkar, V.; Phillips, M. Ventral Striatum Functional Connectivity during Rewards and Losses and Symptomatology in Depressed Patients. *Biol. Psychol.* **2017**, *123*, 62–73. [CrossRef] [PubMed]

37. Hwang, J.W.; Xin, S.C.; Ou, Y.M.; Zhang, W.Y.; Liang, Y.L.; Chen, J.; Yang, X.Q.; Chen, X.Y.; Guo, T.W.; Yang, X.J.; et al. Enhanced default mode network connectivity with ventral striatum in subthreshold depression individuals. *J. Psychiatry Res.* **2016**, *76*, 111–120. [CrossRef] [PubMed]

38. Zhang, A.; Ajilore, O.; Zhan, L.; Gadelkarim, J.; Korthauer, L.; Yang, S.; Leow, A.; Kumar, A. White matter tract integrity of anterior limb of internal capsule in major depression and type 2 diabetes. *Neuropsychopharmacology* **2013**, *38*, 1451–1459. [CrossRef]

39. Alonso, P.; Cuadras, D.; Gabriels, L.; Denys, D.; Goodman, W.; Greenberg, B.D.; Jimenez-Ponce, F.; Kuhn, J.; Lenartz, D.; Mallet, L.; et al. Deep Brain Stimulation for Obsessive-Compulsive Disorder: A Meta-Analysis of Treatment Outcome and Predictors of Response. *PLoS ONE* **2015**, *10*, e0133591. [CrossRef]

40. Matsumoto, M.; Hikosaka, O. Lateral habenula as a source of negative reward signals in dopamine neurons. *Nature* **2007**, *447*, 1111–1115. [CrossRef]

41. Meng, H.; Wang, Y.; Huang, M.; Lin, W.; Wang, S.; Zhang, B. Chronic deep brain stimulation of the lateral habenula nucleus in a rat model of depression. *Brain Res.* **2011**, *1422*, 32–38. [CrossRef]

42. Sartorius, A.; Henn, F.A. Deep brain stimulation of the lateral habenula in treatment resistant major depression. *Med. Hypotheses* **2007**, *69*, 1305–1308. [CrossRef]

43. Ranft, K.; Dobrowolny, H.; Krell, D.; Bielau, H.; Bogerts, B.; Bernstein, H.G. Evidence for structural abnormalities of the human habenular complex in affective disorders but not in schizophrenia. *Psychol. Med.* **2010**, *40*, 557–567. [CrossRef]

44. Sartorius, A.; Kiening, K.L.; Kirsch, P.; von Gall, C.C.; Haberkorn, U.; Unterberg, A.W.; Henn, F.A.; Meyer-Lindenberg, A. Remission of major depression under deep brain stimulation of the lateral habenula in a therapy-refractory patient. *Biol. Psychiatry* **2010**, *67*, e9–e11. [CrossRef] [PubMed]

45. Lee, D.J.; Dallapiazza, R.F.; De Vloo, P.; Elias, G.J.B.; Fomenko, A.; Boutet, A.; Giacobbe, P.; Lozano, A.M. Inferior thalamic peduncle deep brain stimulation for treatment-refractory obsessive-compulsive disorder: A phase 1 pilot trial. *Brain Stimul.* **2019**, *12*, 344–352. [CrossRef] [PubMed]

46. Velasco, F.; Velasco, M.; Jimenez, F.; Velasco, A.L.; Salin-Pascual, R. Neurobiological background for performing surgical intervention in the inferior thalamic peduncle for treatment of major depression disorders. *Neurosurgery* **2005**, *57*, 439–448, Discussion 439–448. [CrossRef] [PubMed]

47. Schlaepfer, T.E.; Bewernick, B.H.; Kayser, S.; Madler, B.; Coenen, V.A. Rapid effects of deep brain stimulation for treatment-resistant major depression. *Biol. Psychiatry* **2013**, *73*, 1204–1212. [CrossRef]

48. Schoene-Bake, J.C.; Parpaley, Y.; Weber, B.; Panksepp, J.; Hurwitz, T.A.; Coenen, V.A. Tractographic analysis of historical lesion surgery for depression. *Neuropsychopharmacology* **2010**, *35*, 2553–2563. [CrossRef]

49. Fenoy, A.J.; Schulz, P.; Selvaraj, S.; Burrows, C.; Spiker, D.; Cao, B.; Zunta-Soares, G.; Gajwani, P.; Quevedo, J.; Soares, J. Deep brain stimulation of the medial forebrain bundle: Distinctive responses in resistant depression. *J. Affect. Disord.* **2016**, *203*, 143–151. [CrossRef]

50. Neumann, W.J.; Huebl, J.; Brucke, C.; Gabriels, L.; Bajbouj, M.; Merkl, A.; Schneider, G.H.; Nuttin, B.; Brown, P.; Kuhn, A.A. Different patterns of local field potentials from limbic DBS targets in patients with major depressive and obsessive compulsive disorder. *Mol. Psychiatry* **2014**, *19*, 1186–1192. [CrossRef]

51. Bagby, R.M.; Ryder, A.G.; Schuller, D.R.; Marshall, M.B. The Hamilton Depression Rating Scale: Has the gold standard become a lead weight? *Am. J. Psychiatry* **2004**, *161*, 2163–2177. [CrossRef]

52. Kennedy, S.H.; Giacobbe, P.; Rizvi, S.J.; Placenza, F.M.; Nishikawa, Y.; Mayberg, H.S.; Lozano, A.M. Deep brain stimulation for treatment-resistant depression: Follow-up after 3 to 6 years. *Am. J. Psychiatry* **2011**, *168*, 502–510. [CrossRef]

53. Bewernick, B.H.; Hurlemann, R.; Matusch, A.; Kayser, S.; Grubert, C.; Hadrysiewicz, B.; Axmacher, N.; Lemke, M.; Cooper-Mahkorn, D.; Cohen, M.X.; et al. Nucleus accumbens deep brain stimulation decreases ratings of depression and anxiety in treatment-resistant depression. *Biol. Psychiatry* **2010**, *67*, 110–116. [CrossRef]

54. Bewernick, B.H.; Kayser, S.; Sturm, V.; Schlaepfer, T.E. Long-term effects of nucleus accumbens deep brain stimulation in treatment-resistant depression: Evidence for sustained efficacy. *Neuropsychopharmacology* **2012**, *37*, 1975–1985. [CrossRef] [PubMed]

55. Malone, D.A., Jr.; Dougherty, D.D.; Rezai, A.R.; Carpenter, L.L.; Friehs, G.M.; Eskandar, E.N.; Rauch, S.L.; Rasmussen, S.A.; Machado, A.G.; Kubu, C.S.; et al. Deep brain stimulation of the ventral capsule/ventral striatum for treatment-resistant depression. *Biol. Psychiatry* **2009**, *65*, 267–275. [CrossRef] [PubMed]

56. Lozano, A.M.; Mayberg, H.S.; Giacobbe, P.; Hamani, C.; Craddock, R.C.; Kennedy, S.H. Subcallosal cingulate gyrus deep brain stimulation for treatment-resistant depression. *Biol. Psychiatry* **2008**, *64*, 461–467. [CrossRef] [PubMed]

57. Puigdemont, D.; Perez-Egea, R.; Portella, M.J.; Molet, J.; de Diego-Adelino, J.; Gironell, A.; Radua, J.; Gomez-Anson, B.; Rodriguez, R.; Serra, M.; et al. Deep brain stimulation of the subcallosal cingulate gyrus: Further evidence in treatment-resistant major depression. *Int. J. Neuropsychopharmacol.* **2012**, *15*, 121–133. [CrossRef]

58. Lozano, A.M.; Giacobbe, P.; Hamani, C.; Rizvi, S.J.; Kennedy, S.H.; Kolivakis, T.T.; Debonnel, G.; Sadikot, A.F.; Lam, R.W.; Howard, A.K.; et al. A multicenter pilot study of subcallosal cingulate area deep brain stimulation for treatment-resistant depression. *J. Neurosurg.* **2012**, *116*, 315–322. [CrossRef]

59. Holtzheimer, P.E.; Kelley, M.E.; Gross, R.E.; Filkowski, M.M.; Garlow, S.J.; Barrocas, A.; Wint, D.; Craighead, M.C.; Kozarsky, J.; Chismar, R.; et al. Subcallosal cingulate deep brain stimulation for treatment-resistant unipolar and bipolar depression. *Arch. Gen. Psychiatry* **2012**, *69*, 150–158. [CrossRef]

60. Crowell, A.L.; Riva-Posse, P.; Holtzheimer, P.E.; Garlow, S.J.; Kelley, M.E.; Gross, R.E.; Denison, L.; Quinn, S.; Mayberg, H.S. Long-Term Outcomes of Subcallosal Cingulate Deep Brain Stimulation for Treatment-Resistant Depression. *Am. J. Psychiatry* **2019**, *176*, 949–956. [CrossRef]

61. Merkl, A.; Schneider, G.H.; Schonecker, T.; Aust, S.; Kuhl, K.P.; Kupsch, A.; Kuhn, A.A.; Bajbouj, M. Antidepressant effects after short-term and chronic stimulation of the subgenual cingulate gyrus in treatment-resistant depression. *Exp. Neurol.* **2013**, *249*, 160–168. [CrossRef]

62. Accolla, E.A.; Aust, S.; Merkl, A.; Schneider, G.H.; Kuhn, A.A.; Bajbouj, M.; Draganski, B. Deep brain stimulation of the posterior gyrus rectus region for treatment resistant depression. *J. Affect. Disord.* **2016**, *194*, 33–37. [CrossRef]

63. Berlim, M.T.; McGirr, A.; Van den Eynde, F.; Fleck, M.P.; Giacobbe, P. Effectiveness and acceptability of deep brain stimulation (DBS) of the subgenual cingulate cortex for treatment-resistant depression: A systematic review and exploratory meta-analysis. *J. Affect. Disord.* **2014**, *159*, 31–38. [CrossRef]

64. Merkl, A.; Aust, S.; Schneider, G.H.; Visser-Vandewalle, V.; Horn, A.; Kuhn, A.A.; Kuhn, J.; Bajbouj, M. Deep brain stimulation of the subcallosal cingulate gyrus in patients with treatment-resistant depression: A double-blinded randomized controlled study and long-term follow-up in eight patients. *J. Affect. Disord.* **2018**, *227*, 521–529. [CrossRef] [PubMed]

65. Holtzheimer, P.E.; Husain, M.M.; Lisanby, S.H.; Taylor, S.F.; Whitworth, L.A.; McClintock, S.; Slavin, K.V.; Berman, J.; McKhann, G.M.; Patil, P.G.; et al. Subcallosal cingulate deep brain stimulation for treatment-resistant depression: A multisite, randomised, sham-controlled trial. *Lancet Psychiatry* **2017**, *4*, 839–849. [CrossRef]

66. Morishita, T.; Fayad, S.M.; Higuchi, M.A.; Nestor, K.A.; Foote, K.D. Deep brain stimulation for treatment-resistant depression: Systematic review of clinical outcomes. *Neurotherapeutics* **2014**, *11*, 475–484. [CrossRef] [PubMed]

67. Eitan, R.; Fontaine, D.; Benoit, M.; Giordana, C.; Darmon, N.; Israel, Z.; Linesky, E.; Arkadir, D.; Ben-Naim, S.; Iserlles, M.; et al. One year double blind study of high vs low frequency subcallosal cingulate stimulation for depression. *J. Psychiatry Res.* **2018**, *96*, 124–134. [CrossRef]

68. Dougherty, D.D.; Rezai, A.R.; Carpenter, L.L.; Howland, R.H.; Bhati, M.T.; O'Reardon, J.P.; Eskandar, E.N.; Baltuch, G.H.; Machado, A.D.; Kondziolka, D.; et al. A Randomized Sham-Controlled Trial of Deep Brain Stimulation of the Ventral Capsule/Ventral Striatum for Chronic Treatment-Resistant Depression. *Biol. Psychiatry* **2015**, *78*, 240–248. [CrossRef] [PubMed]

69. Peichel, D. A Clinical Evaluation of Different Device Parameters for the Management of Patients with Treatment Resistant Major Depressive Disorder, Single or Recurrent Episode, with Deep Brain Stimulation. Available online: https://clinicaltrials.gov/ct2/show/NCT01331330 (accessed on 24 August 2020).

70. Rezai, A. Feasibility, Safety and Efficacy of Deep Brain Stimulation of the Internal Capsule for Severe and Medically Refractory Major Depression. Available online: https://clinicaltrials.gov/ct2/show/NCT00555698 (accessed on 24 August 2020).

71. Nuttin, B.J.; Gabriels, L.A.; Cosyns, P.R.; Meyerson, B.A.; Andreewitch, S.; Sunaert, S.G.; Maes, A.F.; Dupont, P.J.; Gybels, J.M.; Gielen, F.; et al. Long-term electrical capsular stimulation in patients with obsessive-compulsive disorder. *Neurosurgery* **2003**, *52*, 1263–1272, Discussion 1264–1272. [CrossRef]

72. Abelson, J.L.; Curtis, G.C.; Sagher, O.; Albucher, R.C.; Harrigan, M.; Taylor, S.F.; Martis, B.; Giordani, B. Deep brain stimulation for refractory obsessive-compulsive disorder. *Biol. Psychiatry* **2005**, *57*, 510–516. [CrossRef]

73. Van Laere, K.; Nuttin, B.; Gabriels, L.; Dupont, P.; Rasmussen, S.; Greenberg, B.D.; Cosyns, P. Metabolic imaging of anterior capsular stimulation in refractory obsessive-compulsive disorder: A key role for the subgenual anterior cingulate and ventral striatum. *J. Nucl. Med.* **2006**, *47*, 740–747.

74. Bergfeld, I.O.; Mantione, M.; Hoogendoorn, M.L.; Ruhe, H.G.; Notten, P.; van Laarhoven, J.; Visser, I.; Figee, M.; de Kwaasteniet, B.P.; Horst, F.; et al. Deep Brain Stimulation of the Ventral Anterior Limb of the Internal Capsule for Treatment-Resistant Depression: A Randomized Clinical Trial. *JAMA Psychiatry* **2016**, *73*, 456–464. [CrossRef]

75. Loonen, A.J.; Ivanova, S.A. Circuits Regulating Pleasure and Happiness-Mechanisms of Depression. *Front. Hum. Neurosci.* **2016**, *10*, 571. [CrossRef]

76. Goodman, W. A Clinical Pilot Study Examining Bilateral Inhibition of the Lateral Habenula as a Target for Deep Brain Stimulation in Intractable Depression. Available online: https://clinicaltrials.gov/ct2/show/NCT01798407 (accessed on 24 August 2020).

77. Rolls, E.T. A non-reward attractor theory of depression. *Neurosci. Biobehav. Rev.* **2016**, *68*, 47–58. [CrossRef] [PubMed]

78. Raymaekers, S.; Luyten, L.; Bervoets, C.; Gabriels, L.; Nuttin, B. Deep brain stimulation for treatment-resistant major depressive disorder: A comparison of two targets and long-term follow-up. *Transl. Psychiatry* **2017**, *7*, e1251. [CrossRef] [PubMed]

79. Price, J.L.; Drevets, W.C. Neural circuits underlying the pathophysiology of mood disorders. *Trends Cogn. Sci.* **2012**, *16*, 61–71. [CrossRef]

80. Barcia, J.A.; Avecillas-Chasin, J.M.; Nombela, C.; Arza, R.; Garcia-Albea, J.; Pineda-Pardo, J.A.; Reneses, B.; Strange, B.A. Personalized striatal targets for deep brain stimulation in obsessive-compulsive disorder. *Brain Stimul.* **2019**, *12*, 724–734. [CrossRef] [PubMed]

81. Beijers, L.; Wardenaar, K.J.; van Loo, H.M.; Schoevers, R.A. Data-driven biological subtypes of depression: Systematic review of biological approaches to depression subtyping. *Mol. Psychiatry* **2019**, *24*, 888–900. [CrossRef]

82. Drysdale, A.T.; Grosenick, L.; Downar, J.; Dunlop, K.; Mansouri, F.; Meng, Y.; Fetcho, R.N.; Zebley, B.; Oathes, D.J.; Etkin, A.; et al. Resting-state connectivity biomarkers define neurophysiological subtypes of depression. *Nat. Med.* **2017**, *23*, 28–38. [CrossRef]

83. Riva-Posse, P.; Choi, K.S.; Holtzheimer, P.E.; Crowell, A.L.; Garlow, S.J.; Rajendra, J.K.; McIntyre, C.C.; Gross, R.E.; Mayberg, H.S. A connectomic approach for subcallosal cingulate deep brain stimulation surgery: Prospective targeting in treatment-resistant depression. *Mol. Psychiatry* **2018**, *23*, 843–849. [CrossRef]

84. Clark, D.L.; Johnson, K.A.; Butson, C.R.; Lebel, C.; Gobbi, D.; Ramasubbu, R.; Kiss, Z.H.T. Tract-based analysis of target engagement by subcallosal cingulate deep brain stimulation for treatment resistant depression. *Brain Stimul.* **2020**, *13*, 1094–1101. [CrossRef]

85. Gormezoglu, M.; van der Vlis, T.B.; Schruers, K.; Ackermans, L.; Polosan, M.; Leentjens, A.F.G. Effectiveness, Timing and Procedural Aspects of Cognitive Behavioral Therapy after Deep Brain Stimulation for Therapy-Resistant Obsessive Compulsive Disorder: A Systematic Review. *J. Clin. Med.* **2020**, *9*, 2383. [CrossRef]

86. Hacimusalar, Y.; Esel, E. Suggested Biomarkers for Major Depressive Disorder. *Noro Psikiyatr Ars* **2018**, *55*, 280–290. [CrossRef]

87. MacDonald, K.; Krishnan, A.; Cervenka, E.; Hu, G.; Guadagno, E.; Trakadis, Y. Biomarkers for major depressive and bipolar disorders using metabolomics: A systematic review. *Am. J. Med. Genet. B Neuropsychiatr. Genet.* **2019**, *180*, 122–137. [CrossRef] [PubMed]

88. Schmidt, H.D.; Shelton, R.C.; Duman, R.S. Functional biomarkers of depression: Diagnosis, treatment, and pathophysiology. *Neuropsychopharmacology* **2011**, *36*, 2375–2394. [CrossRef] [PubMed]

89. Kennis, M.; Gerritsen, L.; van Dalen, M.; Williams, A.; Cuijpers, P.; Bockting, C. Prospective biomarkers of major depressive disorder: A systematic review and meta-analysis. *Mol. Psychiatry* **2020**, *25*, 321–338. [CrossRef]

90. Rosin, B.; Nevet, A.; Elias, S.; Rivlin-Etzion, M.; Israel, Z.; Bergman, H. Physiology and pathophysiology of the basal ganglia-thalamo-cortical networks. *Parkinsonism Relat. Disord.* **2007**, *13* (Suppl. S3), S437–S439. [CrossRef]

91. Redgrave, P.; Rodriguez, M.; Smith, Y.; Rodriguez-Oroz, M.C.; Lehericy, S.; Bergman, H.; Agid, Y.; DeLong, M.R.; Obeso, J.A. Goal-directed and habitual control in the basal ganglia: Implications for Parkinson's disease. *Nat. Rev. Neurosci.* **2010**, *11*, 760–772. [CrossRef] [PubMed]

92. Panksepp, J. The basic emotional circuits of mammalian brains: Do animals have affective lives? *Neurosci. Biobehav. Rev.* **2011**, *35*, 1791–1804. [CrossRef] [PubMed]

93. Abelaira, H.M.; Reus, G.Z.; Quevedo, J. Animal models as tools to study the pathophysiology of depression. *Braz. J. Psychiatry* **2013**, *35* (Suppl. S2), S112–S120. [CrossRef] [PubMed]

94. Lim, L.W.; Prickaerts, J.; Huguet, G.; Kadar, E.; Hartung, H.; Sharp, T.; Temel, Y. Electrical stimulation alleviates depressive-like behaviors of rats: Investigation of brain targets and potential mechanisms. *Transl. Psychiatry* **2015**, *5*, e535. [CrossRef]

95. Verhagen, S.J.; Hasmi, L.; Drukker, M.; van Os, J.; Delespaul, P.A. Use of the experience sampling method in the context of clinical trials. *Evid. Based Ment. Health* **2016**, *19*, 86–89. [CrossRef]

96. Kramer, I.; Simons, C.J.; Hartmann, J.A.; Menne-Lothmann, C.; Viechtbauer, W.; Peeters, F.; Schruers, K.; van Bemmel, A.L.; Myin-Germeys, I.; Delespaul, P.; et al. A therapeutic application of the experience sampling method in the treatment of depression: A randomized controlled trial. *World Psychiatry* **2014**, *13*, 68–77. [CrossRef]

97. Davidson, K.W.; Peacock, J.; Kronish, I.M.; Edmondson, D. Personalizing Behavioral Interventions Through Single-Patient (N-of-1) Trials. *Soc. Pers. Psychol. Compass* **2014**, *8*, 408–421. [CrossRef] [PubMed]

Permissions

All chapters in this book were first published by MDPI; hereby published with permission under the Creative Commons Attribution License or equivalent. Every chapter published in this book has been scrutinized by our experts. Their significance has been extensively debated. The topics covered herein carry significant findings which will fuel the growth of the discipline. They may even be implemented as practical applications or may be referred to as a beginning point for another development.

The contributors of this book come from diverse backgrounds, making this book a truly international effort. This book will bring forth new frontiers with its revolutionizing research information and detailed analysis of the nascent developments around the world.

We would like to thank all the contributing authors for lending their expertise to make the book truly unique. They have played a crucial role in the development of this book. Without their invaluable contributions this book wouldn't have been possible. They have made vital efforts to compile up to date information on the varied aspects of this subject to make this book a valuable addition to the collection of many professionals and students.

This book was conceptualized with the vision of imparting up-to-date information and advanced data in this field. To ensure the same, a matchless editorial board was set up. Every individual on the board went through rigorous rounds of assessment to prove their worth. After which they invested a large part of their time researching and compiling the most relevant data for our readers.

The editorial board has been involved in producing this book since its inception. They have spent rigorous hours researching and exploring the diverse topics which have resulted in the successful publishing of this book. They have passed on their knowledge of decades through this book. To expedite this challenging task, the publisher supported the team at every step. A small team of assistant editors was also appointed to further simplify the editing procedure and attain best results for the readers.

Apart from the editorial board, the designing team has also invested a significant amount of their time in understanding the subject and creating the most relevant covers. They scrutinized every image to scout for the most suitable representation of the subject and create an appropriate cover for the book.

The publishing team has been an ardent support to the editorial, designing and production team. Their endless efforts to recruit the best for this project, has resulted in the accomplishment of this book. They are a veteran in the field of academics and their pool of knowledge is as vast as their experience in printing. Their expertise and guidance has proved useful at every step. Their uncompromising quality standards have made this book an exceptional effort. Their encouragement from time to time has been an inspiration for everyone.

The publisher and the editorial board hope that this book will prove to be a valuable piece of knowledge for researchers, students, practitioners and scholars across the globe.

List of Contributors

Jeremy Watts, Anahita Khojandi and Oleg Shylo
Department of Industrial and Systems Engineering, University of Tennessee, Knoxville, TN 37996, USA

Ritesh A. Ramdhani
Department of Neurology, Donald and Barbara Zucker School of Medicine at Hofstra/Northwell, Hempstead, NY 11549, USA

Julia K. Steffen, Hannah Jergas, Jan N. Petry-Schmelzer, Till A. Dembek, Tabea Thies, Stefanie T. Jost, Haidar S. Dafsari, Josef Kessler and Michael T. Barbe
Department of Neurology, Faculty of Medicine and University Hospital Cologne, University of Cologne, 50937 Cologne, Germany

Jochen Wirths and Veerle Visser-Vandewalle
Department of Stereotactic and Functional Neurosurgery, Faculty of Medicine and University Hospital Cologne, University of Cologne, 50937 Cologne, Germany

Gereon R. Fink
Department of Neurology, Faculty of Medicine and University Hospital Cologne, University of Cologne, 50937 Cologne, Germany
Cognitive Neuroscience, Research Center Jülich, Institute of Neuroscience and Medicine (INM-3), 52428 Jülich, Germany

Yongzhi Huang, Binith Cheeran, Alexander L. Green and Tipu Z. Aziz
Oxford Functional Neurosurgery Group, Nuffield Departments of Surgical Sciences, University of Oxford, Oxford OX3 9DU, UK

Timothy J. Denison
Institute of Biomedical Engineering, University of Oxford, Oxford OX3 7DQ, UK

Nicolas Favez and Michalina Radomska
Faculty of Psychology and Educational Sciences, University of Geneva, Boulevard du Pont-d'Arve 40, 1205 Geneva, Switzerland

Marc Baertschi
Faculty of Psychology and Educational Sciences, University of Geneva, Boulevard du Pont-d'Arve 40, 1205 Geneva, Switzerland
Nant Foundation, Service of General Psychiatry and Psychotherapy, Avenue des Alpes 66, 1820 Montreux, Switzerland

João Flores Alves Dos Santos
Service of Liaison Psychiatry and Crisis Intervention, Geneva University Hospitals, Rue Gabrielle-Perret-Gentil 4, 1205 Geneva, Switzerland

François Herrmann
Division of Geriatrics, Geneva University Hospitals, Chemin du Pont-Bochet 3, 1226 Thônex, Switzerland

Pierre R. Burkhard
Service of Neurology, Geneva University Hospitals, Rue Gabrielle-Perret-Gentil 4, 1205 Geneva, Switzerland

Alessandra Canuto and Kerstin Weber
Faculty of Medicine, University of Geneva, Rue Michel Servet 1, 1206 Geneva, Switzerland

Paolo Ghisletta
Faculty of Psychology and Educational Sciences, University of Geneva, Boulevard du Pont-d'Arve 40, 1205 Geneva, Switzerland
Swiss Distance Learning University, Überlandstrasse 12, 3900 Brig, Switzerland
Swiss National Centre of Competence in Research LIVES—Overcoming Vulnerability: Life Course Perspectives, Universities of Lausanne and of Geneva, CH-1015 Lausanne, Switzerland

Sharafuddin Khairuddin, Fung Yin Ngo, Man-Lung Fung and Ying-Shing Chan
Neuromodulation Laboratory, School of Biomedical Sciences, Li Ka Shing Faculty of Medicine, The University of Hong Kong, L4 Laboratory Block, 21 Sassoon Road, Hong Kong, China

Wei Ling Lim and Lee Wei Lim
Neuromodulation Laboratory, School of Biomedical Sciences, Li Ka Shing Faculty of Medicine, The University of Hong Kong, L4 Laboratory Block, 21 Sassoon Road, Hong Kong, China
Department of Biological Sciences, School of Science and Technology, Sunway University, Bandar Sunway 47500, Malaysia

Luca Aquili
School of Psychological and Clinical Sciences, Charles Darwin University, NT0815 Darwin, Australia

Naveed Ahmed Khan
Department of Biology, Chemistry and Environmental Sciences, College of Arts and Sciences, American University of Sharjah, Sharjah 26666, UAE

Yasin Temel
Departments of Neuroscience and Neurosurgery, Maastricht University, 6229ER Maastricht, The Netherlands
Department of Experimental Neurosurgery, Maastricht University Medical Center, 6202 AZ Maastricht, The Netherlands

Jordan Prosky
Department of Anesthesiology (Pain Management), University of California San Francisco, San Francisco, CA 94143, USA

Kristin K. Sellers, Ashlyn Schmitgen, Isabella Joseph, Philip A. Starr and Edward F. Chang
Department of Neurological Surgery, University of California San Francisco, San Francisco, CA 94143, USA

Prasad Shirvalkar
Department of Anesthesiology (Pain Management), University of California San Francisco, San Francisco, CA 94143, USA
Department of Neurological Surgery, University of California San Francisco, San Francisco, CA 94143, USA
Department of Neurology, University of California San Francisco, San Francisco, CA 94143, USA

Hye Ran Park
Department of Neurosurgery, Soonchunhyang University Seoul Hospital, Seoul 04401, Korea

Yong Hoon Lim, Eun Jin Song and Sun Ha Paek
Department of Neurosurgery, Seoul National University Hospital, Seoul 03080, Korea

Jae Meen Lee
Department of Neurosurgery, Pusan National University Hospital, Busan 49241, Korea

Kawngwoo Park
Department of Neurosurgery, Gachon University Gil Medical Center, Incheon 21565, Korea

Kwang Hyon Park
Department of Neurosurgery, Chuungnam National University Sejong Hospital, Sejong 30099, Korea

Woong-Woo Lee
Department of Neurology, Nowon Eulji Medical Center, Eulji University, Seoul 01830, Korea

Han-Joon Kim and Beomseok Jeon
Department of Neurology, Seoul National University Hospital, Seoul 03080, Korea

Meltem Görmezoğlu
Department of Psychiatry, Ondokuz Mayıs University, 55270 Samsun, Turkey
Department of Neurosurgery, Maastricht University Medical Centre, 6229 Maastricht, The Netherlands

Tim Bouwens van der Vlis
Department of Neurosurgery, Maastricht University Medical Centre, 6229 Maastricht, The Netherlands

Koen Schruers and Albert F.G. Leentjens
Department of Psychiatry and Neuropsychology, Maastricht University Medical Center, 6229 Maastricht, The Netherlands
School of Mental Health and Neuroscience, Maastricht University, 6229 Maastricht, The Netherlands

Linda Ackermans
Department of Neurosurgery, Maastricht University Medical Centre, 6229 Maastricht, The Netherlands
School of Mental Health and Neuroscience, Maastricht University, 6229 Maastricht, The Netherlands

Mircea Polosan
Grenoble Institute of Neurosciences, University of Grenoble Alpes, 38058 Grenoble, France

Anneke Alkemade and Birte U. Forstmann
Integrative Model-based Cognitive Neuroscience Research Unit, University of Amsterdam, 1018 WS Amsterdam, The Netherlands

Bethany R. Isaacs
Integrative Model-based Cognitive Neuroscience Research Unit, University of Amsterdam, 1018 WS Amsterdam, The Netherlands
Department of Experimental Neurosurgery, Maastricht University Medical Center, 6202 AZ Maastricht, The Netherlands

Max C. Keuken
Municipality of Amsterdam, Services & Data, Cluster Social, 1000 AE Amsterdam, The Netherlands

Pierre-Louis Bazin
Integrative Model-based Cognitive Neuroscience Research Unit, University of Amsterdam, 1018 WS Amsterdam, The Netherlands
Max Planck Institute for Human Cognitive and Brain Sciences, D-04103 Leipzig, Germany

Frederick L. Hitti, Andrew I. Yang and Gordon H. Baltuch
Department of Neurosurgery, Pennsylvania Hospital, University of Pennsylvania, 800 Spruce St, Philadelphia, PA 19107, USA

Mario A. Cristancho
Department of Psychiatry, University of Pennsylvania, 3535 Market Street, Philadelphia, PA 19104, USA

Carlo Alberto Artusi and Leonardo Lopiano
Department of Neuroscience 'Rita Levi Montalcini', University of Torino, 10126 Torino, Italy

Francesca Morgante
Neurosciences Research Centre, Molecular and Clinical Sciences Research Institute, St George's University of London, London SW17 0RE, UK
Department of Clinical and Experimental Medicine, University of Messina, 98125 Messina, Italy

Milaine Roet, Jackson Boonstra and Ali Jahanshahi
Department of Neurosurgery, Maastricht University Medical Center, P. Debyelaan 25, 6202 AZ Maastricht, The Netherlands

European Graduate School of Neuroscience (EURON); 6229 ER Maastricht, The Netherlands

Erdi Sahin
Department of Neurology, Istanbul Faculty of Medicine, Istanbul University Capa, Istanbul 34093, Turkey

Anne E.P. Mulders
Department of Neurosurgery, Maastricht University Medical Center, P. Debyelaan 25, 6202 AZ Maastricht, The Netherlands
European Graduate School of Neuroscience (EURON); 6229 ER Maastricht, The Netherlands
Department of Psychiatry and Psychology, Maastricht University Medical Center, P. Debyelaan 25, 6202 AZ Maastricht, The Netherlands

Index

Printed in the USA
CPSIA information can be obtained
at www.ICGtesting.com
JSHW051357091023
49903JS00006B/180